A Century of Surgeons and Surgery

The American College of Surgeons

1913–2012

David L Nahrwold, MD, FACS

and

Peter J Kernahan, MD, PhD, FACS

Book design by Mary Beth Cohen

© Copyright 2012 The American College of Surgeons, David L Nahrwold, and Peter J Kernahan

American College of Surgeons
633 N. Saint Clair Street
Chicago, IL 60611-3211

www.facs.org

ISBN: 978-1-880696-99-6

Library of Congress Control Number: 2012941481

Printed in the United States of America

PAGE

Foreword

In 2006, Dr. Thomas Russell, then the Executive Director of the American College of Surgeons, organized an exploratory meeting to discuss the possibility of a book celebrating the Centennial of the College in 2012–2013. The group was chaired by Dr. George Sheldon, a Past President of the College and editor-in-chief of its Web portal, and included Dr. C Rollins Hanlon, Executive Consultant; Dr. Paul Collicott, Director of Member Services; Ms. Linn Meyer, Director of Communications; Ms. Susan Rishworth, archivist; Dr. J Patrick O'Leary, then the First Vice President; Fred Holtzrichter, Chief Development Officer; and Ms. Barbara Dean, Director of Executive Services. Dr. Virginia Dawson, a historian, was present as an advisor. Subsequently other historians were also consulted. Later, Dr. Peter J Kernahan, a surgeon and medical historian, and Dr. David L Nahrwold, the retired chair of surgery at Northwestern University, were added to the group.

Members of the group reviewed histories published by other medical organizations and discussed previous histories of the College, including *The Joy of Living*, the autobiography of College founder Dr. Franklin H Martin published in 1933 by Doubleday, Doran & Co. Dr. Loyal Davis, Past President of the College and for 13 years editor of its journal, wrote *Fellowship of Surgeons: A History of the American College of Surgeons*, originally published by the College in 1960, and reprinted seven times. *The American College of Surgeons at 75*, written by Dr. George W Stephenson, who served the College in many executive positions for 48 years, was published by the College in 1990 as a companion piece to Davis's work. Eventually, the need for a scholarly narrative encompassing the entire first century of the College's existence became obvious. We—Drs. Kernahan and Nahrwold—were asked to write that first century narrative, and this book is the result. Peter Kernahan wrote the first four chapters; we collaborated on the fifth; and David Nahrwold wrote the remaining 18 chapters. Some of the events in the first five chapters have also been discussed in Peter Kernahan's doctoral dissertation *Franklin Martin and the Standardization of American Surgery, 1890–1940* (University of Minnesota, 2010).

A major source of material was the College's archives, which contain the minutes, agendas, and supporting materials for the meetings of most of the College committees, records of education programs, the papers of the founder, Franklin Martin, and thousands of photographs. A special resource was the 26 three-ring binders compiled by Miss Eleanor K Grimm, Martin's secretary, who after his death functioned as the Chief Administrative Officer of the College. She compiled clippings and tear sheets from College publications, the minutes of College committees, and her own notes into a historical compendium that eventually became Davis' *Fellowship of Surgeons*.

The minutes of the Board of Regents and its Executive Committee were an indispensible source of information because they contain all the supplemental information provided to the Regents before and at their meetings. These materials included reports, background papers, correspondence, statistical and demographic information, and summaries of the issues presented to the Regents for discussion and decisions. Because these materials, usually three or more inches thick, were part of the official minutes of the Board of Regents, they are cited frequently. Until the mid-1950s the minutes were transcribed verbatim, giving unique insights to the personalities and thinking of the participants.

The authors are indebted to the many individuals who provided material, information, and advice. They are especially indebted to Ms. Susan Rishworth, the College archivist, and Ms. Delores Barber, assistant archivist. Dr. C Rollins Hanlon critiqued most of the manuscript until his death in May 2011. Others who read and critiqued portions of the book were Drs. George Sheldon, J Patrick O'Leary, LaMar McGinnis, David Hoyt, Kevin Mitchell, and Mss. Linn Meyer, Caitjan Gainty, Anne Richter, Carolyn Nahrwold, and Susan Rishworth.

Members of the College staff were very helpful in supplying information. Ms. Gay Vincent, Ms. Barbara Dean, Dr. Ajit Sachdeva, and Dr. David Hoyt provided important insights. Drs. Thomas Russell and past presidents R Scott Jones and George Sheldon consented to interviews, as did past Board Chairman Dr. Josef Fischer. Dr. Patricia Numann, president in 2011–12, provided valuable information. Others who were especially helpful were Dr. Kathleen Casey, Dr. Clifford Ko, Mr. Christian Shalgian, Mss. Maxine Rogers, Rhonda Peebles, Mary Fitzgerald, Patricia Sprecksel, Diane Mazmanian, Kathryn Matousek, and Donna Coulombe. We are also grateful to Mss. Cynthia Brown, Christine Shiffer, Caroline Foote, Jessica Sault, Debra Scarborough, and Marian Taliaferro.

This book would not have been possible without the assistance and courtesy of many others across the country. Grateful thanks are extended to the Wangensteen Historical Library of Biology and Medicine, University of Minnesota, Minneapolis MN; the Mayo Historical Unit, Mayo Clinic, Rochester MN; Archives and Rare Books, Becker Library, Washington University, St. Louis MO; the Western Reserve Historical Society, Cleveland OH; the Center for the History of Medicine, Countway Library, Harvard University, Boston MA; the History of Medicine Division, National Library of Medicine, Bethesda MD; the Alan Mason Chesney Medical Archives, Johns Hopkins University, Baltimore MD; Manuscripts and Archives, Yale University, New Haven CT; the Franklin D Roosevelt Presidential Library, Hyde Park, NY; and the Osler Library of the History of Medicine, McGill University, Montreal, PQ. A particular debt is owed by one of the authors (PJK) to Professors John Eyler and Jennifer Gunn of the University of Minnesota.

We thank our editor, Ms. Wendy Cowles Husser, who corrected our errors and improved the manuscript while allowing us to keep our voices. Ms. Caitjan Gainty, then a graduate student in history at the University of Chicago, compiled lists of the College's officers, Regents, and members of the Executive Committee of the Board of Governors by year, a great resource. She also provided invaluable help in bringing archival material to our attention. Ms. Linn Meyer and her successor as ACS Director of Integrated Communications, Ms. Lynn Kahn, were our invaluable liaisons with the College. Ms. Nancy Puckett provided the final editing touches and helped bring the book to fruition.

David L Nahrwold, MD, FACS
Chicago, IL

Peter J Kernahan, MD, PhD, FACS
Minneapolis, MN

CHAPTER 1
The Context
of the College:
1880–1910

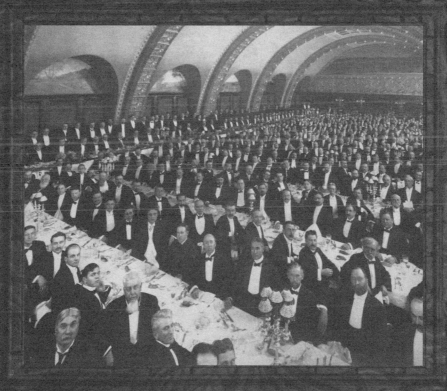

Nicholas Senn Memorial Banquet, Auditorium Hotel, November 11, 1905

The American College of Surgeons (ACS) grew out of an unstable medical environment and a crisis in surgical care. Three factors—scientific, regulatory, and economic—combined to produce this crisis. After the general adoption of antisepsis and asepsis, the scope of surgery expanded rapidly between 1880 and 1910. New areas of the body—the abdomen, chest, and even brain—became the subjects of surgical interest. At the same time, North American physicians, beyond basic medical licensing, worked in an essentially unregulated medical marketplace. This turn-of-the-century marketplace could be brutally competitive.

An overcrowded profession (many inadequately educated), the increasing importance of hospitals, and two major economic depressions meant struggle and declining incomes for many practitioners. Only a small minority would obtain wealth and they tended to do so as specialists. Surgeons featured prominently among these fortunate few. For the ambitious general practitioner or recent graduate, therefore, surgery offered both the excitement and prestige of the scientifically new and the chance of financial success. Additionally, no regulatory authority existed to prevent any physician, even the inadequately trained or the incompetent, from embarking on a career in surgery. In this environment, a cadre of leading surgeons, led by the dynamic Franklin H Martin of Chicago, attempted to bring order out of surgical chaos by creating the American College of Surgeons.

The Transformation of Surgery

Anesthesia, asepsis, and a changing understanding of disease would transform surgery and surgical careers in the second half of the 19th century. The introduction of anesthesia in 1846 provided an escape from the pain of operation but did not immediately produce a rapid expansion in either the number of operations or the scope of surgery. Apart from more frequent attempts at limb salvage rather than amputation, little else changed in surgery.[1] Surgeons continued to largely confine their work, apart from the infrequently performed and controversial ovariotomy, to the exterior of the body and to the extremities. Not all patients even received anesthesia—the Irish laborer was far more likely to have to endure the pain of operation than was the refined lady.[2] Anesthesia alone could not produce a surgical revolution.

Even the introduction of antisepsis from the late 1860s did not immediately change this conservative attitude. The controversies surrounding the introduction of Listerism have been extensively discussed by historians of medicine, with hagiography giving way to more nuanced assessments.[3] Even many of Lister's "opponents"—surgeons who had difficulty accepting Lister's theory of airborne germs as the cause of the postoperative septic complications collectively known as hospitalism—adopted some form of "cleanliness" into their practices.[4] Although more patients now underwent operation, the field of surgery did not immediately expand. John Erichsen, president of the Royal College of Surgeons and author of a textbook issued to all Union Army surgeons, reflected this surgical conservatism in 1876 when he stated flatly that the abdomen, chest, and brain would "forever remain closed to the wise and humane surgeon."

The transformation of surgery would require a transformation in the understanding of disease. Without this change, operations on internal organs, even if technically feasible, made no sense. This change would require overturning long held views about disease. From the days of Hippocrates and Galen, physicians understood disease to be highly individualistic. In any given patient, an illness was the result of multiple factors, including the environment and the patient's own moral and physical characteristics; no two patients ever had quite the same disease process. By the 1870s, two 19th century developments—anatomic pathology and the germ theory—combined to change this view and justify an expanded surgery.

In the waning years of the 18th century and the first decades of the 19th, physicians, particularly at the great Paris hospitals, had begun to correlate antemortem symptoms with postmortem findings. Increasingly, diseases began to be recognized as originating in local, organ-based phenomena. Improvements in microscopy and the work of researchers like Rudolf Virchow brought this localization of disease down to the cellular level.[5]

The germ theory, with its emphasis on a single, specific cause—the entry of the germ as the cause of the disease—reinforced this localization. Increasingly, a disease began to be understood as an entity in its own right, as a thing apart from any individual patient, what the philosopher of science K Codell Carter has called an ontologic view of disease.[6] Reginald Fitz of Boston epitomized these new understandings of disease when he described appendicitis in 1886. Through his work, a generalized inflammatory process of the colon (typhlitis) became a localized disease of the appendix (appendicitis). Before this transformation, removing the appendix would have made no sense.[7] After, appendectomy became one of the operations that would define the new, aggressive surgery.

Once surgeons had convinced themselves, physicians, and the public of the benefits of this aggressive intervention, surgery expanded rapidly.[8] In the 1880s alone, surgeons devised more than one hundred new operations.[9] The number of operations performed also increased dramatically.[10] Thus, the transformation of surgery in the last 20 years of the 19th century had required both new ideas and new techniques.

≈≈ ✳ ≈≈

Surgeons and the New Surgery

The question remained, one that the ACS would attempt to answer: Who should perform this new surgery? And with the new operations, even established surgeons were essentially self-taught. In Europe, surgery had long existed as a separate branch of the medical profession. Nowhere was this tradition stronger than in the United Kingdom, with its tripartite division of the profession into physicians, surgeons, and surgeon-apothecaries (general practitioners), each with its own institutional structure. This demarcation, as the historian Rosemary Stevens has observed, had never extended to North America.[11] Specialties, surgery in particular, would develop in the absence of any pre-existing institutional framework of the sort provided by the Royal Colleges.

Beginning in the mid-19th century, these specialties arose from an egalitarian profession proud of its generalist traditions. The general practitioner performed such surgery as might be necessary.[12] Even into the early years of the 20th century, the authors of many surgery texts wrote explicitly for the "practitioner of general medicine who rarely takes up the scalpel."[13] In the country's oldest and most medically sophisticated cities—Boston, New York, and Philadelphia—practices limited to surgery do not appear until at least the 1880s.[14] For many in the profession, including America's preeminent surgeon, Philadelphia's Samuel Gross, generalism was a source of pride, an affirmation of American individualism and Yankee ingenuity.[15] In the United States, basic medical licensing, which slowly returned in the last three decades of the century after disappear during the Jacksonian Era, designated all medical practitioners as both "physicians and surgeons."

So by the end of the century, as more and more physicians turned their attention toward surgery, no formal mechanisms existed to either train or to identify them. Many graduates of North America's often inadequate, if not deplorable, medical schools had never served even an internship. The fortunate minority received a year or two of hospital instruction and perhaps a form of apprenticeship with a prominent surgeon. The customary route to specialization, gradually limiting one's practice, provided a sort of market-based evaluation, but on-the-job-training might not be an altogether desirable way of selecting the aspiring surgeon. Additionally, the prestige and, as we will see, the financial rewards of surgery caused many inadequately trained young graduates to avoid the traditional route and to go directly into surgery, as the editor of *American Medicine* lamented in 1908.[16] But even at the nation's most prestigious hospitals, training could be vague, as Harvey Cushing reflected many years later.[17] In many cities, few if any surgeons had served an apprenticeship.[18] While leading surgeons, like Chicago's flamboyant John B Murphy, called for longer training and William Halsted established a residency at Johns Hopkins based on German models, many decades would elapse before the formal residency system became widespread.[19]

In 1913, the year the College was founded, a small-town physician in Minnesota, Ludwig Sogge, undertook a survey of surgery in country hospitals. Writing to physicians in towns of 1,500–3,000 people with 5–15 bed hospitals, he received 11 responses.[20] On average, his respondents had one year of internship and six years in practice and performed one major operation per week—a result that supports contemporary arguments that it was the younger physician who practiced surgery. Sogge, a defender of the general practitioner-surgeon, went on to argue that the local operator, watched by the whole community and with his reputation at stake, was likely to be more careful than the big-city surgeon. He also pointed out that local surgery offered other advantages to the patient—no railroad fare, a lower fee, and comparable care in the local hospital. The country doctor was "entitled to do some surgical work, and he will do it successfully."[21]

Leading "big city" surgeons could be unsympathetic to such claims, whether advanced by the country doctor or the occasional operator in the city. As William Haggard, professor of surgery at Vanderbilt, warned the American Medical Association's (AMA) Section on Surgery in 1913, "the most dangerous operator is the occasional operator, the general practitioner without special training and the young man" newly graduated.[22] That year Haggard would join the effort to remedy this situation by becoming a Founder and one of the first Regents of the new American College of Surgeons.

The early careers of the original 17 Regents and officers of the College illustrate the varied and inconstant training behind most surgical careers of the period. Only five held undergraduate degrees. Graduating as physicians between 1877 and 1894, most had attended one of the better North American medical schools, those beginning to reform and establish a three-year graded curriculum. But not all; George Crile graduated in 1887 from one of the country's weakest schools. Wooster Medical College had no microscope, occupied a building condemned as unfit for an elementary school, and required only two short summer sessions for the MD degree. From these unpromising beginnings he would rise to an international reputation for pioneering research on shock, serve for many years as Chair of the Board of Regents, and found the Cleveland Clinic.

All of these future leaders of the ACS had taken an internship of one to two years, itself uncommon at the time. William Haggard of Nashville and Robert McKechnie of Vancouver took additional hospital training before beginning their careers in surgery. John B Murphy started as a general practitioner and built his practice from there. Albert J (AJ) Ochsner in Chicago and George Crile in Cleveland served as assistants to

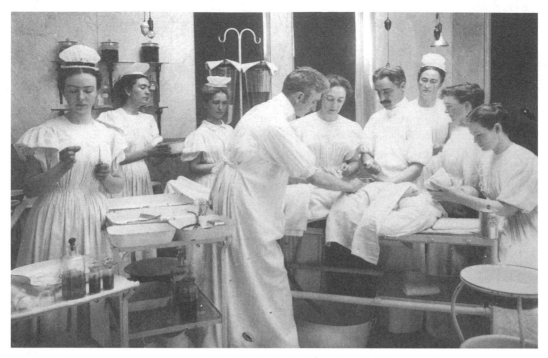

FIGURE 1.1 A young and still red-haired Franklin H Martin, the College's Founder, in the operating room.

established surgeons. Seven, including Murphy, Crile, and Ochsner, at one time or another went to Europe for varying lengths of time. On the other hand, Charles Mayo, with his brother Will, had learned surgery from their father and by visiting clinics in Chicago and the East. Franklin Martin learned by observation during a two year internship at Mercy Hospital in Chicago. JMT Finney, who would eventually succeed Halsted, began his surgery career staffing the dispensary at Johns Hopkins after eighteen months as house surgeon at the Massachusetts General Hospital. (Figure 1.1)

Only Canadian Walter Chipman of Montreal and McGill University followed what would become by the mid-20th century the standard sequential path to a surgical career: undergraduate degree, medical degree, several years of graded hospital training, and then certification. And he did so by taking all of his medical training in the United Kingdom and passing the fellowship exam of the Royal College of Surgeons of Edinburgh. Yet despite all these obstacles, by the 1910s, leading North American surgeons including the Mayos, Crile, and Finney were beginning to equal if not surpass their European counterparts, and even visiting German surgeons, the international leaders in the profession, found much to admire in American surgery.[23]

The Economics of Practice

The transformation of surgery allowed a fortunate few to prosper. On the other hand most general practitioners, who comprised the great majority of physicians, struggled in an over-crowded marketplace; a struggle exacerbated by the pervasive economic insecurity and instability of the period. The severe depressions of 1873-1879 and 1882-1885 were followed by financial crises and panics in 1890, 1893 (another decade of depression), and 1907. The resulting large scale labor unrest and populist movements across rural America added to the sense of instability. Both the medical marketplace and the general economy took their toll on the majority of physicians.

The rewards of practice varied greatly. A 1902 survey suggested that 75 percent of American physicians made less than $1,500 a year.[24] In a similar survey in 1907 of an unidentified Midwestern city, 80 percent of the city's doctors had fairly marginal practices.[25] By comparison, skilled railroad workers (engineers, firemen, conductors, and others) earned between $900 and $1,200 a year.[26] In Chicago, physicians were no more likely to own a home than was the population as a whole.[27] Even among the successful, surgeons' incomes were two to four times higher than those of medical practitioners. In 1914, the $25,000 that Frank Billings earned as Chicago's leading medical specialist paled by comparison to John B Murphy's $80,000.[28] The discrepancies in charges did not escape public attention. Ambition, greed, or sheer economic necessity could drive a general practitioner into the operating room.

Actually, most surgeons outside an elite few in the major cities still did some general practice. To refer a patient in these circumstances was to risk losing the entire family.[29] The surgeon needed referrals; the general practitioner wanted his patients back and a little more money. An *ad hoc* solution soon developed, encouraged by the huge discrepancy in fees—fee splitting. By dividing the fee, the two parties established a mutually beneficial referral relationship. The generalist received some of the rewards of operating while retaining his patients. The specialist gained referrals at the expense of competitors so long as he cooperated.[30] At least in theory, the patient might even benefit because the generalist had less incentive to attempt an operation.[31] Indeed, many physicians saw nothing wrong with the practice, particularly if the patient had been informed.[32] Unfortunately, as a practical matter, it also tended to encourage unnecessary surgery; both the surgeon and the referring physician had a financial incentive to recommend operation.

In the absence of any action on the part of the medical profession, state legislatures and courts intervened with limited effect. A few states, among them Minnesota, Nebraska, and Wisconsin, outlawed fee splitting. The appellate court in Michigan held that the physician had a fiduciary responsibility to the patient, one broken by fee splitting.[33] These efforts had little practical effect. The practice often occurred in secret and few physicians were willing to challenge the system, particularly where the practice was widespread. The medical societies and the AMA took no action. Founded in part to reform the ethics of surgeons, the College would quickly learn just how insidious and hard to eliminate the practice was.

≈✳≈

The Surgeon's Workplace

As ideas about disease changed the scope of surgery, the site of surgical practice also changed from the home to the hospital. More complex operations placed greater demands on the infrastructure of surgery. Exploring the abdomen or chest required better lighting and a greater variety of instruments. Postoperative care put more demands on nurses. In an age devoted to efficiency, traveling from house to house to operate wasted time (and money).[34] The hospital became the preferred site for the new surgery.

In many cities the character of the hospital also began to change. Even in the 1870s, the relatively few hospitals in the United States had been sites of charity care for the indigent. Most medical care took place within the home and, as late as 1878, the nation had only 178 hospitals.[35] For the expanding urban population, whether in the tenements of the immigrant poor or the apartment houses of the growing middle class, the home became an increasingly unsatisfactory site for care. And hospital administrators saw middle class paying patients as a way out of budgetary difficulties precipitated by a series of financial panics and recessions. Hospitals expanded and competed to attract paying patients.[36]

By 1909 the number of hospitals in the United States had reached 4,359.[37] At the time, founding a hospital required only a modest investment. An old house or mansion could be converted into a hospital relatively easily.[38] Even if a town already possessed a hospital, these low capital requirements allowed ambitious or excluded physicians to establish their own rival institution. Small and often proprietary, many of the new hospitals, particularly in the South and West, tended to be dominated by surgery.[39] As we have seen, however, the qualifications and training of many "surgeons" left much to be desired. The hospital could be no better than its medical staff, and, at times, much worse.

Reform and the Rise of Franklin Martin

"Will the profession," demanded the editor of the *Journal of the Minnesota State Medical Association* in 1913, "meet the challenges of the day, which verge closely upon a crisis?"[40] Precipitated by the rapid expansion of surgery, four immediate challenges confronted the profession and the public: defining the qualified surgeon, eliminating financial graft, improving the hospital, and making those reforms national in scope. The fifth challenge would be establishing the legitimacy of any organization that presumed to undertake the first four tasks. In the absence of effective action by existing medical organizations or legislative bodies, these challenges would be taken up by a new organization—the American College of Surgeons.

Many physicians recognized the need for surgical reform, just as they recognized the need for reform of medical education epitomized by the Flexner Report. No existing organization, however, was in a position to act. The various specialty societies, founded between 1864 and 1887, represented a tiny self-selected elite. The American Surgical Association (ASA), the one national surgery body, had only 146 members largely drawn from the leading medical schools and centers of the East. With a correspondingly small budget, its members had neither the resources nor the interest to sponsor a reform campaign, whatever the inclination of individual members. Even the national umbrella organization of specialty societies, the Congress of American Physicians and Surgeons had, at its founding in 1888, eschewed any interest in matters of policy. There would not be "even the least interference with the American Medical Association," its first chairman promised.[41]

But the AMA leadership had more pressing interests and little political will to take on such divisive issues. Despite its venerable name and age, the organization had only recently expanded to a national level, increasing from 8,400 members in 1900 to more than 70,000 by 1910. Professional unity and the reform of education, its first priorities, had the support of all its constituents—the value of their degrees would increase as reform limited the number of new entrants and unity increased the influence of the profession. On the other hand, neither the recently constituted House of Delegates, the association's representative body, nor the specialty "sections" would be likely to support any restrictions on their members' individual freedom to practice as they saw fit.[42]

The second option, legislative action, a response to growing public concerns, proved equally problematic. Federal action in either the United States or Canada was out of the question, even if some progressives called for a national health department and Congress had briefly considered national medical licensing.[43] At the state level, basic medical licensing had only slowly begun to return to the United States in the 1870s and still remained controversial.[44] By the 1920s, of 57 states and provinces, only Alberta had a system of specialty licensing, one administered by the University of Alberta's Faculty of Medicine.[45] Elsewhere, physicians, who had supported basic licensing, vigorously and successfully opposed specialty licensing as an unwarranted intrusion into medical practice.

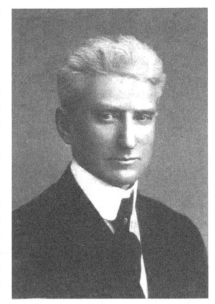

FIGURE 1.2 Dr. Franklin H Martin, circa 1910.

Given the above, did the circumstances call for a new organization? The idea began to circulate among leading surgeons. Addressing the ASA in 1909, its president, Dudley Allen of Cleveland, called for "annual exams" and a National College of Surgeons to administer them and award fellowships.[46] The rather conservative organization had not been stirred to action by his words. Several of its younger members, however, had already formed a new society, the Society of Clinical Surgery (SCS) in 1903. With 40 members, the new society replaced papers with operative clinics. Reflecting Progressive Era beliefs in active learning, George Crile of Cleveland would later describe it as a "society with a minimum of proceedings and a maximum of ideas."[47] Several members of the Society of Clinical Surgery, including the Mayo brothers, George Crile, Edward Martin, and Ernest Codman featured prominently in the organization and early years of the College. The society itself would provide the inspiration for the Clinical Congress of Surgeons of North America (CCSNA). The Clinical Congress would in turn provide the starting point for the American College of Surgeons. Linking all three would be Franklin H Martin of Chicago, a gynecologic surgeon who used his journal *Surgery, Gynecology, and Obstetrics* (now the *Journal of the American College of Surgeons*) to promote reform.

Born in rural Wisconsin in 1857, Martin grew up on farms and would become part of the great movement of ambitious youth from agrarian America to the growing cities. His formal education was sketchy—something to which he remained sensitive and his enemies condescending throughout his life. After attending country schools, at fifteen he apprenticed as a clerk and millwright in his uncle's Minneapolis flour mill. He then attended the Elroy Seminary in Elroy, Wisconsin for a few semesters. Local seminaries and academies like Elroy dotted the countryside and provided some opportunity for a secondary education before public high schools became commonplace. (Figure 1.2)

Like many similarly educated young men and women, including John B Murphy, George Crile, and Albert Ochsner, Martin spent time as a country school teacher. He returned to the fields and brick-making during the summer, where the sight of a prosperous physician in his fine buggy convinced him to become a doctor.[48] In the fashion of the day, after an apprenticeship with a local physician, he entered the Chicago Medical College (Northwestern University Medical School) in 1877 and graduated in 1880. After two years as an intern at Mercy Hospital, Martin became one of the young men who rapidly took up surgery. Ambitious, talented, and confident, he soon developed a successful practice despite his dismay at the death of his first surgical patient.[49]

By the second decade of the century, Martin already had a well-established reputation, not only as a successful gynecologic surgeon, but also as an institutional entrepreneur. First, dissatisfied with a conservative, existing organization, Martin and a colleague opened the Chicago Post-Graduate Medical School in 1889. Although proprietary, such schools met a demand for continuing medical education at a time of rapid increase in specialty knowledge and no formal residencies.[50] While the fortunate could devote a year or two to study in Europe, for many physicians the post-graduate schools with their short courses offered a path to specialization. In creating his school, the 31-year-old Martin for the first time displayed his formidable organizational skills. Within seven months his first project moved from an idea to a functioning, fully-staffed institution and opened on April 1, 1889.

Martin then moved on to medical journalism and, in 1905, he began editing and publishing *Surgery, Gynecology, and Obstetrics* (*SGO*)—a journal by and for "practical men dealing with facts, actually engaged in the work of the day."[51] *SGO* would play an important role in the College's early history. First, it provided a means of reaching the continent's surgeons and would-be surgeons. Second, its emphasis on the practical and the practicing surgeon rather than an academic elite would be reflected in College policy throughout Martin's leadership. Third, Martin began, through his choice of editors and collaborators, a closer association with several key future College allies: Allen B Kanavel, John B Murphy, Frederic Besley, and William and Charles Mayo. Fourth, it exacerbated the ill-feeling toward Martin on the part of three powerful figures in the AMA and Chicago medical politics: surgeons Malcolm L Harris and Arthur Dean Bevan, and George H Simmons, a physician and editor of the *Journal of the American Medical Association*. Years later, Martin's loyal secretary, Eleanor K Grimm, recalled that Bevan became "the arch enemy" of Martin from this moment on.[52] In his rise Martin had made allies but also enemies among Chicago's medical elite, and these enmities would have important consequences for the College.

Martin next created a national educational forum for surgeons. Unlike the Surgical Section of the AMA, Martin's Clinical Congress of Surgeons of North America would, like the very small Society of Clinical Surgery, use active demonstrations rather than papers. Participants would view actual operations and attend clinical demonstrations hosted by leading surgeons. "It was far better," wrote Martin later, "to have a practicing surgeon demonstrate his work than to have him tell about it."[53] (Figure 1.3)

The speed with which he moved again spoke to Martin's organizational abilities and drive. Having drawn up his plans on a Mediterranean cruise in the summer of 1910, Martin announced the Congress in the September issue of *SGO*. Just two months later the Congress opened on November 7 and ran through November 19, 1910. Martin had hoped to attract 200 physicians. Reflecting the great interest in surgery (for all the reasons discussed earlier), 1,300 attended. Growing ever larger, the Congress became a permanent organization and moved on to Philadelphia in 1911 and New York in 1912, where almost 3,000 physicians attended. Out of the New York Clinical Congress arose the American College of Surgeons (ACS). While Martin's previous projects had sought to educate, the College would represent an attempt to reform and exert control over the practice of surgery in North America.

Dudley Allen's suggestion of a national college, while not acted on by the ASA, had not gone unnoticed. Members of the younger SCS continued to discuss the idea among themselves.[54] When the SCS met in London in the summer of 1910—at the same time as Franklin Martin's Mediterranean cruise—two of its members, Ernest A Codman of Boston and Edward Martin of Philadelphia (no relation to Franklin Martin), shared a hansom cab.[55] Both had an interest in medical reform.

Codman, of a Brahmin family and a surgeon at the Massachusetts General Hospital, had a growing interest in improving the quality of hospital care. Influenced by the efficiency movement in industry, Codman had begun to advocate what he styled the "end-result system." Surgeons and hospitals would monitor and improve their clinical outcomes through long-term follow-up of their patients. At a time when even basic medical record keeping was rudimentary, this was a novel idea. During their cab ride, Codman attempted to interest Martin in his ideas.

In Edward Martin, a prominent Philadelphia surgeon and clinical professor at the University of Pennsylvania's medical school, Codman found a receptive audience. As the cab made its way through the streets of London, Edward Martin began to tell Codman of his own interest in establishing a college of surgeons. Further discussions with other members of the society, including Harvey Cushing, George Crile, and AJ Ochsner, produced general agreement among the society's members on the need for reform and for the idea of a college. But like the ASA, the SCS took no direct action.

Franklin Martin's organizational genius would turn these rather vague ideas into an operational plan. Martin, while not a member of either the ASA or the SCS, had close contacts with several members of both organizations. These included fellow Chicagoans John B Murphy and AJ Ochsner together with George Crile and the Mayos. His CCSNA,

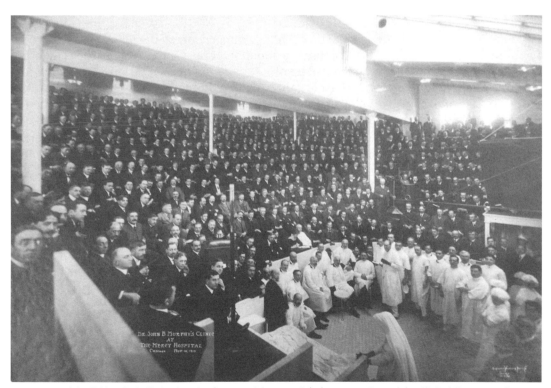

FIGURE 1.3 John B Murphy's Clinic, showing how participants might have experienced the Clinical Congress of Surgeons of North America.

as the one organization, apart from the surgical section of the AMA, that drew surgeons from across the continent, would provide the opportunity.

This opportunity would occur at the New York Congress in November 1912 when Edward Martin assumed the presidency of the CCSNA. Codman, in his autobiographical sketch, speculated that "Martin of Chicago," in Codman's words, "had appointed Martin of Philadelphia as President of the Congress so that he of Philadelphia could appoint him of Chicago to organize the College."[56] Given Franklin Martin's close control of the organizations that he founded and his contacts, Codman's coy suggestion is not unreasonable. Franklin Martin's diaries and surviving correspondence, however, provide no evidence one way or the other. In fact, Martin, in his memoirs, placed the origins of the College in a sudden inspiration as he rode the *Twentieth Century Limited* to New York City that November.

In any event, Martin of Chicago drew up a proposal for a college of surgeons during the train trip. By the time he arrived in New York, the train's stenographer had a typed copy ready. Martin's plan called for:

- A standard of professional, ethical, and moral requirements for every authorized graduate in medicine who practices general surgery or one of its specialties, in so far as feasible along the lines of the Royal Colleges of Surgeons of England, Ireland, and Scotland.
- A supplemental degree for operating surgeons.
- Special letters to indicate fellowship in the college.
- A published list of members of the college.
- The appointment of a committee of twelve members of the Clinical Congress with full power to proceed with the plan, if careful consideration proved its worth.[57]

John B Murphy and Edward Martin of Philadelphia endorsed the plan enthusiastically. Franklin Martin presented the proposal as a motion at the Congress's business meeting on Friday, November 15. Seconded by Murphy, the motion passed unanimously. Edward Martin, as President, appointed an organizational committee (the Committee on the Standardization of Surgery) charged with defining a minimum standard for surgeons and then considering each of the points raised in Martin's proposal. The Congress then established three-member local committees in the major cities of the United States and Canada. Speaking before the Massachusetts Medical Society in July 1913, Dr. Homer Gage of Worcester, Massachusetts joined many others when he called the decision "the most significant and important result of that congress."[58]

Overlooked by Gage and many other commentators, a second, equally important committee had been appointed. Allen Kanavel, one of Franklin Martin's young Chicago associates, presented a resolution calling for the standardization of hospital work and equipment. The resolution passed easily and the Clinical Congress appointed a committee on hospital standardization under the direction of Ernest Codman. Both the ACS and its hospital standardization program had their origins in the CCSNA. In the next five years the College would subsume both hospital standardization and the Congress itself.

The committee on organization promptly convened its first meeting. Its 11 members (two ex officio) represented some of the leading surgeons of their generation with an average age of 51. At 56, Franklin Martin and John B Murphy were the oldest members and among the five Midwesterners on the committee. George Crile of Cleveland, Charles Mayo from Minnesota, and fellow Chicagoan AJ Ochsner completed the Midwestern contingent. The others included one Canadian (Walter Chipman of Montreal), one Southerner (Rudolph Matas of New Orleans and Tulane), one New Englander (Frederic

Cotton of the Massachusetts General Hospital, the youngest at 44), and three from the Mid-Atlantic States (JMT Finney of Johns Hopkins, George Brewer of New York, and Edward Martin).

This geographic diversity was politically important during the organization of the College. Both Murphy and Franklin Martin were concerned that the College not appear to be a Chicago operation, particularly as they were both controversial figures. Murphy would turn down the first presidency of the College for that same reason. Eight of the 11 were members of the Society of Clinical Surgery. As George Crile would later write "the Society of Clinical Surgery furnished the idea, Franklin Martin and his journal furnished the spark."[59]

While no record remains of this first meeting, four actions resulted. First, Franklin Martin immediately obtained a charter for an "American College of Surgeons" from the State of Illinois. Second, committee members began work on a set of bylaws for the proposed organization. Third, the Committee agreed to reconvene on May 5, 1913 in Washington, DC at the annual Congress of Physician and Surgeons of North America, where a larger organizational meeting of invited surgeons would be called at the New Willard Hotel. Fourth, Franklin Martin and other members of the committee made a series of journeys across North America to the larger cities with medical schools. In each of these, three-member committees chosen by the CCSNA had arranged meetings with an invited group of surgeons.

Martin began on January 20, 1913 with a "preliminary canvas of the eastern seaboard cities" traveling from Chicago to Baltimore, Washington, Philadelphia, New York, Brooklyn, and Boston.[60] Baltimore, Philadelphia (despite Edward Martin's enthusiasm), and New York provided a poor welcome. Martin's Midwestern tendency to boosterism may have offended some Eastern sensibilities. Further, with a longer history of surgical specialization, some well-established surgeons in the East may also have been less interested in the problems of surgery elsewhere or in a more democratic surgical organization. In light of this, somewhat to his surprise, Martin received an encouraging response from Harvey Cushing and other Boston surgeons.

After returning from the East and briefly resuming his surgical practice, Martin traveled west on March 6. He made his way up the West Coast via Los Angeles, San Francisco, Portland, Seattle and Vancouver. From there he traveled inland to Winnipeg (then the third largest city in Canada), Minneapolis, St. Paul, Kansas City, and St. Louis. In these cities he generally received enthusiastic support, although medical politics in San Francisco required that his supporters be discreet.[61] In fact, San Franciscan Phillip Mills Jones, editor of the *California State Journal of Medicine*, would prove one of the College's most vociferous critics. Martin himself did not visit the South: organization there depended on the work of local committees.

With his transcontinental travels completed, Martin journeyed to Washington, DC to meet with the other members of the organizing committee on the morning of May 5, 1913 at the Willard Hotel. Occurring at the same time as the Congress of Physicians and Surgeons, this second meeting established the efficient practice of holding meetings of the Regents during major national conferences, one which persisted for many years. At 2:30 pm the organizing committee met with a somewhat larger, representative body of surgeons from around the country. The final meeting of that busy day would occur in the evening when the organizing committee presented its report to those surgeons who had been invited to be founders of the new College and had accepted the invitation. Of the 500 invited, 450 accepted and of those about 300 were in Washington, DC that evening.

Edward Martin, as chair, set the tone of the afternoon meeting by describing the new College's mission as "the standardization of surgery for the benefit of the profession and the protection of the public."[62] Martin of Philadelphia had chosen his words advisedly.

"Standardization" had strongly positive connotations during the Progressive Era as organizations grew larger and more complex. Rhetorically, "standardization" also reflected a reaction to the apparent social chaos of rapid industrialization, immigration, urbanization, and recurrent economic crisis. For good reason a classic history of the Progressive Era bears the title *The Search for Order*.[63] Order was what the committee hoped to bring to surgery.

Franklin Martin, as secretary, next presented the proposed bylaws. The introduction to the bylaws made the College's goals explicit. The new organization, to be named the College of Surgeons, would raise the standard of surgery by defining fellowship and "formulat[ing] a plan which will indicate to the public and to the profession that the surgeon possessing such a fellowship is specially qualified to practice surgery as a specialty."[64] In other words, as the historian Rosemary Stevens observed, the College would be the first organization to offer the North American public a definition of a qualified specialist.[65]

Significantly for the College's future, much of the responsibility for the management of the College was invested in the 12 member Board of Regents to be elected from the Board of Governors. Of the Governors, 50 in number, 30 would be elected from surgeons nominated by the 13 major surgical societies and the surgical sections of the American and Canadian Medical Associations (three nominees each), and the United States Army and Navy (one nominee each). The remaining 20 would be elected at large. After a transition period both Regents and Governors would serve three-year terms. The Governors would also elect a President, First and Second Vice Presidents, a Treasurer, and a General Secretary. All but the Vice Presidents would be members of the Board of Regents. The bylaws, to an uncommon degree, invested much of the decision making and governing authority in the Board of Regents. Ostensibly, this elaborate structure would prevent the College from being captured by a particular faction. In practice it would mean that the Regents often "micromanaged" to a degree unusual in a board.

Martin also discussed the criteria for selecting Fellows. The bylaws laid out the basic prerequisites for membership: a valid medical license, endorsement by three Fellows (one a Governor), and meeting the qualification standards established by the Regents. The latter would prove to be an ongoing source of discussion and controversy for the next 50 years. To simplify their initial task, Martin and the organizing committee had divided potential members into four classes, A to D. The first three classes were filled through professional networks. The As consisted of the Founders; the Bs were nominees from the constituent surgical societies and the surgical section of the AMA; Cs were "surgeons of prominence" with 10 years' experience and the approval of the Credentials Committee to be admitted without examination. The Ds would require an examination. For an organization already accused of elitism and monopoly, this classification, while useful and purely functional, seemed to confirm the worst fears of the College's critics.

Apart from some objections about the under-representation of the Pacific Northwest and Canada on the Board of Governors, the afternoon meeting approved the bylaws. That evening the bylaws received the unanimous endorsement of the assembled Founders. Also unanimously approved was the strong stand made by a venerable Indiana surgeon, Miles F Porter, against admitting the many known fee splitters into the College. Porter had reminded the meeting that the College existed to judge the morals as well as the technical abilities of North American surgeons. The meeting then approved the officers of the new College: JMT Finney, President; Walter Chipman, First Vice President; Rudolph Matas, Second Vice President; AJ Ochsner, Treasurer; and Franklin Martin, General Secretary.

The new President addressed the Founders. Significantly, his remarks directly addressed critics of the College and reflected some of the controversy and medical politics surrounding the creation of the College. He reassured the audience that the College "was no surgical trust" and not "run by any one man or group of men ... for personal gain or aggrandizement."[66] (Franklin Martin's critics always believed that Martin established his organizations for his own benefit. Aware of these innuendos Finney took the precaution of getting an undated letter of resignation from Martin—one that he never needed to use and later quietly destroyed.)[67] Finney concluded his remarks by paying a handsome tribute to Martin, introducing him as the man "who after thirty years of hand-wringing and talking made this possible in six months."[68] Martin's drive, determination, and entrepreneurship had made the College a reality. In the coming years these qualities would prove both a boon and a handicap for the new organization.

Despite some reservations, many medical editors welcomed the new College. For example, the editor of the *Journal of the Michigan State Medical Society* "urge[d] the hearty and earnest support of the profession in Michigan to this College of Surgeons."[69] In general, those who supported the College drew attention to the need for reform and tended to see the College as part of a larger reform movement within medicine, one exemplified by the Flexner Report. In turn, this medical reform was part of the broader current of institutional reform that characterized the Progressive Era.

Those who opposed the College focused on its presumed "undemocratic" and thus "un-American" character. In particular, Phillip Mills Jones of the *California State Journal of Medicine* conducted a vigorous campaign against, as he termed it, the "American Royal College of Surgeons."[70] Jones spoke for many others. One letter writer to the *Illinois Medical Journal* referred to the College as an attempt "to engraft upon the democratic tree of free American medicine a royal sprout of would-be aristocracy."[71] The unfortunate categorization of surgeons as A, B, C, and D provided ammunition for critics like Jones. "Think of the state of mind of the poor man with a bellyache" Jones wrote "and finds that he has got a "B" Fellow or a "D" Fellow instead of an "A" Fellow! Shocking! Oh you Fellow [a play on a popular catch phrase]."[72] The classification suggested that undemocratic, elitist, and invidious distinction would occur even inside the new College.

The critics reflected a tension in American medicine. Jones and others like him, while supporting licensing that restricted competition *with* physicians, became fervent advocates of laissez-faire policies when it came to competition *between* physicians. In the critics' view, specialists were those who were implicitly recognized as such in the medical marketplace and no self-selected group had the right to make that distinction explicit or public. They also, like Jones, regarded the AMA as the only legitimate representative of the American medical profession. If reform was needed, then the AMA was the appropriate place for the medical profession to debate the question.

Even the editor of the *American Journal of Surgery* worried that the College might seek legislation establishing surgical licenses—a not unreasonable concern in an era that had seen a rapid expansion of professional and occupational licensing.[73] In fact, the Clinical Congress had endorsed just such a policy. Although the Regents seem to have briefly discussed this, no serious action was ever undertaken. Essentially, the College would rely on establishing itself as a brand.

The ASA officially distanced itself from the new organization. Although all but four of the Regents were ASA members, the minutes of the Association made no mention of the new College until 1915. At that year's annual meeting, the Secretary reported that the council had received a request from the ACS to appoint three members to the College's Board of Governors. While commending the purposes of the College, the council rejected the request on the grounds that these purposes were "totally" different from the ASA's and that no precedent existed for appointing members to the board of another society.[74] Nonetheless, despite this official indifference, a comparison of ASA and ACS membership lists shows that by 1920 almost all of the ASA's active members had joined the College.

The *Journal of the American Medical Association* (*JAMA*) confined itself to factual reporting. Powerful figures within the AMA's Chicago-based leadership and in Illinois medical politics disliked Franklin Martin. In fact, the Illinois delegation would introduce a motion condemning the College in the House of Delegates at the AMA's 1914 meeting. Martin and the College, however, did not lack allies among Illinois's medical politicians. A second, contradictory motion introduced by the Illinois delegation asked that the AMA "recognize the [the ACS] as filling a long-felt want which the American Medical Association has hitherto failed to meet." [75] The House of Delegates, wisely, tabled both motions. [76] The episode reflected the strong and divided reactions that Martin and the new College provoked.

Further, the jealousies aroused by Martin's successful foray into medical journalism still rankled with *JAMA*'s editor, George H Simmons. In April 1914 Simmons privately lectured Martin about the shortcomings of the new College and its organizers. [77] Beyond personalities, however, the new College represented a potential challenge to the AMA. At a time when the AMA was attempting to unify medicine and reform the profession's image and education, here was a new and independent organization that claimed the right to identify and represent an important specialist constituency.

REFERENCES

1. Brieger, G. H. (1992). From conservative to radical surgery in late nineteenth-century America. In C. Lawrence (Ed.), *Medical Theory, Surgical Practice: Studies in the History of Surgery* (pp. 216–229). New York, NY: Routledge.

2. Pernick, M. S. (1985). *A Calculus of Suffering: Pain, Professionalism, and Anesthesia in Nineteenth-century America*. New York, NY: Columbia University Press.

3. Wangensteen, O. H. (1965). Preludes to Lister and the interdependence of the sciences. *Surgery*, 58(5), 931-4. Granshaw, L. (1992). Upon this principle I have based a practice: The development and reception of antisepsis in Britain, 1867–90. In J. V. Pickstone (Ed.), *Medical Innovations in Historical Prospective* New York, NY: St. Martin's Press. Gariepy, T. S. (1994). The introduction and acceptance of Listerian antisepsis in the United States. *Journal of the History of Medicine and Allied Sciences*, 49(2), 167-206. Gaw, J. L. (1999). A Time to Heal: The Diffusion of Listerism in Victorian Britain. Darby, PA: Diane. Worboys, M. (2000). *Spreading Germs: Disease Theories and Medical Practice in Britain, 1865–1900*. Cambridge, UK: Cambridge University Press.

4. Greenwood, A. (1998). Lawson Tait and opposition to germ theory: Defining science in surgical practice. *Journal of the History of Medicine and Allied Sciences*, 53(2), 99–131. Kernahan, P. J. (2008). Causation and cleanliness: George Callender, wounds, and the debates over Listerism. *Journal of the History of Medicine and Allied Sciences*, 64(1), 1-37.

5. Temkin, O. (1951). The role of surgery in the rise of modern medical thought. *Bulletin of the History of Medicine*, 25, 248–59.

6. Carter, K. C. (2003). *The Rise of Causal Concepts of Disease: Case Histories, the History of Medicine in Context*. Burlington, VT: Ashgate. Temkin, O. (1977). The scientific approach to disease specific entity and individual sickness. In *The Double Face of Janus and Other Essays in the History of Medicine* (pp. 441–455). Baltimore, MD: Johns Hopkins University Press.

7. Smith, D. C. (1996). Appendicitis, appendectomy, and the surgeon. *Bulletin of the History of Medicine*, 70(3), 414–41. Sachs, M. (2004). Erfahrung und handeln in der geschichte der chirurgie, dargestellt am beispiel der sog. blinddarmoperation (appendektomie). *Sudhoffs Arch Z Wissenschaftsqesch Beih*, 54, 239–50.

8. Bulander, R. E. (2007). A sharp knife and a clean pair of hands: Surgical debates on the role of laparotomy, 1880–1900. *Journal of the American College of Surgeons*, 204(3), 498–504. Trohler, U. (1991). To operate or not to operate? Scientific exchanges and extraneous factors in therapeutic controversies within the Swiss Society of Surgeons, 1913–1988. *Clio Medica, 22*, 89–113. Wilde, S. (2004). See one, do one, modify one: Prostate surgery in the 1930s. *Medical History, 48*(3), 351–366. Wilde, S. (2009). Truth, trust, and confidence in surgery, 1890–1910: Patient autonomy, communication, and consent. *Bulletin of the History of Medicine, 83,* 302–31.

9. Fogelman, M. J. & Reinmiller, E. (1968). 1880–1890: A creative decade in world surgery. *American Journal of Surgery, 115*, 812–824.

10. Howell, J. D. (1995). *Technology in the Hospital: Transforming Patient Care in the Early Twentieth Century* (p. 57). Baltimore, MD: Johns Hopkins University Press.

11. Stevens, R. A. (1998). *American Medicine and the Public Interest: A History of Specialization* (2nd ed., p. 27). Berkeley, CA: Johns Hopkins University Press.

12. Ibid., p. 80.

13. Lilienthal, H. (1900). *Imperative Surgery for the General Practitioner, the Specialist, and the Recent Graduate* (p. vii). New York, NY: MacMillan.

14. Kernahan, P. (2010). *Franklin Martin and the standardization of American surgery 1890–1940*. (p. 46; Doctoral dissertation, University of Minnesota). Available from CIC Institutions. (Publication No. AAT 3422569)

15. Kernahan, P. J. (2008). A condition of development: Muckrakers, surgeons, and hospitals, 1890–1920. *Journal of the American College of Surgeons, 206*(2), 378. Lawrence, C. (1992). Democratic, divine and heroic: The history and historiography of surgery. In C. Lawrence (Ed.), *Medical Theory, Surgical Practice: Studies in the History of Surgery* (pp. 1–47). New York, NY: Routledge.

16. Editorial: The surgical fledgling [Editorial]. (1908). *American Medicine, 14*, 383.

17. Cushing, H. (1921). The personality of the hospital. *Boston Medical and Surgical Journal, 185*, 529–536.

18. American Medical Association. (1912). Abstract of discussion, section on hospitals, 63rd annual meeting of the AMA. *JAMA, 59*, 1677.

19. Murphy, J. B. (1912). Relation of the physician to the hospital. *JAMA, 59*, 1675. Firor, W. M. (1965). Residency training in surgery: Birth, decay and recovery. *Review of Surgery, 22*, 153–157. Kernahan, P. J. (2008). A condition of development: Muckrakers, surgeons, and hospitals, 1890–1920. *Journal of the American College of Surgeons, 206*(2), 378.

20. Sogge, L. (1913). Surgery in country hospitals. *Journal–Lancet, 33*(11), 313–314.

21. Ibid., p. 314.

22. Haggard, W. D. (1913). The qualifications of the surgeon. *Journal of the American Medical Association, 61*(3), 162.

23. Bonner, T. N. (1963). *American Doctors and German Universities: A Chapter in International Intellectual Relations, 1870–1914* (pp. 139–56). Lincoln, NE: University of Nebraska Press.

24. Burrow, J. G. (1977). *Organized Medicine in the Progressive Era: The Move Toward Monopoly*. Baltimore, MD: Johns Hopkins University Press.

25. Forbes, E. A. (1907). Is the doctor a shylock? Facts and figures about medical fees and incomes. *World's Work, 14*, 8892–6.

26. Dawson, A. (1979). The paradox of dynamic technological change and the labor aristocracy in the United States, 1880–1914. *Labor History, 20*(3), 336

27. Goebel, T. (1996). The uneven rewards of professional labor: Wealth and income in the Chicago professions, 1870–1920. *Journal of Social History, 29*(4), 754.

28. Ibid., p. 759.

29. Ghent, M. M. (1913). Who should do surgery? *The Journal–Lancet, 33*(22), 626–631.

30. Stevens, R. A. (1998). *American Medicine and the Public Interest: A History of Specialization* (2nd ed.; p. 82). Berkeley, CA: Johns Hopkins University Press.

31. Pauly, M. V. (1979). The ethics and economics of kickbacks and fee splitting. *The Bell Journal of Economics, 10*(1), 334–352.

32. Konold, D. E. (1962). *A History of American Medical Ethics, 1847–1912* (p. 66). Madison, WI: State Historical Society of Wisconsin. Grip of the specialist. (1907). *Living Age, 255*, 312–15.

33. Recent important decisions: Contracts—public policy-splitting fees by doctors. (1914). *Michigan Law Review, 12*(3), 227–8.

34. Rosenberg, C. E. (1987). *The Care of Strangers: the Rise of America's Hospital System* (p. 247). Baltimore, MD: Johns Hopkins University Press.

35. The figure for 1873 includes mental institutions. Ibid., p. 5. The figure for 1924 is from Morris, R. T. (1935). *Fifty Years a Surgeon* (p. 86). New York, NY: E P Dutton.

36. Rosenberg, C. E. (1987). *The Care of Strangers: the Rise of America's Hospital System* (pp. 237–61). Baltimore, MD: Johns Hopkins University Press.

37. Ibid., p. 249.

38. Kernahan, P. J. (2008). A condition of development: Muckrakers, surgeons, and hospitals, 1890–1920. *Journal of the American College of Surgeons, 206*(2), 380.

39. Starr, P. (1982). *The Social Transformation of American Medicine* (p. 171). New York, NY: Basic Books.

40. Jones, W. A. (1913). Medical Chaos and Crime. *Journal of the Minnesota State Medical Association and the Northwestern Lancet, 31*(5), 115–116.

41. Congress of American Physicians and Surgeons. (1888, September 18–20). *Minutes, First Triennial Session, Washington DC September 18–20, 1888*. Transactions of the Congress of American Physicians and Surgeons (p. xxiv).

42. Stevens, R. A. (1998). *American Medicine and the Public Interest: A History of Specialization* (2nd ed.; p. 89). Berkeley, CA: Johns Hopkins University Press.

43. Schieffelin, W. J. (1911). Work of the committee of one hundred on national health. *Annals of the American Academy of Political and Social Science, 37*(2), 77–86.

44. Shryock, R. H. (1967). *Medical Licensing in America* (p. 59; n2). Baltimore, MD: Johns Hopkins University Press. Petrina, S. (2008). Medical liberty: Drugless healers confront allopathic doctors, 1910–1931. *Journal of Medical Humanities 29*(4), 205–230.

45. Lewis, D. S. (1962). *The Royal College of Physicians and Surgeons of Canada, 1920–1960* (pp. 144–5). Montreal, CAN: McGill University Press.

46. Allen, D. P. (1907). The teaching of surgery. *Transactions of the American Surgical Association, 25*, 1–14.

47. Crile, G. W. & Crile, G. M. (1947). *George Crile: An Autobiography, vol. 1* (p. 141). Philadelphia, PA: J. B. Lippincott.

48. Martin, F. H. (1934). *Fifty Years of Medicine and Surgery: An Autobiographical Sketch* (p. 3). Chicago: The Surgical Publishing Company.

49. Ibid., p. 140.

50. Peitzman, S. J. (1980). Thoroughly practical: America's polyclinic medical schools. *Bulletin of the History of Medicine, 54*, 166–187.

51. Martin, F. H. (1905). Surgery, gynecology, and obstetrics [Editorial]. *Surgery, Gynecology, and Obstetrics, 1*(1), 62.

52. Grimm, E. K., *Dr. Franklin H. Martin, Criticism During WW1*. n.d., Eleanor Grimm Notebooks XXIV, Archives of the American College of Surgeons, Chicago.

53. Martin, F. H. (1934). *Fifty Years of Medicine and Surgery: An Autobiographical Sketch* (p. 293). Chicago: The Surgical Publishing Company.

54. Crile, G. W. & Crile, G. M. (1947). *George Crile: An Autobiography, vol. 2* (p. 232). Philadelphia, PA: J. B. Lippincott.

55. Codman, E. A. (1934). *Rupture of the Supraspinatus Tendon and Other Lesions In or About the Subacromial Bursa* (p. xiii). Boston, MA: Thomas Dodd.

56. Ibid., xvii.

57. Martin, F. H. (1934). *Fifty Years of Medicine and Surgery: An Autobiographical Sketch* (p. 300). Chicago: The Surgical Publishing Company.

58. Gage, H. (1914). Some abuses in surgical practice. *Boston Medical and Surgical Journal, 169*(1), 3.

59. Crile, G. W. & Crile, G. M. (1947). *George Crile: An Autobiography, vol. 1* (pp. 232–3). Philadelphia, PA: J. B. Lippincott.

60. Martin, F. H. (1934). *Fifty Years of Medicine and Surgery: An Autobiographical Sketch* (p. 303). Chicago: The Surgical Publishing Company.

61. Martin, F. H. (1933). *The Joy of Living: An Autobiography, vol. 1* (pp. 413–422). New York, NY: Doubleday, Doran & Co. Davis, L. (1960). *Fellowship of Surgeons: A History of the American College of Surgeons* (pp. 71–7). Springfield, IL: Charles C. Thomas.

62. American College of Surgeons. (1913, May 5). *Board of Regents: Minutes May 5, 1913*. Complete Minute Book 1. Archives of the American College of Surgeons, Chicago.

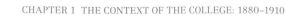

63. Wiebe, R. H. (1967). *The Search for Order, 1877–1920.* The Making of America, editor: David Donald. New York: Hill and Wang.

64. American College of Surgeons (1913, May 5). *Board of Regents: Minutes May 5, 1913.* Complete Minute Book 1. Archives of the American College of Surgeons, Chicago.

65. Stevens, R. A. (1998). *American Medicine and the Public Interest: A History of Specialization.* (2nd ed.; p. 96). Berkeley, CA: Johns Hopkins University Press.

66. American College of Surgeons. (1913, May 5). *Meeting of the Organization Committee of the College of Surgeons.* Complete Minute Book 1, Archives of the American College of Surgeons, Chicago.

67. Finney, J. M. T. (1940). *A Surgeon's Life: the Autobiography of J. M. T. Finney* (p. 134–5). New York, NY: G. P. Putnam's Sons.

68. American College of Surgeons. (1913, May 5). *Meeting of the Organization Committee of the College of Surgeons.* Complete Minute Book 1, Archives of the American College of Surgeons, Chicago.

69. Editorial: The American College of Surgeons [Editorial]. (1913). *J. Michigan State Medical Society,* 338. Eleanor Grimm Notebooks V, Archives of the American College of Surgeons, Chicago.

70. Jones, P. M. (1913). The American Royal College of Surgeons. *California State Medical Journal, 11*(5), 175–6.

71. Noble, W. L. (1913). [Letter]. *Illinois Medical Journal, 25*(5), 308–9.

72. Jones, P. M. (1913). THE College. *California State Medical Journal, 11*(7), 254–5.

73. Editorial: The College of Surgeons [Editorial]. (1913). *American Journal of Surgery, 27,* 234–5. Hogan, D. B. (1983). The effectiveness of licensing: History, evidence, and recommendations. *Law and Human Behavior, 7*(2/3), 120.

74. American Surgical Association. (n.d.). *Annual meeting minutes 1905–1920.* American Surgical Association (MSC 379, Box 1, Folder 2, p. 735). National Library of Medicine.

75. American Medical Association. (1914). Proceedings of the Atlantic City session. *Journal of the American Medical Association, 63*(1), 104.

76. Ibid.

77. American College of Surgeons. (1914, April 11). *Board of Regents: Minutes April 11, 1914.* Complete Minute Book 1. Archives of the American College of Surgeons, Chicago.

CHAPTER 2
Who Is a Surgeon?
1912–1920

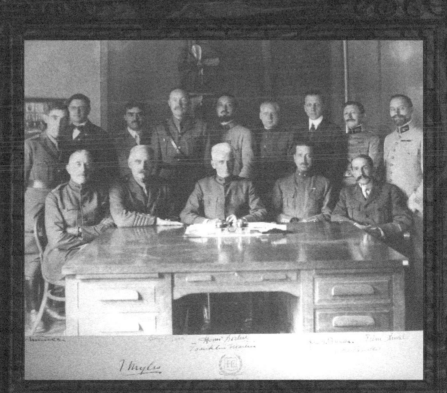

Visiting Doctors from Abroad, 1918: Foreign surgeons who visited the United States during World War I

Late in the evening of that busy May 5 in Washington, DC, the Regents of the new College of Surgeons met for the first time. In the emotionally charged atmosphere they prepared for the task ahead. Over the course of the next eight years, they would attempt to standardize both surgeon and hospital. World War I would see most of the College principals and many Fellows engaged in war work. The war would also strengthen ties with the Royal College of Surgeons. A permanent home for the College would be selected and an uneasy relationship established with the American Medical Association (AMA).

≈✳≈

Defining the Surgeon

The new College existed to define and designate the qualified surgeon and to combat fee splitting. Assessing the fitness of an individual to practice surgery requires a close evaluation of training, experience, clinical and basic science knowledge, technical skill, and ethical fitness. The bylaws prescribed the basic minimums: license, medical school, and endorsement by three Fellows. The question of a suitable evaluation or examination remained open. For the A, B, and C Fellows admitted in the 1913 cohort, reputation sufficed for the evaluation. For those in the D category who fell outside of elite networks, the new Regents quickly recognized that some form of examination would be required in addition to criteria defining adequate training and experience.

The task would prove a difficult one. In the initial optimism surrounding the founding of the College, the new Regents hoped to develop criteria for the unfortunately named Class D surgeons by the time of the first convocation in October of 1913. In fact it would be 1915 before the final criteria for admission would be published. (The Regents' meetings lacked a formal agenda until 1935, which probably contributed to the sometimes wandering and indecisive nature of debates on controversial matters.) Even so, within 10 years individuals both within and outside the College would argue that standards were too lax—an argument that precipitated the first serious critique of the College's leadership.

Perhaps unsurprisingly, the Regents vacillated over the question of what constituted an appropriate examination. How much should the exam measure academic knowledge and how much should it evaluate practical experience? Did their only existing model, the examinations of the Royal Colleges, place too much emphasis on academic knowledge and too little on technical knowledge and experience? Should the exam be a formal written examination and, if so, who should administer it and where should it be held? How should experience (essentially technical skill and judgment) be measured? How could adequate training be determined at a time when most surgeons had little formal training?

Given the realities of medical practice in North America, should the fellowship be restricted to surgeons who limited their practice entirely to surgery? The fact that the Regents had to set a standard for those already in practice and those who would be entering practice compounded their difficulties. All told, the Regents faced a formidable task while under close and sometimes hostile scrutiny from the profession and existing institutions.

The difficult task fell to Edward Martin as chair of the committee on examinations. Like the discussions of the Regents, his recommendations fluctuated back and forth. His first report to the Regents in October 1913 defined the problem as "certifying that a man is fit to practice surgery—not going to be fit" and gave some general requirements.[1] He left open the type of examination. At that point the sense of the meeting seemed to favor some form of academic exam. As Edward Martin put it, the requirements represented "an entering wedge for a special examination" one perhaps ultimately given by the U.S. and Canadian governments.[2] With this and other flights of fancy, to which Franklin Martin proved particularly prone, the discussion at times became unfocused as the Regents debated what form an examination should take.

As the debate continued into 1914, the Regents weighed the pros and cons of judging a surgeon by experience or by formal examination. Herbert Bruce, a fellow of the Royal College of Surgeons, recommended that the College take a two-stage approach.[3] For the moment, admission of existing surgeons could be based on experience. This, in his mind, would correspond to the category of Member of the Royal College of Surgeons. In later years, as the problem shifted from identifying the qualified surgeon among those already in practice to the surgeon preparing to enter practice, a higher academic qualification could be introduced corresponding to the Fellowship of the Royal College.

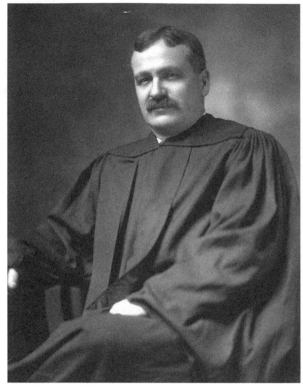

FIGURE 2.1 Dr. JMT Finney, first ACS President, 1913–16.

John B Murphy and JMT Finney both supported this approach and, as Finney observed, "the sooner we get to the double examination [experience and testing] the better."[4] Given the democratic ethos of American medicine and the fact that even the operational categories of A, B, C, and D surgeons had generated controversy, such a two-tiered system would have aroused even greater criticism of the College. For better or worse, the Regents ultimately rejected Bruce's suggestion. (Figure 2.1)

In June 1914, Edward Martin presented his committee's final report to the Regents and to a mass meeting of the Fellows at the Bellevue Stratford in Philadelphia.[5] In it, they recommended an experience-based standard rather than a written academic examination. After a year of internship, the prospective candidate would need a year as a first assistant or three years as a second assistant to "an active surgeon of recognized ability" and exposure to at least 100 cases. Also required were evidence of visiting other clinics, a list of publications, some evidence of work done to advance surgery, and a report of 50 consecutive major operations followed up to the date of application to the College. Drawing on 19th century stereotypes of the pragmatic American, Edward Martin regarded this as "a simple American solution" for an organization of practical surgeons.[6] Unlike the unmentioned Royal Colleges, the candidate would need to expend no time "preparing for foolish examinations."[7] A modified version of the plan, described as "tentative" and requiring only abstracts of cases, appeared in the 1914 Year Book.[8]

The College finally published the formal requirements for fellowship in the 1915 Year Book, almost two years after the Regent's original November 1913 deadline. Without ever taking a definite vote, a consensus seems to have been reached that the case reports (50 in detail and 50 in summary) submitted to the Central Credentials Committee would constitute the examination. Franklin Martin first suggested the idea of case reports as a way to assess the competency of the surgeon in the smaller community, from which many applications in Class D would come. These surgeons stood outside of more elite and urban networks, and their work was less subject to professional scrutiny.

The plan bore some resemblance to medical reformer Ernest Codman's end-result system that would influence the other great standardization project—the inspection of hospitals. As first suggested by Martin, however, the case reports would have been as a preliminary evaluation before a formal examination.[9] As the debate went forward, case reports became the examination. The number 50 first appeared as an impromptu aside by Charlie Mayo.[10] From this somewhat haphazard process emerged the requirements for fellowship.

As finally published, the qualified surgeon would be one who had (a) graduated from an approved medical school, (b) served one year as an intern at a "creditable" hospital, (c) served two years as a surgical assistant or gave evidence of an equivalent apprenticeship, (d) had five to eight years of practice experience, (e) did not split fees and signed the pledge against fee-splitting (ethical fitness), and (f) in a city of under 50,000 devoted at least a 50 percent of the practice to surgery and in a larger city at least 80 percent of the practice to surgery. The Regents established an examination of 100 case records, 50 in detail and an additional 50 in summary. Having met these criteria and been recommended by the local committee, the successful applicant could use the post-nominal letters of FACS.

Given the circumstances prevailing at the time, the Regents' own training, and the logistical difficulties of arranging a formal examination, the plan can be defended as a reasonable compromise to evaluate surgeons already in practice. It left open the question of a more rigorous examination for future candidates, one the Regents discussed in October 1915.[11] But despite slight amendments to the fellowship criteria, throughout Martin's tenure as Director General the College never readdressed this question. As a result, the College would lose the opportunity to remain the certifying authority in surgery to the American Board of Surgery in 1937 (see chapter 6).

The post-nominal letters went through several iterations between the initial proposal of FACS and the final acceptance of FACS. Out of concern for presumed Canadian sensitivities the "American" had been briefly dropped from the College's name. Fellows would be identified as FCSA or FCSC (Fellow of the College of Surgeons of America or Canada respectively). Others objected that FACS spelled 'facts,' a trivial objection in Franklin Martin's view, not least because it appears to have originated from his longtime opponent Chicago surgeon Arthur Bevan of the AMA. After some delay, and after Canadian reassurances that "American" was to be understood in its broadest sense, the initials FACS met with the Regents' approval.

This was not a trivial matter. At a time when custom condemned advertising by physicians the initials would be the identifying mark of the qualified surgeon. Perhaps surprisingly, the AMA did not officially object to the use of the initials.[12] A number of editorialists did, reflecting the profession's discomfort with such undemocratic distinctions. As the editor of Minnesota's *Journal-Lancet* commented, "the use of titles does not make much of an impression on an American, he is too democratic."[13] But without a mechanism to identify the qualified surgeon to the public and the profession, and in the absence of any legal authority, the College's reform program could not succeed.

This reform agenda extended to the moral character of surgeons. Ethical surgery, in the minds of the Regents and many other leading surgeons, meant an end to fee splitting. Combating fee splitting generated considerable discussion among the Regents in those early meetings. At times the discussion became very frank and sensitive, but the Regents remained united in their condemnation of the practice. In the absence of any legal authority, the College would attempt to eliminate fee splitting by a three-fold strategy: (a) denying admission to known fee splitters (hence the importance of the local knowledge of the state and provincial credentials committees), (b) making hospital accreditation contingent on eliminating fee splitters from the staff, and (c) requiring applicants to sign an oath (the Fellowship Pledge) renouncing fee splitting. While the latter action made a strong rhetorical point and its violation defensible grounds for revoking a fellowship, the Regents' recognized its limitations. As JMT Finney ruefully noted during a discussion of the Pledge, the dishonest would sign and break it, just as dishonest bridegrooms swore fidelity at the altar.[14]

Having defined the qualifications (training, experience, and ethics) required to be recognized as a surgeon, the Regents also needed to define the borders of surgery as a discipline. At a time of growing specialization, which specialties counted as "surgical"? In 1913, 53 percent of the first class of Fellows gave their specialty as 'surgery' (the term "general surgery" as a category of surgeon does not appear in the Directory until 1965). Forty-three percent listed one of the special branches of surgery, including ophthalmology, otolaryngology, gynecology, orthopaedics, and genito-urinary surgery.[15] There had initially been some debate over otolaryngology and urology about whether these were truly surgical specialties given their outpatient focus at the time. The Regents answered in the affirmative for those who operated, but drew the line at dermatology.[16] In other words, the Regents answered the question broadly—the operating room defined the discipline.

The bylaws gave each of the major surgical specialty societies, including the Surgical Sections of the AMA and the Canadian Medical Association (CMA), the right to nominate representatives to the Board of Governors. After some debate, the Regents included the American Institute of Homeopathy (AIH) among the 16 nominating societies with the understanding that this did not constitute an endorsement of homeopathy.[17] At the time, graduates of the homeopathic medical schools represented about 10 percent of all physicians and the AIH remained a nominating society until the late 1940s. Additionally, the Regents established the tacit policy of reserving three seats on the Board of Regents for Canadians—one that persisted into 1950s.[18] Later the College briefly considered offering the fellowship to anesthesiologists in the early 1950s.[19] While this later suggestion came to nothing, the new College would represent a broadly defined North American surgery.

In drawing up their criteria for admission to the College, the Regents had not considered either gender or race. While no women appear among the original 500 Founders, by the end of 1913 five women had received fellowships. All were from Boston. Here women made up a significant part of the medical workforce, and the New England Hospital for Women and Children helped provide an important support network. Despite the small number of women, male and female Fellows represented remarkably similar proportions of the medical workforce—a little less than one percent of the physicians of each gender.[20]

By 1930, the College had at least 60 women members and six had served on the Board of Governors. Lillian K P Farrar and Agnes C Vietor became the first in 1925.[21] The women Fellows practiced primarily in the Northeast and upper Midwest, reflecting the overall distribution of women doctors at the time. Boston and Philadelphia contributed the largest numbers. Bertha Van Hoosen, a nationally prominent surgeon and professor of gynecology at Loyola University in Chicago, believed that the College admitted men and women on equal terms.[22] In responding to critics in the 1930s, the Regents would specifically refer to "the men and women of the College"—an inclusiveness rarely demonstrated in medical writings of the period.

For African American surgeons, admission would be difficult for more than a generation—the founding of the College occurred as Jim Crow became entrenched. Professionals, including physicians, faced particular hardships.[23] In this setting, the prominent Chicago surgeon, Daniel Hale Williams, founder of Chicago's interracial Provident Hospital, one of the first surgeons in the world to operate on a stab wound to the heart, and, like Franklin Martin and Charles Mayo, a graduate of Northwestern University, became the first African American to receive the fellowship—but only after a heated debate among the Regents.

Williams' application had been strongly endorsed by Martin and eight other leading Chicago surgeons, and he was among those who would be inducted at the 1913 Convocation. Significantly, no objection was made to Williams' inclusion until Regent William Haggard of Nashville raised the issue when the Regents met the night before the convocation. As the Regents reviewed the list of candidates, Haggard called attention to Williams, having learned "that he is a colored man."[24] The presence of a "negro" would, Haggard argued, pose an intolerable social problem for the wives of Southern surgeons; result in an "enormous number of negroes" applying; and cause Southern surgeons to reject the College. Haggard threatened to resign over the issue.

A heated exchange between Haggard and AJ Ochsner then ensued in which Ochsner championed Williams' cause. Significantly, during the debate JMT Finney (a Southerner by birth) and George Brewer stated firmly that as a scientific organization the College should have no color line. Without expressing a personal opinion on a matter that concerned the American members, Robert McKecknie of Vancouver pointed out that the Royal College of Surgeons, so often used as a model by the Regents in their deliberations, admitted "Hindoos (sic) [and] negroes as well as different white races" as Fellows.[25] When John B Murphy offered a compromise that would have deferred action, Ochsner threatened to resign himself. Faced with such strong opposition Haggard retreated. Ochsner had won the debate.

The Regents' decision drew a favorable response from African American publications. The *Chicago Defender*, the city's leading African American newspaper, and the *Journal of the National Medical Association* (*JNMA*) wrote enthusiastically about the College's decision.[26] But within a year, the editor of the latter journal had become aware of the debate that accompanied Williams' admission and with regret informed his readers of this fact. The debate also affected College headquarters. Fearful of controversy and of losing an entire region, it would be another two decades before "MERIT and not RACE," to use the words of *JNMA*'s editor, "would be the countersign at the portals of the American College of Surgeons."[27] The memory of Haggard's threat of a Southern boycott lingered on. Not until the 1940s would the College really address the color line.

JNMA's editor had also identified a structural flaw in the fellowship process—the potential that "membership goes by local favor not by merit."[28] Using a standard based on experience, while reasonable at the time, required local knowledge of a candidate's fitness. This gave the local committees, however, the ability to block applicants for a variety of reasons beyond competence and ethical character, itself a slippery concept. The editor of the *New York Medical Journal* expressed similar concerns while generally supporting the aims of the College, as did many others.[29] The Regents themselves had recognized the potential for local prejudice in their discussion of the entrance exam.[30] In the coming years, the Regents would receive many appeals from candidates blocked by their local committees.

John G Bowman Joins the College

When the Regents met on June 22, 1914, Franklin Martin recommended that a permanent director be hired. At the time, all of the Regents, including Martin, continued in the active practice of surgery while the administrative demands of the College grew. By the end of 1914, the Regents had formed a Committee on Administrative Policy, chaired by JMT Finney and including Martin. Out of this came a recommendation to the Regents that the College hire a full-time director to oversee its programs, particularly its educational activities. Although some of the Regents, notably Rudolph Matas, argued that the director should be a surgeon, Martin felt strongly that, as an educational institution, the College required an educator.

The Regents subsequently considered two candidates: John G Bowman, the former president of the University of Iowa, and Charles R van Hise, the president of the University of Wisconsin. As the younger of the two at age 39, Bowman became the clear choice with relatively little debate. Franklin Martin met with Bowman and came away highly impressed, as did Finney, Surgeon General Stokes, and Edward Martin. Finney favorably described Bowman as a "straight, clean fellow."[31] Given the importance attached to combating fee splitting, Bowman's uncompromising if ultimately unsuccessful campaign against the practice at the University of Iowa's medical school recommended him highly. (Iowa would remain an area of particular concern to the College for many years.)

Also, Bowman's previous position as secretary of the Carnegie Foundation and the strong endorsement of the Foundation's president, Henry S Pritchett, worked in Bowman's favor, particularly because the Regents looked to Carnegie as a possible source of funding. Martin had exclaimed earlier that the College "should have a $12,000 man and not a $7,000 man."[32] The more down to earth Pritchett recommended that the College offer Bowman $5,000 per annum and settle for $6,000. The Regents' offered $6,000. Bowman promptly accepted the offer and joined the College as Director of Education in February 1915.

He took up his new duties with enthusiasm. He traveled extensively and made the College's cause his own. Addressing the Fellows attending the annual AMA meeting in San Francisco in June 1915, he compared the fellowship to a master's degree in surgery.[33] Perhaps reflecting his academic background Bowman introduced the Certificate of Fellowship at this meeting. Like the academic gowns that Martin chose for the College in 1913, the new certificates emphasized the College as a *fellowship* and as an educational organization. Like the post-nominal FACS, the certificate provided a distinguishing mark in the medical marketplace and, as the office display of diplomas did not contravene professional ethics, an acceptable form of advertising.

Bowman's travels brought him into contact with the local committees as they selected members, bringing an additional measure of central oversight to the process. Writing from San Francisco, he informed Martin that, in the case of two candidates, "I am inclined to hesitate…rather than take the judgment of the San Francisco Fellows."[34] In Halifax, Nova Scotia, as in many other cities, he met with business leaders, "the governor [sic] of the province," hospital trustees, and the local credentials committee.[35] These travels would be important in developing the hospital standardization program and in increasing the public profile of the new organization as the arbiter of surgical quality and the qualified surgeon.

The Regents' hopes that he would provide a liaison with the Carnegie Foundation proved true. Bowman remained in close contact with Pritchett and, after a dinner with

Pritchett shortly after taking up his duties with the College, Bowman could reassure Martin that the latter had Pritchett's goodwill.[36] The question of how the Secretary and the Director would share responsibility for the College's management remained open—at this time Martin continued to maintain his private practice and would soon be caught up in preparations for U.S. entry into World War I.

≈ ✳ ≈

The College, the Great War, and the "Battle of Chicago"

With a membership representing surgeons of the United States and Canada, the American College of Surgeons entered WWI twice. First, the British Government's declaration of war on August 4, 1914 brought all of the Empire, including Canada, into the conflict. Second, the United States declared war on the Central Powers on April 7, 1917. But the intervening years saw the College, and particularly Franklin Martin, preparing for the conflict. These wartime activities gave the new College a greater national prominence but would lead to a rift between the College and the AMA. Additionally, the war greatly strengthened the ties between the new American College and the Royal College of Surgeons.

As United States entry into the war became increasingly likely in 1916, Martin, together with several other ACS principals including the Mayo brothers, established the Committee of American Physicians for National Preparedness. Among 80 members, the AMA had one lone official representative. At the same time, Martin offered the services of the new College to Army Surgeon General William C Gorgas.

Martin's interest in preparedness reflected his Anglophilia, his ambitions to be at the center of national affairs, and his own war-time adventures. In August 1914, he had helped organize the repatriation of members of the Clinical Congress (held that summer in London) stranded in England by the outbreak of war. Subsequently, he made a dramatic trip across Germany to bring his niece safely home from Munich, a feat reported nationally.[37] In December 1914, Martin, JMT Finney, and Charles Mayo helped found a relief organization for the physicians and pharmacists of occupied Belgium.[38] In 1916, by seizing the initiative and organizing the profession's preparedness committee, Franklin Martin brought himself and the College to the attention of the highest levels of government.

Meanwhile, President Woodrow Wilson established his war cabinet—the Council on National Defense (CND)—consisting of the Secretaries of War, Navy, Interior, Agriculture, Commerce, and Labor. In the same flurry of preparedness, Congress authorized a six-member civilian Advisory Council for the CND to represent finance, industry, retail, transportation, labor, and education.

Through lobbying, Martin's ally Dr. Frank Simpson, secretary of the Committee of America Physicians for Medical Preparedness, obtained a seventh representative for medicine—an appointment Martin then occupied; one the leadership of the AMA, not unreasonably, thought should have been given to their organization. In doing so, Martin joined Julius Rosenwald, Sears Roebuck's vice president and Chicago philanthropist; Daniel Willard, president of the Baltimore and Ohio Railroad; Bernard Baruch, an influential financier; Hollis Godfrey of the Drexel Institute; Howard Coffin of the Hudson Motor Car Company; and Samuel Gompers, president of the American Federation of

Labor. When a subsidiary General Medical Board was established in April 1917 to oversee medical mobilization, Martin became its chair. The College, an institution that had not existed five years earlier and which represented less than one percent of the nation's medical manpower, had risen, through Martin, to national prominence.

But the outcome did nothing to improve relations with the AMA, setting the stage for what George Crile, returning from active service in France in October 1917, called "The Second Battle of Chicago."[39] (The first was his attempt to reorganize the Army's medical services.) Recognizing the undesirability of friction between the AMA, representative of the profession as a whole, and the College, Crile and William Mayo, now President of the College, attempted a rapprochement between the AMA's leadership and Martin. Encouraged by an initial meeting with the AMA, Crile attempted to convince Martin "that he must learn to love these American Medical Association men and take them into his organization [the General Medical Board] as brothers." Martin, ill with influenza, raised himself from his sick-bed long enough to say "Never!" before collapsing back on the bed in a "state of rigor mortis." Grudgingly, Martin accepted the proposal. Crile, Edward Martin, and Regent Frank Simpson then met in several days of at times tense negotiations with Bevan and other senior AMA officials and convinced them to accept Franklin Martin's leadership. But as we will see later collaboration for the war effort was one thing; the relationship between the AMA and the ACS would remain fraught. (Figure 2.2)

In all, 90 percent of the fellowship participated in some way in the war effort. Forty percent of Fellows were on active service in either the U.S. or Canadian armies, with an additional 10 percent in the U.S. Navy Medical Corps. Another 40 percent registered with the Volunteer Medical Service Corps, organized by Martin through the Advisory Council, prepared for emergency service in the U.S. Army, Navy, or Public Health Service. Fellows of the College commanded the majority of the U.S. Army base hospitals in France.[40]

The war brought British, Canadian, and American surgeons into closer contact and also brought the leaders of the Royal and American Colleges together. At the 1917 Convocation, Sir Berkeley Moynihan, one of Britain's most prominent surgeons serving as a Colonel in the British Army, delivered the Fellowship Address, "What Is the War About?" The next year with the Clinical Congress and Convocation cancelled because of the influenza epidemic, Martin arranged a tour of leading medical centers for an Allied delegation led by Moynihan.

At casualty clearing stations and base hospitals, American surgeons provided care for British and Canadian casualties, among them Edward Revere Osler, only son of Sir William Osler; the great-great-great grandson of Paul Revere; and a 21-year-old officer in the British artillery. (Tragically, even the combined efforts of Founders Harvey Cushing, George Crile, William Darrach, and George Brewer could not save the young man's life.)[41] In recognition of this wartime collaboration, in 1920 the Royal College of Surgeons presented the ACS with the ceremonial Great Mace. (Figure 2.3)

The inscription reads: "From the Consulting Surgeons of the British Armies to the American College of Surgeons in memory of mutual work and good fellowship in the Great War 1914–1918."

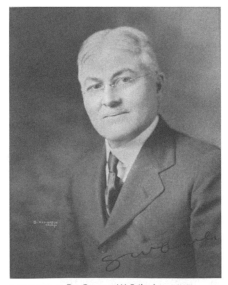

FIGURE 2.2 Dr. George W Crile, longtime chairman of the Board of Regents, in 1920.

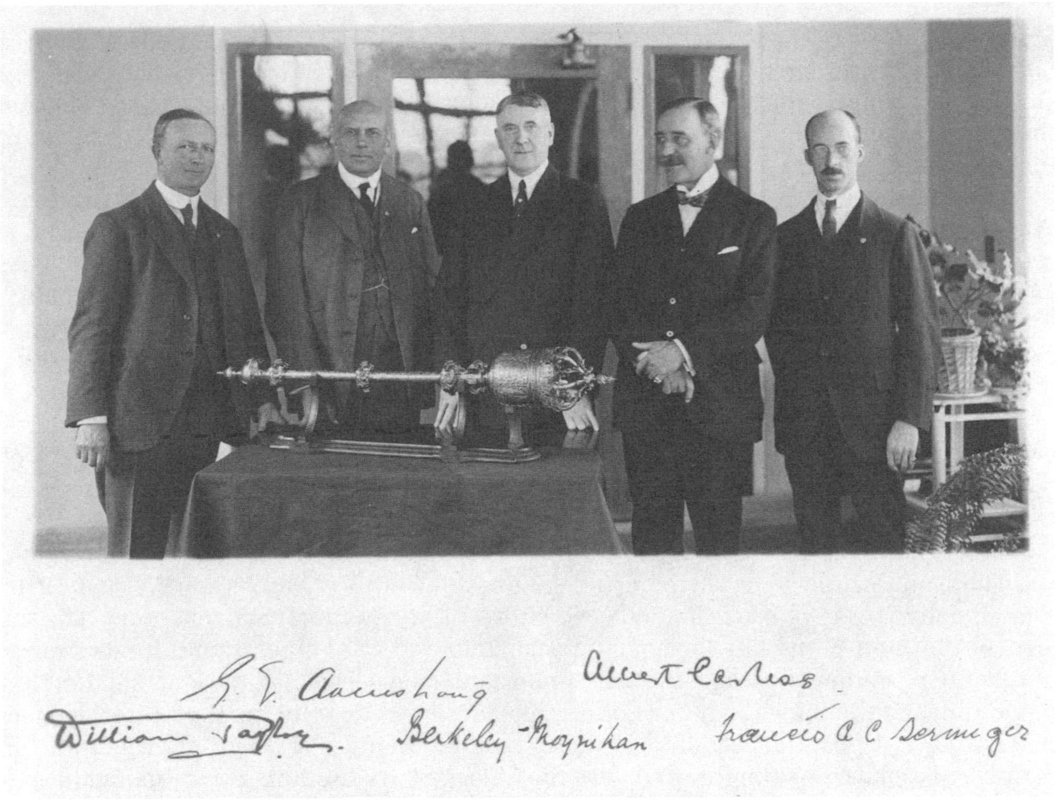

G. E. Armstrong   Albert Carless

William Taylor   Berkeley Moynihan   Francis A C Bermingez

FIGURE 2.3 The Great Mace, presented to the College by the Royal College of Surgeons.

The College Finds a Home

Throughout this time, Martin and his fellow officers remained in surgical practice. Much of the initial College business was conducted from their private offices and at their own expense. As Ochsner noted, handling the more than 15,000 letters of inquiry about fellowship had monopolized the time of one young man in his office while Martin kept four clerks busy in his.[42] The College used Martin's own office as its headquarters until 1917 when the College rented an office on East Washington Street in Chicago. From the beginning, the Regents recognized that the College would need a more satisfactory arrangement than shared space or a rented office.

As early as November 1913, Franklin Martin and JMT Finney, the College's President, discussed the question of a permanent home. The uneasy relationship with the AMA complicated the search. Finney and Martin agreed that the presence of the AMA in Chicago made that city a difficult location for the new College. While subsequently presented by Martin to the Regents as a "matter of equity [that] another city should have the honor of housing this new and important organization," it is clear from the subsequent discussion that the Regents were sensitive to the AMA's reaction to the new organization and to Martin's fraught relationship with its Chicago-based leadership.[43] Also, opposition to the College had been particularly intense in Illinois, where the Illinois

State Medical Society had passed a resolution condemning the College as undemocratic.[44] Similar resolutions had been passed by various branches of the Chicago Medical Society.[45] "It is my absolute conviction," Martin told the Regents, "that this is the wrong place for the American College of Surgeons."[46] The Regents then appointed a committee to study the question.

The Regents continued their discussion of a permanent home during the next year. Washington, DC became an early favorite, but the large Midwestern cities offered a central location and reasonable railway connections from both coasts and Canada. Thus, as Crile noted, Chicago "would be the natural center were it not for other influences." His suggestion that Cleveland made a good substitute was dismissed by Navy Surgeon General Stokes, who believed the dignity of the College would not be helped by locating it in Cleveland rather than in Washington, his personal choice.[47] Murphy suggested Minneapolis and argued that it was better to stay away from Washington with its potential for malign political influence.[48] At this time, William Mayo, as a Regent of the University of Minnesota, apparently thought that he could persuade the university to donate land and money for a College headquarters. This somewhat parochial and inconclusive discussion continued into 1916 with Washington remaining the leading site.

The issue would be resolved after the death of John B Murphy in August 1916. The Murphy family offered the College a substantial donation in his memory. Martin formed the John B Murphy Memorial Association and raised additional funds from a number of prominent Chicagoans. More importantly, he persuaded the Regents that this made Chicago the logical site for College headquarters despite his (and their) earlier reservations. A postal ballot of the Fellows resulted in an overwhelming vote in favor of Chicago. Delayed by the war and with the Chicago Park Commission refusing the use of lake-front land, Martin, with the approval of the Regents, purchased the Nickerson Mansion property on the northwest corner of Erie Street at Cass (now Wabash) in 1919. The Murphy Memorial Auditorium would be built, not without controversy, next to the mansion on Erie and dedicated on June 11, 1926. A symbol of Martin's at times grandiose ideas and excess with its $15,000 brass doors from Tiffany & Company, the building cost more than $500,000. Only a last minute appeal by Martin to the three Murphy daughters produced the final $30,000 that allowed completion of the project.[49] The baronial auditorium with its raised dais and throne-like chairs for the Regents proved too small for the Convocations and was rarely used.

The editorial office of *Surgery, Gynecology, and Obstetrics (SGO)* subsequently moved to a property adjacent to the auditorium on the northeastern side of the Erie block. Owned by the Surgical Publishing Company, in which the Martins held 51 percent of the shares, *SGO* had become the College's official organ in 1919 and the move helped consolidate the relationship with the College. (Martin rejected Will Mayo's suggestion that *SGO* be renamed the *Journal of the American College of Surgeons*, an idea adopted 75 years later.)[50] As part of Martin's astute investment in Chicago real estate, the College subsequently acquired the land on the south side of Erie. The Nickerson Mansion remained College headquarters until 1963, when the College built a new building across Erie Street on the land Martin had acquired.

What Is a Hospital? The Beginnings of the Hospital Standardization Program

After the standardization of the surgeon, the standardization of the surgeon's workplace, the hospital, became the second great arm of the College's reform program. Having defined a "minimum standard" to identify the qualified surgeon, the College would do the same for the hospital. Indeed, concerns about the quality of hospital care had been as great as those about surgeons. For this reason, the 1912 Clinical Congress of Surgeons of North America (CCSNA) meeting saw the appointment of two committees: one headed by Franklin Martin and charged with creating a college, the second, headed by Boston surgeon Ernest A Codman, charged with reforming the hospital. In the coming years the College would assume the work of Codman's committee.

Codman, a surgeon at the Massachusetts General Hospital, had a keen interest in improving the quality of hospital care. He argued forcefully, if not always tactfully, for his "end-result system"—hospitals should measure outcomes through long-term patient follow-up and make this information public.[51] Unfortunately, Codman lacked Franklin Martin's executive abilities. His committee produced two reports that confirmed the need for hospital improvement, but left any action to the AMA or the Carnegie Foundation.[52] The AMA had no interest in taking on a project that might lead to conflict with local members.[53] Codman's attempts to interest the Carnegie Foundation in a survey of hospitals were unsuccessful. (Pritchett in fact went to some lengths to avoid meeting Codman even when Codman arrived unannounced in his office.)[54] At the same time, Codman had managed to alienate much of Boston's medical establishment. With his own political troubles mounting, Codman resigned from the committee in late 1915. With that, the CCSNA's committee disbanded and the College took up the task of hospital standardization.

The case reports required from applicants had confirmed that significant problems existed in many hospitals. As Martin observed, "We had early evidence that much surgical work was being done in hospitals that lacked many facilities essential in the scientific care of the patient."[55] By January 1916, Martin had raised $526,000 from the Fellows to support the College's program and an additional $30,000 from the Carnegie Foundation specifically for hospital standardization. The College established an International (i.e., U.S. and Canadian) Committee on Standards and local state and provincial Committees on Standards. While this engaged local Fellows as community leaders, much of the work on standardization was carried out at College headquarters, principally by Allen Kanavel and John Bowman. Bowman remained in contact with Codman who had now opened his own private hospital to put his end-result system into practice.

The war delayed the implementation of the hospital standardization program. A "Joint Session of the International, State, and Provincial Committees on Standards" did not occur until October 19 and 20, 1917. No representatives from Canada, now in the fourth year of war, came. Sixty hospital superintendents attended, demonstrating both the increasing professionalization of hospital management and their interest in standardization. Significantly, the College secured the cooperation of Charles B Moulinier, SJ, director of the Catholic Hospital Association, which represented about half of the hospital beds in North America. In December 1917, the Regents approved an initial questionnaire, from which a final set of standards could be drawn.

Bowman, who organized the conference and drew up both the questionnaire and the standardization plan, had an unenviable job. Criticized by Franklin Martin, Edward Martin, and George Crile for being dilatory, he was rebuked by William Mayo for being too inquisitorial in the early drafts of the questionnaire.[56] Bowman, who would go on to become the powerful chancellor of the University of Pittsburgh, held the unenviable position of being buffeted between strong egos.

By March 1918, Bowman had completed the minimum standard and travelled extensively to explain the College's program at local meetings. The original detailed and potentially controversial questions about hospital accounts and finances had been dropped. The questionnaire sought only "to define the few factors which are imperative in any hospital for the proper care of patients."[57] The minimum standard itself called for (1) an organized medical staff—which also increased the voice of the physicians in coordinating the affairs of the hospital; (2) that the staff be licensed medical graduates, competent in their respective fields and worthy in character—while no specific mention was made of the fellowship, the implication was clear, and character spoke to fee splitting (the fraught question of whether or not a hospital should be open to all licensed qualified physicians in a community was not addressed); (3) staff meetings at least monthly with analysis of cases—a nod to Codman's end-result system and a way of exposing the incompetent operator; (4) the keeping of accurate medical records—the College provided preprinted forms to facilitate all aspects of record keeping; and (5) clinical lab and x-ray facilities under the charge of trained technicians—the support systems that modern "scientific" surgery increasingly required.[58]

After two years of effort, Bowman had produced a practical and workable plan. While not as rigorous as Codman's idealized system, hospital standardization as adopted would be accepted by Fellows and hospital superintendents, which was vital for its success in the absence of any legally enforceable mandate. In fact, it would be the first national system of hospital inspection in the world. In April, the first survey of hospitals with more than 100 beds began.

Scheduled for release at the October 1919 Clinical Congress in New York City, the report horrified the Regents when they met at the Waldorf Astoria during the Congress. Of 671 hospitals surveyed, only 89 met the minimum standard. Several of the nation's most famous hospitals failed the inspection. Convinced by Bowman that the hospitals would blame wartime conditions for the dismal results, the Regents also recognized that publication would probably end any future chances of cooperation. Discretion seemed the better plan, particularly as Bowman had information that almost 200 of the hospitals had already begun making improvements.[59] Pursued by reporters, Mrs. MT Farrow, the Board's secretary, carried the report to the hotel's furnace room at midnight and "solemnly cremated" every copy.[60]

≈ ✳ ≈

The AMA and the ACS

By the second decade of the 20th century, the AMA had begun to consolidate its position as the "voice of organized medicine."[61] Its four great Councils—Medical Education (1904), Medical Legislation (1904), Pharmacy and Chemistry (1905), and Health and Public Institutions (1910)—would wield enormous influence over health care and policy in the ensuing decades. Its specialty sections offered a forum for the majority of full- or part-time specialists who did not belong to one of the small, elite societies. Its House of Delegates functioned as a representative body for the county medical societies. The sudden appearance of a new organization that claimed the right to both certify and represent an important specialty constituency was bound to cause alarm, particularly when that organization appeared to have its own national ambitions. As Arthur Bevan, chair of the powerful Council on Medical Education, told William Mayo, in the AMA's view the College had only two legitimate functions—conducting the Clinical Congress and defining the training of surgical specialists. Anything more suggested that "there is something fundamentally wrong with the organization and management of the [ACS]."[62] Bevan's remarks reflected the over-riding importance that the AMA placed on professional unity. For his part, Franklin Martin firmly believed that the "the College of Surgeons has as great a function as the Royal College or there is no reason for its existence at all."[63] The clash would be both personal and political.

Attempting to end this animosity, William Mayo, as President of the College from November 1916 to November 1918, tried to involve Bevan, a Fellow, in College affairs and co-opt him onto the Board of Regents. The sensitive topic of the College's and the CCSNA's finances (and the rumor that Martin used his projects for personal financial gain) offered Mayo an opportunity. Mayo appointed Bevan to a committee to examine the ACS's and CCSNA's accounts in December 1917. The five-member committee began its work with Bevan and one other member openly hostile to Martin, one member "rather critical," and Mayo and the fifth member "open to conviction."[64] By the end of the month, its five members had concluded that all accounts were correct. The report ended in handsome praise for Martin's organizational efforts. In Mayo's words the report provided "as complete a vindication of Martin as could be desired."[65] A vindication that he hoped would "end the warfare" between the AMA and the ACS.[66]

This did not occur. So while brother Charles Mayo, the outgoing AMA president, publically deplored the bickering and disunity of the profession, Arthur Bevan used his 1918 AMA presidential address, 'The Organization of the Medical Profession for War,' to attack the College. "A small coterie of specialists … no matter how eminent or how successful they have been as promoters and exploiters of special societies, can in no way in this great emergency and in this great democracy represent the medical profession."[67] Following words with action, Bevan denounced Martin in a long letter to President Wilson.[68] This clumsy attempt to force Martin out of government service failed. Instead of dismissal, Martin received a letter of commendation from the President and a promotion to colonel.[69]

The next year, Bevan intensified the competition by publically urging that the AMA publish a surgery journal.[70] Martin understandably saw the 1920 creation of the *Archives of Surgery* as both a personal affront and a deliberate attempt to undermine his *SGO*, the College's official journal. As AJ Ochsner, Chicago surgeon and Regent, dryly observed, "At the present time, one of the chief ambitions of the present president of the American Medical Association [Bevan] is the destruction of the American College of Surgeons."[71]

Hospital standardization exacerbated the conflict. By late 1918, the AMA and Bevan, whose Council on Medical Education approved hospitals for internships, refused all cooperation with the College.[72] Will Mayo, in the face of resistance from Martin and despite his view that the "Chicago crowd" of the AMA had ill-used his brother, organized a meeting between the AMA's Trustees and the College on February 7, 1919. Notwithstanding the apparently harmonious tone, little came of the meeting beyond a vague statement about cooperation and avoiding duplication.[73] Mayo's attempt to engineer the election of JMT Finney as "harmony candidate" for president-elect of the AMA that summer also ended in failure.[74]

Meanwhile, behind the scenes Bevan worked to gain control of hospital standardization through a new umbrella organization, the American Hospital Conference. His efforts ultimately proved unsuccessful and only succeeded in further antagonizing Franklin

Martin. One observer described the "bellicose attitude" in Chicago by 1920 as having the character of a "rural feud" between wholly incompatible personalities.[75] At the same time, however, both the Mayo brothers and George Crile had become convinced that the hospital standardization project placed too heavy a burden on the College. After a "good clearing up report," as Charles Mayo described it, the task of on-going inspection should be passed to the AMA.[76] Distrustful of the AMA, Martin opposed the idea and the College withdrew from the American Hospital Conference. The College continued the program alone for 30 years until a new collaborative organization of the ACS, AMA, and AHA—the Joint Commission on Accreditation of Hospitals—assumed the responsibility in 1950.

Convocations and Surgical Identity

By 1920, the College had held eight Convocations at the annual Clinical Congresses. The first, a product of Martin's careful stage management and showmanship, had established the pattern. As a North American institution, the first Convocation opened with "God Save the King" (or "America") which, like the Union Flag on the stage, acknowledged the Fellows from the Dominion of Canada and honored the Convocation's guest, Sir Rickman Godlee, Lister's nephew and president of the older English College. JMT Finney, the College President, led the guest and a formal procession of the Regents, all dressed in the College's new academic robes, to the dais. The candidates for fellowship, the majority of whom had purchased the new gown, were sworn in. Godlee gave a flattering address and the assembly closed with the singing of the "Star-Spangled Banner." Newspapers across the country and the *Times* of London carried coverage of the Convocation, favorably comparing the new College to the Royal College of Surgeons and referring to its members as "leading" surgeons.[77] Many papers also published the names of local Fellows. The editor of the *Chicago Medical Reporter* rightly attributed the success of the meeting and the promise of the new College to the "great organizational ability and the indefatigable labor of Dr. Franklin H Martin of Chicago."[78]

Critics saw all of this ceremony as further evidence of the College's undemocratic tendencies. The *Journal of the American Medical Association*, previously confined to factual reporting, published a satirical article by "Samuel Pepys, M.D., F.A.C.O.D." "Received notice of election as a Fellow in ye American College of Ordinary Doctors... each fellowe doth require a special raiment—ye collegiate gown and cap."[79] The Regents, too, had initially opposed Martin's plans for academic dress—relatively new even to American universities—until their opposition lost all credibility in London in August 1913. There, at the Royal College of Surgeons, Martin beheld Regents Crile and Murphy, along with Harvey Cushing and William Mayo receiving Honorary Fellowships "in the glorious regalia" of the older College.[80] The next day Martin had Ede and Ravenscroft, robe makers to the King, design a gown for the American College.

Even one historian has commented on Martin's "unfortunate" Anglophilia and the College's "pretentiousness" for its academic robes and ceremonial mace.[81] Unrecognized by the critics, the ceremonial aspects of the Convocation served an important function. By inventing a tradition, Martin gave an appearance of solidity and stability to a new organization and helped create an identity for its members.

Until this time the majority of surgeons in North America had had no distinct professional or institutional identity. In a highly competitive market, by introducing the ceremonial forms of the Royal College of Surgeons, Martin helped change this. First, the College offered a competitive advantage by identifying its members as qualified surgeons, represented by the post-nominal FACS. Second, through the ceremonial regalia and ritual, however undemocratic or pretentious to some, the College gave its members an identity as part of a centuries-old tradition that distinguished the surgeon from the physician and transcended the realities of a competitive, laissez-faire marketplace.

REFERENCES

1. American College of Surgeons. (1913, October 9). *Board of Regents: Minutes October 9, 1913*. Complete Minute Book 1. Archives of the American College of Surgeons, Chicago.
2. Ibid.
3. American College of Surgeons. (1914, January 9). *Board of Regents: Minutes January 9, 1914*. Complete Minute Book 1. Archives of the American College of Surgeons, Chicago.
4. Ibid.
5. Martin, E. (1914). Committee on examinations. *Surgery, Gynecology, and Obstetrics, 19*, 265.
6. Ibid.
7. Ibid.
8. American College of Surgeons. (1914) Admission by examination. In *Year Book of the American College of Surgeons: 1914* (pp. 12–13). Chicago: American College of Surgeons.
9. American College of Surgeons. (1914, January 9). *Board of Regents: Minutes January 9, 1914*. Complete Minute Book 1. Archives of the American College of Surgeons, Chicago.
10. American College of Surgeons. (1914, April 11). *Board of Regents: Minutes April 11, 1914*. Complete Minute Book 1. Archives of the American College of Surgeons, Chicago.
11. American College of Surgeons. (n.d.). *Board of Regents: Minutes October 29, 1915*. Complete Minute Book 1. Archives of the American College of Surgeons, Chicago.
12. Stevens, R. A. (1999). The challenge of specialism in the 1900s. In *The American Medical Ethics Revolution* (p. 86). Baltimore, MD: Johns Hopkins University Press.
13. Anonymous. (1914). A conducted tour for doctors: Its amusing side. *The Journal–Lancet, 34*(18), 471.
14. American College of Surgeons. (1913, June 7). *Board of Regents: Minutes June 7, 1913*. Complete Minute Book 1. Archives of the American College of Surgeons, Chicago.
15. Kernahan, P. (2010). *Franklin Martin and the standardization of American surgery 1890–1940* (p. 102; Doctoral dissertation, University of Minnesota). Available from CIC Institutions. (Publication No. AAT 3422569).
16. American College of Surgeons. (1913, October 9). *Board of Regents: Minutes October 9, 1913*. Complete Minute Book 1. Archives of the American College of Surgeons, Chicago.
17. American College of Surgeons. (1913, November 13). *Board of Regents: Minutes November 13, 1913*. Complete Minute Book 1. Archives of the American College of Surgeons, Chicago. American College of Surgeons. (1914, April 11). *Board of Regents: Minutes April 11, 1914*. Complete Minute Book 1. Archives of the American College of Surgeons, Chicago.
18. American College of Surgeons. (1913, May 7). *Board of Regents: Minutes May 7, 1913*. Complete Minute Book 1. Archives of the American College of Surgeons, Chicago. Hawley, P. R., *Letter to O. W. Wangensteen*. October 6, 1954, Papers of the University of Minnesota Department of Surgery, University Archives, University of Minnesota, Twin Cities, Minneapolis, MN.
19. Hawley, P. R. (1955). Fellowship for anesthesiologists. *Bulletin of the American College of Surgeons, 40*(5), 302.
20. Kernahan, P. (2010). *Franklin Martin and the standardization of American surgery 1890–1940* (p. 103; Doctoral dissertation, University of Minnesota). Available from CIC Institutions. (Publication No. AAT 3422569).

21. Kernahan, P. (2010). *Franklin Martin and the standardization of American surgery 1890–1940* (pp. 162–4; Doctoral dissertation, University of Minnesota). Available from CIC Institutions. (Publication No. AAT 3422569) Van Hoosen, B. (1930). The woman surgeon. *Medical Women's Journal, 37*(1), 13. Rishworth, S. (2002). A short history of women surgeons in the college. *Bulletin of the American College of Surgeons, 87*(5), 34–5.

22. Van Hoosen, B. (1929). Women doctors as members of medical societies. *Medical Women's Journal, 36*(10), 276.

23. Litwak, L. F. (1998). *Trouble in Mind: Black Southerners in the Age of Jim Crow* (pp. 317,318–9). New York, NY: Alfred A. Knopf.
Savitt, T. L. (1987). Entering a white profession: Black physicians in the new south, 1880–1920. *Bulletin of the History of Medicine, 61*(4), 507–40.

24. American College of Surgeons. (1913, November 13). *Board of Regents: Minutes November 13, 1913*. Complete Minute Book 1. Archives of the American College of Surgeons, Chicago.

25. Ibid.

26. Dr. Daniel H. Williams gets national degree: Dr. Daniel H. Williams honored; and through him ten million negroes. (1913, November 22). *The Chicago Defender* [Big Weekend Edition, p. 1]. Retrieved November 11, 2011 from ProQuest Historical Newspapers: The Chicago Defender (1910–1975). Document ID: 1003860942.
Editorial: The American College of Surgeons [Editorial]. (1914). *Journal of the National Medical Association 6*(1), 30.

27. Editorial: Progress and prejudice [Editorial]. (1915). *Journal of the National Medical Association 7*(4), 287.

28. Ibid.

29. Sees flaws in plan to mark surgeons: Cliques could withhold the letters F.C.S. out of personal pique. (1913, August 10). *New York Times (1857–1922)*, p. 11. Retrieved November 11, 2011 from ProQuest Historical Newspapers: The New York Times (1851–2007). Document ID: 100273387.

30. American College of Surgeons. (1914, January 9). *Board of Regents: Minutes January 9, 1914*. Complete Minute Book 1. Archives of the American College of Surgeons, Chicago.

31. American College of Surgeons. (1915, February 6). *Board of Regents: Minutes February 6, 1915*. Complete Minute Book 1. Archives of the American College of Surgeons, Chicago.

32. American College of Surgeons. (1914, June 22). *Board of Regents: Minutes June 22, 1914*. Complete Minute Book 1. Archives of the American College of Surgeons, Chicago.

33. Davis, L. (1960). *Fellowship of Surgeons: A History of the American College of Surgeons* (p. 169). Springfield, IL: Charles C. Thomas.

34. Bowman, J. G., *Letter to F H Martin*. June 19, 1916, Archives of the American College of Surgeons, Chicago.

35. Bowman, J. G., *Letter to F H Martin*. May 25, 1920, Eleanor Grimm Papers, Archives of the American College of Surgeons, Chicago.

36. Bowman, J. G., *Letter to F H Martin*. April 30, 1915, Archives of the American College of Surgeons, Chicago.

37. Chicago doctor rescues niece: Franklin Martin makes wild auto dash from Munich; safe in London. (1914, August 22). *Chicago Daily Tribune (1872–1922)*, p.3. Retrieved November 11, 2011 from ProQuest Historical Newspapers: Chicago Tribune (1849–1987). Document ID: 383331451.

Into Germany by automobile: Chicago man reaches Munich in search of niece. (1914, August 22). *Los Angeles Times (1886–1922)*, p. I5. Retrieved November 11, 2011 from ProQuest Historical Newspapers: Los Angeles Times (1881–1987). Document ID: 334322622.

Sped through German lines as German royalty: Flag on auto of Chicago surgeon enabled him to go from Holland to Munich and back. (1914, August 22). *New York Times (1857–1922)*, p. 3. Retrieved November 11, 2011 from ProQuest Historical Newspapers: The New York Times (1851–2007). Document ID: 100678078.

38. American doctors to aid Belgians: Organize to help brothers of their profession in war-ridden land. (1914, December 15). *Los Angeles Times (1886–1922)*, p. I1. Retrieved November 11, 2011 from ProQuest Historical Newspapers: Los Angeles Times (1881–1987). Document ID: 749484442.

39. Crile, G. W., *Diary: The Second Battle of Chicago*. October 23, 1917, George W. Crile Papers (MSS 2806), Container 35, Folder 112, Manuscript Collections, Western Reserve Historical Society, Cleveland, OH.

40. Martin, F. H. (1930). Peace jubilee: Address of the retiring President. *Surgery, Gynecology, and Obstetrics, 50*, 288.

41. Bliss, M. (2005). *Harvey Cushing: A Life in Surgery* (pp. 326–7). Oxford, UK: Oxford University Press.

42. American College of Surgeons. (1913, May 7). *Board of Regents: Minutes May 7, 1913*. Complete Minute Book 1. Archives of the American College of Surgeons, Chicago.

43. American College of Surgeons. (1913, November 13). *Board of Regents: Minutes November 13, 1913*. Complete Minute Book 1. Archives of the American College of Surgeons, Chicago.

44. Anonymous. (1914, May 30). *Chicago Medical Society Bulletin*, p. 2.

45. Eleanor K. Grimm. (1914). *Excerpts from the Chicago Medical Society Bulletin, 1914*. n.d., Eleanor Grimm Notebooks V/22A, Archives of the American College of Surgeons, Chicago.

46. American College of Surgeons. (1913, November 13). *Board of Regents: Minutes November 13, 1913*. Complete Minute Book 1. Archives of the American College of Surgeons, Chicago.

47. American College of Surgeons. (1914, January 9). *Board of Regents: Minutes January 9, 1914*. Complete Minute Book 1. Archives of the American College of Surgeons, Chicago.

48. Ibid.

49. American College of Surgeons. (1925, October 27). *Board of Regents: Minutes October 27, 1925*. Complete Minute Book 3. Archives of the American College of Surgeons, Chicago.

50. Martin, F. H., *Letter to W J Mayo*. December 29, 1919, W. J. Mayo Papers, Box 1, Folder "American College of Surgeons, 1919," Mayo Historical Unit, Mayo Clinic, Rochester, MN.

51. Codman, E. A. (1996). *A Study in Hospital Efficiency: As Demonstrated by the Case Report of the First Five Years of a Private Hospital (p. 1917)*. Oakbrook Terrace, IL: Joint Commission on Accreditation of Healthcare Organizations. Reverby, S. (1981) Stealing the golden eggs: Ernest Amory Codman and the science and management of medicine. *Bulletin of the History of Medicine, 552*(2), 156–71. Crenner, C. (2001). Organizational reform and professional dissent in the careers of Richard Cabot and Ernest Amory Codman. *Journal of the History of Medicine and Allied Sciences, 56*(3), 211–237.

52. Codman, E. A., *Report from the Committee on the Standardization of Hospitals*. October 31, 1913, Ernest A. Codman Papers (B MS c60), Box 1, Folder 11, Boston Medical Library in the Francis A. Countway Library of Medicine, Boston, MA. Codman, E. A., *Report of the Committee on Standardization of Hospitals (1914)*. November 11, 1914, Ernest A. Codman Papers (B MS c60), Box 1, Folder 13, Boston Medical Library, Francis A. Countway Library of Medicine, Boston, MA. The report, accepted by the Clinical Congress was sent on to Bevan at the AMA. Kanavel, A. B., *Letter to Codman*. January 4, 1914, Ernest A. Codman Papers (B MS c60), Box 2, Folder 29, Boston Medical Library, Francis A. Countway Library of Medicine, Boston, MA.

53. Ochsner, A. J., *Letter to W J Mayo*. Letter December 10, 1918, n.d., W. J. Mayo Papers, Box 1, Folder "American College of Surgeons, 1913–1918," Mayo Historical Unit, Mayo Clinic, Rochester, MN.

54. *Carnegie Foundation 1913–16: Correspondence with Henry S. Pritchett*. n.d., Ernest A. Codman Papers (B MS c60), Box 1, Folder 8, Boston Medical Library, Francis A. Countway Library of Medicine, Boston, MA.

55. Martin, F. H. (1934). *Fifty Years of Medicine and Surgery: An Autobiographical Sketch* (p. 337). Chicago: The Surgical Publishing Company.

56. Crile, G. W., *Diary*. October 20, 1917, George W. Crile Papers (MSS 2806), Container 35, Folder 112, Manuscript Collections, Western Reserve Historical Society, Cleveland, OH. Mayo, W. J., *Letter to J G Bowman*. January 13, 1918, W. J. Mayo Papers, Box 1, Folder ACS 1913–1918, Mayo Historical Unit, Mayo Clinic, Rochester, MN.

57. Bowman, J. G. (1918). Standards of efficiency: First hospital survey of the college. *Bulletin of the American College of Surgeons, 3*(3), 1.

58. Anon (1920). The minimum standard. *Bulletin of the American College of Surgeons, 4*(4), 4.

59. American College of Surgeons. (1919, October 23). *Board of Regents: Minutes October 23, 1919*. Complete Minute Book 1. Archives of the American College of Surgeons, Chicago.

60. Grimm, E. K., *Eleanor K. Grimm Notebooks*. n.d., Reel B/13/14, 8, Archives of the American College of Surgeons, Chicago.

61. Burrow, J. G. (1963). *AMA: Voice of American Medicine*. Baltimore, MD: Johns Hopkins University Press.

62. Bevan, A. D., *Letter to W J Mayo*. December 24, 1918, W. J. Mayo Papers, Mayo Historical Unit, Mayo Clinic, Rochester, MN.

63. Martin, F. H., *Letter to W J Mayo*. January 30, 1919, W. J. Mayo Papers, Box 1, Folder American College of Surgeons 1919, Mayo Historical Unit, Mayo Clinic, Rochester, MN.

64. Mayo, W. J., *Letter to W W Pearson*. January 2, 1918, W. J. Mayo Papers, Box 1, Folder American College of Surgeons 1913–1918, Mayo Historical Unit, Mayo Clinic, Rochester, MN.

65. Ibid.

66. Mayo, W. J., *Letter to G W Crile*. January 2, 1918, W. J. Mayo Papers, Box 1, Folder American College of Surgeons 1913–1918, Mayo Historical Unit, Mayo Clinic, Rochester, MN.

67. Bevan, A. D. (1918). The organization of the medical profession for war. *JAMA, 70*(24), 1806.

68. Grimm, E. K., *Dr. Franklin H. Martin, Criticism During WW1*. Eleanor Grimm Notebooks XXIV, Archives of the American College of Surgeons, Chicago.

69. Ibid.

70. Fishbein, M. (1947). *A History of the American Medical Association, 1847–1947* (p. 308). Philadelphia, PA: W. B. Saunders.

71. Ochsner, A. J., *Letter to W J Mayo*. December 10, 1918, W. J. Mayo Papers, Box 1, Folder American College of Surgeons 1913–18, Mayo Historical, Unit Mayo Clinic, Rochester, MN.

72. Bowman, J. G., *Letter to W J Mayo*. November 20, 1918, W. J. Mayo Papers, Box 1, Folder "American College of Surgeons 1913–18," Mayo Historical Unit, Mayo Clinic, Rochester, MN.

73. Bowman, J. G., *Conference Between Trustees of the American Medical Association and a Committee Appointed by the President of the American College of Surgeons*. February 7, 1919, W. J. Mayo Papers, Box 1, Folder "American College of Surgeons, 1919," Mayo Historical Unit, Mayo Clinic, Rochester, MN.

74. Martin, F. H., *Diary*. June 9, 1919. Franklin Martin Diary, Archives of the American College of Surgeons, Chicago.

75. Lambert, A. V. S., *Letter to W J Mayo*. March 8, 1920, W. J. Mayo Papers, Box 2, Folder 2, Mayo Historical Unit, Mayo Clinic, Rochester, MN.

76. Mayo, C. H., *Letter to G W Crile*. April 26, 1921, C. H. Mayo Papers, Box 60, Folder 061, Mayo Historical Unit, Mayo Clinic, Rochester, MN.

77. An American college of surgeons: Sir Rickman Godlee's mission. (1913, November 13). *The Times*, sec. News, 4.
    Chicago surgeons made Fellows of American College of Surgery. (1913, November 14). *Chicago Daily Tribune*, p. 4. Retrieved November 11, 2011 from ProQuest Historical Newspapers: Chicago Tribune (1849–1987). Document ID: 404222251.
    3,000 great surgeons assembled in Chicago. (1913, November 13). *Minneapolis Morning Tribune*, p. 2. Retrieved November 11, 2011 from ProQuest Historical Newspapers: Minneapolis Tribune (1867–1922). Document ID: 1527888102.
    32 Minnesotans honored. fellowships in the American College of Surgeons go to 15 Minneapolitans. (1913, November 14). *The Minneapolis Journal*, p. 13.

78. Editorial. (1913, December). *Chicago Medical Recorder*. Eleanor Grimm Notebooks V, Archives of the American College of Surgeons, Chicago.

79. Fishbein, M. (1969). *An Autobiography* (p. 80). New York, NY: Doubleday.

80. Martin, F. H. (1934). *Fifty Years of Medicine and Surgery: An Autobiographical Sketch* (pp. 325–6). Chicago: The Surgical Publishing Company.

81. Bonner, T. N. (1991). *Medicine in Chicago, 1850–1950: A Chapter in the Social and Scientific Development of the City, 2nd ed.* (pp. 96–7). Urbana, IL: University of Illinois Press.

CHAPTER 3
Martin's College, 1920–1930

Mace Presentation Banquet, Montreal, Canada, October 1920

The 1920s represented a period of expansion for the College and established its reputation as an educational institution. With the resignation of John Bowman in 1920, Martin consolidated his position as the executive director of the College. Hospital standardization expanded and by decade's end included even small hospitals of more than 25 beds. Increasing attention was given to improving the quality of care through education and standard setting. Sectional meetings and motion pictures offered new ways of reaching the profession and the public. The College introduced important committees on cancer, trauma, and industrial medicine. During this time the College built an international reputation and membership grew significantly. At the same time, the early years of the decade saw some discontent with the direction in which Martin appeared to be taking the College. Some leading surgeons of Martin's generation hoped quiet persuasion could influence the College's course. A younger generation would adopt a more confrontational approach.

Martin Takes Control

In his years with the College, John Bowman devoted great time and energy to hospital standardization and other projects. He had been hired in 1915 as Director, a position that did not then exist in the bylaws. Further, as a former university president he appears to have, not unnaturally, taken a fairly expansive view of his responsibility for the staff work of the College. This caused relatively few problems as long as Franklin Martin, as Secretary, was involved in his private practice and in his work for the war effort. But the Regents' decision in 1917 to appoint Martin as full-time Secretary-General upset this balance.

The new post represented an attempt by Will Mayo, the incoming President, and George Crile to overcome Martin's resistance to incorporating the Clinical Congress of Surgeons of North America (CCSNA) into the American College of Surgeons (ACS). The CCSNA had become something of an embarrassment to the Regents who believed that Martin continued to sell subscriptions to *Surgery, Gynecology, and Obstetrics*. As a further source of embarrassment, some less scrupulous doctors publically elided "membership" in the Congress with fellowship in the College, muddying the distinction of the latter. In June 1916, under considerable pressure from the Regents, a joint committee was established to study the affiliation between the two organizations.[1]

Unsatisfactorily, the report, written by the manager of the Clinical Congress, Albert D Ballou, effectively left the Clinical Congress as a separate entity.[2] At the October 19, 1917 Regents' meeting, Crile, with the help of Will Mayo and Edward Martin, succeeded in out-maneuvering the protesting Franklin Martin—who had left the item off the agenda—and the Clinical Congress ceased to exist as an independent entity.[3] From Crile's point of view this represented a successful outcome to what he called the "Third Battle of Chicago." Crile and Mayo succeeded in part by offering Martin, who received nothing for his government or College work and whose practice had suffered as a consequence of these commitments, a yearly salary of $10,000 to become the Secretary-General of the College.[4] Crile also seems to have sincerely believed that Martin's genius for organization meant that he could contribute more to surgery through the College than he could by returning to private practice at the war's end.[5] After some deliberation and encouraged by his wife, Isabelle, Martin accepted the offer.[6]

This organizational change meant that the relative status of Martin and Bowman had to be defined. In particular, Bowman thought that the new arrangement placed him in the position of an assistant. Martin, despite claiming that the general executive department and all its activities belonged under the authority of the Secretary-General, insisted that it left Bowman's status as director of educational activities unchanged. Nonetheless, Martin demanded that, in the event of a "showdown," he receive the President's (William Mayo) unequivocal backing.[7] The showdown never came.[8] Bowman and Martin reached a mutually satisfactory agreement by creating two chief executives, a change incorporated into the bylaws. Under the revised bylaws the Secretary-General was to be

> the chief executive of the College ... [with] supervision of all activities and business affairs of the College [while the Director was to be] the chief executive officer of all educational activities of the College ... and have charge of admissions to the fellowship, of hospital standardization and other matters concerned with the educational work of the College.[9]

Bowman also secured the right to "appoint and remove" his subordinates and attend the meetings of the Executive Committee and the Regents.[10] Having two chief executives, however, is not conducive to organizational stability or efficiency.

By 1920, Bowman had been director of the College for six years. Through his efforts, the College's hospital standardization and educational programs became well-established. Further, Bowman had been instrumental in securing the initial $30,000 grant for hospital standardization from the Carnegie Foundation. He had also been, as Loyal Davis observed, an outspoken champion of the College's ideals.[11] Throughout, he remained something of the pedagogue—Martin refers to him in his diary as "Dominie," an old fashioned name with clerical overtones for a schoolmaster. At times Martin was not above gentle teasing, as on a trip west in 1920. "We further confused the interested passengers by asking Dominie if he had prepared his sermon for Sunday. It rather bothered him."[12]

However intended, the teasing disguised a difficult relationship. The Secretary-General had a strong proprietary feeling toward the College, in coming years often referred to by friend and foe alike as "his baby." Although there appears to have been no clear precipitating event, by late 1920 Bowman had begun to consider other offers. On November 3, he informed Martin that the Graduate School of New York had offered him $25,000 a year as its head (he now received $10,000 from the College) and that he had also had an offer from the University of Pittsburgh. "Poor Dominie," wrote Martin in his diary "will have to decide."[13] Six days later Martin learned from Will Mayo that Bowman had accepted the Chancellorship of the University of Pittsburgh. The parting appears to have been reasonably amicable. Some years later, Bowman would tell Martin that he felt more deeply indebted to Martin than the latter could know. "Some of the best times which I ever had were with you."[14] (Figure 3.1)

With Bowman's departure the Regents decided to retain the position of Director and looked for a new candidate. Martin had met and been impressed by Judge Harold M Stephens of Salt Lake City, who had spoken at the hospital standardization meeting held there in 1920. At Martin's urging, Stephens took the position of Director for a five month trial. While he worked actively on hospital standardization, he ultimately declined the position of full-time Director. He would continue to provide the Regents with valuable legal matters throughout the 1920s. With the election of Franklin D Roosevelt, Stephens became an Assistant Attorney General in the new administration and would later be considered for the Supreme Court.

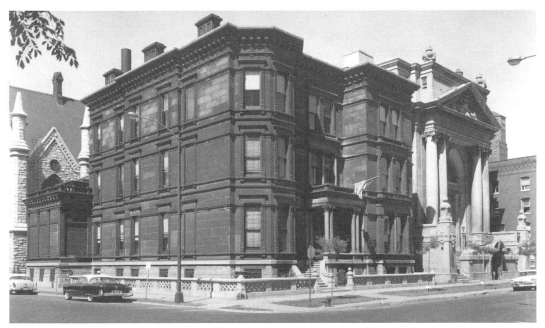

FIGURE 3.1 The Nickerson Mansion and the Murphy Memorial Auditorium as they appeared in the late 1950s.

When Stephens left the directorship, he provided the Regents with a series of recommendations, some of which the Regents would follow.[15] Of these, perhaps most importantly, he recommended a single chief executive—the existing divided government being "foreign to the fundamental principles of executive organization." He also recommended a category for aspiring surgeons to inculcate the values of the College to the next generation; a literary research bureau to assist surgeons without access to a comprehensive medical library; an expansion of hospital standardization to all institutions; and an expansion of public activities (including media and meetings) to enlist the cooperation of the public and identify the College (and its Fellows) as an organization created for public service. All of these initiatives would be put in place during the 1920s.

On the other hand, the College never developed research laboratories (also an enthusiasm of George Crile's) or standardized surgical education (here the initiative would pass to the American Surgical Association). Finally, Stephens warned, the College should never consider membership growth as a source of revenue—a path that would alienate those who identified the College with quality rather than quantity. The size of the membership would, as we will see, prove to be a continuing source of controversy in the coming years.

With Stephens' departure, Martin assumed the new position of Director General. As approved by the Board of Regents and the Governors, the 1922 bylaws made clear that the days of divided government were over:

- The Director General shall be the chief executive officer of the College.
- Under the direction of the Board of Regents he shall have supervision of all activities and business affairs of the College, including the direction of the general executive office.[16]

For better or for worse, it would now be Martin's College.

The Hospital Standardization Program

With Bowman's resignation, the College hired Malcolm MacEachern to direct the hospital standardization program. MacEachern was well qualified for the position. At age 40 he was both a respected surgeon and superintendent of Vancouver General Hospital. Consequently, he had great credibility with both physicians and hospital administrators. Over the next 27 years, his work with the standardization program made him a major figure in hospital management. But on the organizational chart, as director of hospital standardization, he stood clearly subordinate to the Director General.

The size of the hospital standardization department varied over the years. Two young physicians, Doctors Frederich Slibe and LeRoy Sloan, conducted the initial surveys between 1916 and 1921. Both went on to distinguished careers—Slibe as Medical Director for Blue Cross/Blue Shield in Illinois and Sloan as Professor of Medicine at the University of Illinois. As recent medical graduates with a year of internship at Cook County Hospital, they established a pattern of the College using recent graduates to carry out the inspections, a policy that MacEachern would continue. New graduates, MacEachern believed, were both more current in their medical knowledge and perhaps less likely to over-identify with the problems of middle-aged hospital administrators.

The number of surveyors or "visitors" also varied during this time. In the early years of the decade, with a significant backlog of hospitals, up to nine visitors were employed. For the remainder of the decade, four to six visitors conducted the work under the supervision of MacEachern.

The hospital standardization program proved to be as expensive and time-consuming an undertaking as Crile and the Mayos had feared. During the 1920s, the number of new hospitals increased each year. The scope of the program also expanded to encompass hospitals of 50 or more beds and then of 25 or more beds. Finally, each certified hospitals had to be re-inspected. (MacEachern also introduced a revocable certificate for the approved hospital's lobby in 1925.) At a cost of approximately $70,000 per year, the program represented the College's largest single expense and about 40 percent of the College's budget. Despite this, MacEachern would complain that he lacked adequate resources given the size of the task.[17]

For Martin, as Director General, hospital standardization remained central to the College's mission. In the 1924 Annual Report, Martin claimed four benefits for the standardization program: the elimination of incompetent or unnecessary surgery; shortening patient lengths of stay; a reduction in infectious and other complications; and a lowering of the hospital death rate.[18] Drawing on a sample of standardized hospitals, MacEachern confirmed a reduction in length of stay from 14.6 days pre-standardization to 11.9 days after 4 years of standardization and a fall in mortality from 40–60/1,000 to 20–30/1,000.[19] The program had demonstrable results.

College leaders echoed Martin. Despite George Crile's earlier private misgivings, addressing the Hospital Standardization Conference in 1926, he made clear to his audience that "the primary endeavor of the American College of Surgeons has been the standardization of hospitals."[20] By then the College had spent a total of $552,000 on the project, $105,000 of which had been contributed by the Carnegie Foundation.[21] Two years later the retiring College President, George D Stewart of Boston, told attendees at the Clinical Congress that hospital standardization should be continued even if it meant bankruptcy for the College. These hyperbolic remarks reflected both the centrality of the standardization project to the College's identity in the inter-war period and also, tacitly, an ongoing concern among College principals about the costs of the program.

By the end of the decade, MacEachern and his staff had conducted 21,112 surveys with an overall approval rate of 69 percent. The survey results varied with the size of the hospital. In that year (1929), 93 percent of the largest hospitals (100 beds or greater) had met the minimum standard. For intermediate hospitals (50–99 beds), 63 percent met the standard. For the smallest hospitals surveyed (25–49 beds), only 20 percent met the standard.

Local Fellows played an important role in the hospital standardization process and in improving the standard of care. MacEachern encouraged seven actions on their part. These included regular attendance at staff meetings; prompt and accurate completion of records; encouraging consultation ("two heads are better than one"); judicious use of the laboratory and x-ray; studying the hospital's end-results; educating the community about the benefits of the standardized hospital; and keeping the Hospital Department of the ACS informed.[22]

By the end of the decade, hospital accreditation had become increasingly important to communities. MacEachern reported progress even in places like central Illinois, where rampant fee splitting initially had created resistance to the inspectors.[23] In another case, the mayor of Hamilton, Ontario demonstrated the importance of accreditation to the public and public officials. Learning that several municipal hospitals risked removal from the approved list, he ordered their boards to send representatives to Chicago not to appeal but to learn what corrective action was required.[24] Similarly, the hospitals of the U.S. Army, Navy, Public Health Service, and Veterans Bureau proved among the most cooperative with the inspectors. Usefully, the federal government paid for the inspections.[25] Accreditation could even become a condition of issuing bonds for hospital construction.[26]

By 1928, the American Automobile Association's guide for motorists included a list of the approved hospitals in the United States and Canada and recommended that its members seek care in one of them in the event of an accident.[27] In Franklin Martin's words: "if we can visit the small hospital … and get before the small community our program, our propaganda … if we tell them that the list … has been compiled with great care and sent to every newspaper in the country, they will say, 'Why isn't our hospital on the list?'"[28]

As the decade progressed, attention turned from inspection to assisting hospitals. MacEachern described this as emphasizing "the spirit of the movement, as well as the material side."[29] The College issued its first Manual of Hospital Standardization in 1926. Subsequent editions followed almost yearly until 1938 with a tenth edition appearing in 1946. During that time the manual expanded from 18 to 118 pages. In 1926, MacEachern was seconded to Australia and New Zealand for six months at government invitation to advise on hospital standardization. "The work of Dr. Malcolm MacEachern," Sir Louis Barnett, a founder of the Royal Australasian College of Surgeons, would write, "is of world-wide renown."[30] Through the standardization program, Malcolm MacEachern established an international reputation in hospital management, one that reflected well on the College and on Martin's ability to choose subordinates.

The Campaign Against Fee Splitting

Not without controversy, the College had reasonable success in meeting two of its mandates—the standardization of surgeons and the standardization of hospitals. The third goal, the elimination of fee splitting, would prove far more difficult. The Regents would devote significant time to the problem through many years without arriving at an effective solution. This reflected several factors: the difficulty identifying and exposing the fee splitter; the potential liability of the College and Regents in a defamation suit; the College's lack of any legal authority and its consequent reliance on suasion; and a lack of cooperation from the American Medical Association (AMA).

The easiest action would be to deny membership to a known fee splitter, relying on the local knowledge of the state or provincial credentials committees, the Fellowship Pledge, and the bylaws. These committees, however, were not immune to local medical politics. Well-connected fee splitters could still, on occasion, obtain the fellowship or, conversely, a hint of fee splitting could be used by a competitor to derail a worthy applicant. Appeals and counter-appeals in these cases occupied much of the Regents' time. The Fellowship Pledge, which went through several revisions during this time to become a clear and unambiguous statement of principle, carried an obvious weakness. As JMT Finney ruefully noted to the Regents in 1913, the already corrupt would have no moral qualms about making a false declaration. So while the College could deny the fellowship to a known fee splitter and the College's Fellowship Pledge and bylaws could condemn the practice, actually eliminating fee splitting or expelling the Fellow who continued to split fees proved extremely difficult.

The Roeder case in 1924 demonstrated to the Regents the difficulties and legal risks they ran in confronting fee splitting. Charles Roeder, a well-trained Fellow in Omaha, had informed a patient's father that he would not operate on the son at a local proprietary hospital because it tolerated fee splitting. The hospital promptly sued Roeder for libel, demanding $30,000, a significant sum in the day. While the College was never named in the action, which was ultimately dismissed, the College's legal fees amounted to almost $5,000. This salutary lesson ended any thoughts that the Regent's had of publicly expelling fee splitting Fellows. As Judge Stephens warned, given the difficulty of proving fee splitting in court, a retaliatory suit for defamation could expose the Regents and the College to hundreds of thousands of dollars in damages. The courts, in Stephens' opinion, offered little hope in the campaign against fee splitting.[31]

As with other aspects of the College's program, in the absence of a legal mandate, propaganda and the hospital standardization program would be the College's main weapons. In 1917, Martin recognized that a fee splitting surgeon required accomplices and devised a strategy around this.[32] Because splitting fees reduced the surgeon's income, generating an adequate income required more referrals, which in turn required a larger number of complicit referring physicians—by Martin's calculation, six to 20. Consequently, the College would attempt to reform the referring physician.

While the College had no authority over these physicians, it could direct an educational campaign through medical societies on the dangers of fee splitting. When this had relatively little effect, the campaign was redirected toward the public and hospital board members. Such publicity, the Regents hoped, would increase public awareness and bring public pressure to eliminate the practice. These efforts had some limited effect.

Where education and publicity failed, the hospital standardization program remained the only coercive tool available to the College. Hospitals that tolerated fee splitting faced the denial of accreditation or the threat of revocation of accreditation. This approach offered several advantages. It concentrated the minds of hospital trustees. It gave the College some leverage over the medical staff, Fellows and non-Fellows alike. And as an indirect approach that did not accuse any individual, it also offered the Regents and the College some protection from a defamation suit.[33]

The AMA provided little hope of a combined front against fee splitting. The organization at the time took an ambiguous approach to the practice.[34] Many members held that the practice remained ethical if the patient had been "informed." Consequently, the larger medical organization offered the College no cooperation either nationally or at the level of the county medical society where real pressure could have been brought to bear.[35] As with the larger hospital standardization project, throughout the 1920s and the 1930s the College would carry on alone.

During this time, however, despite all of these limitations, the College appeared to be making at least some progress. By 1925, MacEachern believed that distinct progress had been made in Illinois, a particular trouble spot.[36] Decatur and Joliet, Illinois, he reported to the Regents, had recently shown improvement.[37] By 1927, three hospitals in Joliet had been conditionally accepted as a result of the "clean up."[38] The threat of delisting proved a powerful weapon, allowing MacEachern to obtain compliance, as he did in Marshalltown, Iowa, in 1929.[39] Still, it would be many years before earlier optimistic hopes about the elimination of fee splitting would be realized.

To help bring that day about, the College developed one other tool—inculcating aspiring surgeons in the values of the College as they began their training. In 1924, the Regents followed Judge Stephens' recommendation and created the Junior Candidate group. Physicians became eligible two years after graduation on either the recommendation of a Fellow or approval by the local state or provincial credentials committee. Exempt from dues, the candidate was "enjoined to carry out all the requirements of the American College of Surgeons with the same degree of fidelity" as a Fellow.[40] A candidate who failed to qualify as a Fellow would be dropped from the list. Critics would cite the program, officially a plan to impart ideals of the ACS from internship onward and shape the next generation of surgeons, as evidence that the College proselytized to increase membership.

As the body certifying the clinical and ethical standards of surgeons, the College also needed a mechanism to investigate complaints made against Fellows. Most complaints came either directly to the Regents or to College staff, far removed from the practitioner's locality. The Regents took seriously the decision to revoke a fellowship. In some cases, notably that of a Fellow in Hastings, Nebraska who murdered his son-in-law, the decision presented the Regents with little difficulty. Other cases could be far more challenging, particularly those with claims and counter-claims of fee splitting or other unethical behavior. (In fact, the majority of complaints involved either "undue publicity or unethical advertising.")[41] Accused Fellows could also exercise their right to appeal in person to the Board of Regents. Such cases were both time consuming and uncomfortable for the Regents, who usually had no direct knowledge of the circumstances.

To improve the process, in 1926 the Regents, acting on independent suggestions from the Brooklyn chapter and the Indiana state committee, authorized Judiciary Committees for each state or province. The three-to-five member committees had the responsibility, at the request of the College, to "make informal investigations of the rumors [of unethical or poor conduct] and report findings to central office."[42] At the same time, the Regents appointed a Central Judiciary Committee to review the complaint and the evidence. These committees had only an advisory role—the final decision rested with the Regents. Nonetheless, the new committees helped simplify the Regents' task and ensure a more thorough investigation of any complaint.

The Sectional Meetings

The College, having been founded to raise the standards of surgeons, needed ways to reach those surgeons. While the Clinical Congresses remained popular and well-attended, attendance placed a burden on many surgeons. Train travel to and from the host city could consume several days. This and the week devoted to the Congress represented a period without income and presented the risk of losing patients to competitors. In 1919, a Fellow from North Carolina, John Wesley Young, offered Martin a solution, one that was readily adopted by the Regents.[43] Young recommended that the College come to the surgeons through meetings organized by state and provincial chapters. The Regents quickly adopted the plan and not only for its educational benefits. As William Mayo pointed out such meetings also gave visible support to the local Fellows, a support particularly welcomed in areas where fee splitting was rife.[44]

So in September of 1920, Martin, Bowman, and the College staff began essentially a long circuit around the country to attend a series of state meetings. Martin's "travelling circus troupe" apparently provoked some curiosity among fellow passengers.[45] Beginning in Butte, Montana on September 2, by December 2 the group had reached New York. Along the way, state meetings had been held in Idaho, Oregon, Washington, Pennsylvania, Arizona, California, Utah, and Colorado. By October 1921, 38 meetings had been held across North America attended by 80 percent of the College's Fellows. At this point, to ease a punishing travel schedule for College officials and to make it easier to attract prominent speakers, Martin reorganized the states and provinces into geographical sections.[46] Within another eight months, all 48 states and six of the nine provinces had been involved in meetings. (Figure 3.2)

The carefully arranged meetings followed a set pattern to communicate with both the profession and the public. For the profession, the College staff modeled the meetings on the Clinical Congress. Prominent local Fellows and standardized hospitals offered "wet" and "dry" clinics. The College cooperated with the American College of Physicians, establishing a link in the professional and public mind between the two new specialty organizations. Martin and MacEachern (after Bowman's resignation) presided over a hospital standardization section. Nationally prominent Fellows would deliver keynote addresses. The Mayo brothers were particularly active here. A public meeting, usually opened by a leading citizen or political leader, discussed medical subjects and promoted the College's program. In deference to regional sensibilities, in the South the College organized separate meetings for the two races.[47] In the first year of the program alone, perhaps 150,000 people had attended the public meetings and another eight to 12 million reached through the local press.

Dependent on publicity for the success of its programs, the College drew on the techniques of the growing field of public relations to promote the sectional meetings to the public. This expanded significantly after Allan Craig, a McGill University graduate, took over the direction of sectional meetings in 1923. The highly attended Portland, Oregon meeting in 1923 served as a template for the careful preliminary work required for a successful meeting. The campaign included advanced contact with local opinion leaders, including teachers and members of the Rotary; provision of advanced copy to local newspaper editors; a readily available College spokesman for reporters; and local Boy Scouts as ushers at the public meetings. As Dr. Ernst Sommer, chair of the Portland organizing committee, noted, "every Boy Scout that comes as an usher brings his father and mother and sister and brother as they all like to see him out in his uniform."[48] The

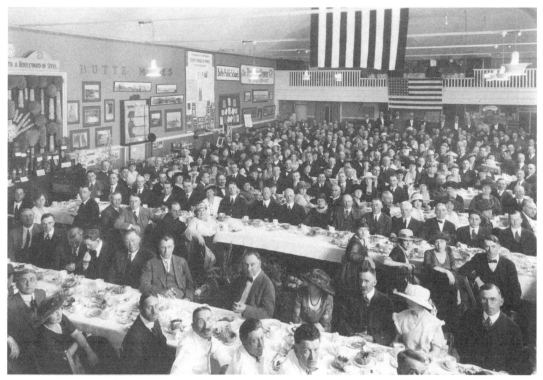

FIGURE 3.2 A banquet during the first sectional meeting in Butte, Montana, 1920.

College provided photographs of the area's approved hospitals to newspaper editors for their Sunday supplements. The attendant publicity helped encourage competing hospitals to seek approval. Each public meeting sought to educate the public about health topics and medical progress and to identify the College with that progress. During the 1920s and 1930s, radio broadcasts during the Clinical Congresses by prominent surgeons served a similar purpose. Reflecting the evolution of advertising in the 1920s, under Craig's direction the College moved from "selling the product" to "selling the benefit."[49]

Committees and Moving Pictures

As part of its efforts to educate both surgeons and the public, the College established a series of committees to improve clinical care and exploited the new medium of motion pictures. Like hospital standardization, the committees grew out of Codman's reformist zeal and his end-result system. Codman recognized that because each clinician's experience was necessarily limited, pooling results would yield greater progress in treatment. Unsurprisingly, given Codman's research interests, the first committee— suggested in 1920, established in 1921, and chaired by Codman—became the Bone Sarcoma Registry.

While sometimes impeded by Codman's impolitic nature, the Registry collected and reviewed cases of bone sarcoma, including the x-rays and microscopic slides of each case. As a result, the committee quickly realized that not only were many of the cases not actually bone sarcomas, but that even among the true cases there was no standard terminology. By circulating the slides, as Codman, Ewing, and Bloodgood noted in their 1923 report, "we shall all have an opportunity to see what Mallory means by osteo-myxo-fibroblastoma or Ewing means by xantho-sarcoma."[50] By 1923, the committee and the American Society of Clinical Pathologists had agreed on a standardized nomenclature. By the end of the decade, the Registry, now under the direction of Dallas Phemister of the University of Chicago (Codman had resigned amid controversy in 1925), received reports from as far away as Hawaii, Korea, China, and New Zealand.[51] While the effort cost the College about $2,500 a year, it represented a significant and singular achievement. For the first time, the nomenclature for a disease had been standardized across institutional and specialty boundaries and treatment outcomes analyzed on an international level.

The Registry became the first of a series of clinical committees. In 1922, the Executive Committee established a Committee on the Treatment of Malignant Disease with Radium and X-ray, often referred to as the Committee on Cancer, under Robert Greenough of the Massachusetts General Hospital. In the same year, the Regents also established a Committee on Fractures under Charles L Scudder and a Committee on Standardization of Clinical Laboratories, chaired by Admiral ER Still. In 1927, a fifth committee was added, the Board on Industrial Medicine and Trauma Surgery. In subsequent years, other committees would attempt standardization of everything from catgut to nomenclature, often in collaboration with other organizations. A reorganization of the College in 1926 recognized the importance of the committees' work by creating a new Department of Clinical Research, headed by a new Associate Director, Bowman C Crowell, to oversee and coordinate their work.

The newer committees followed the model established by the hospital standardization program and the sarcoma registry: standard setting, surveys, inspection, education, and collaboration with other organizations. Both the Committee on Fractures and the Board on Industrial Medicine and Trauma Surgery sought to improve the care of the injured. As a result of the committee's efforts, in 1924 the American Railway Association adopted the fracture committee's recommendations for railroad hospitals receiving accident victims. By 1925, some of the larger railroads had begun centralizing fracture care at designated hospitals. That year the Committee on Fractures surveyed 1,600 hospitals and received 1,050 replies describing a total of 150,989 fractures. Analysis of the data led, at Scudder's urging, to making fracture-care standards part of the minimum standard for hospital accreditation and to educational leaflets for physicians and hospitals.

The Board on Industrial Medicine and Trauma Surgery produced a minimum standard for industrial clinics and by 1932, 84 had been approved. Two of the young hospital "visitors," Drs. EW Williamson and MN Newquist, carried out the surveys, an indication of the close coordination of all of the College's programs. By the following year, despite the Great Depression, 518 of 975 surveyed had been approved.[52] The minimum standard closely paralleled the College's other minimum standards regarding equipment, qualifications of medical staff, and record keeping. In addition, the standard advised that a company's industrial medical department be charged with supervision of plant sanitation and employee health. Synergistically, the standard also required that patients needing hospitalization be sent only to hospitals approved by the American College of Surgeons.[53] Looking beyond industry, the committee recognized that increased mechanization and the increasing speed of automobiles would likely increase demands on hospitals and their staffs. "It is our thought," the committee predicted, "that ultimately it will be possible to assign all accident cases to men especially trained in this department of surgery."[54]

The College secured the interest of both insurers and labor in its efforts at improving the care of the injured worker. An initial grant of $20,000 came from the National Board of Life and Casualty Underwriters. At the same time, the American Federation of Labor, whose longtime leader Samuel Gompers had served on the Advisory Committee with Martin, offered its cooperation, an offer the Regents accepted. Efforts to involve the Federal government followed. With the passage of the National Recovery Act in 1933, Franklin Martin and Frederic Besley, the Board's chair, went to Washington, DC, in an attempt to interest the administration in the College's work as the basis for a national code "that will at least urge industry to do more for their workers."[55] Martin and Besley received a warm welcome in Washington and praise for the College's leadership, which would play an important role in the debate over health insurance (see chapter 4).[56]

The College also turned to moving pictures as an educational medium. Martin held a conference with the Regents and Will Hays, president of the Motion Picture Producers and Distributors of America in May 1925. Hays enthusiastically supported Martin's ideas on the educational value of film. The Regents then established a Motion Picture Advisory Committee headed by J Bentley Squier, a New York urologist and Regent. In October 1926, Hays promised the support of his organization in the distribution of films for both surgical education and the lay public. In May 1927, Martin obtained support from the Eastman Kodak Company. By 1930, eight motion pictures had been approved and prepared for distribution, seven had been approved and were ready to be released, and six were in production. The latter included films on fracture care by the Committee on Fractures and on hospital standardization by MacEachern.[57]

For the Fellows, the Department of Literary Research began operations in 1921 with a goal to become a "connecting link between the surgeon and the research worker."[58] Recognizing that many Fellows either did not have access to an adequate medical library or time for extensive library work, the department offered an extensive research service for Fellows. The staff provided bibliographies, article searches, and packaged copies from its extensive collection of English language reprints free of charge to any Fellow. As the department grew, its services expanded to include translations of foreign language articles. At the same time the College created a library for the use of Fellows visiting Chicago. It also served as a repository for copies of articles and books written by Fellows. Reflecting the orientation of the College to the workplace as well as the surgeon, the library offered its services to and in cooperation with local hospital libraries.[59] Within a few years, the Department of Literary Research received requests from Fellows around the world for its services. Within the United States, Boston, Philadelphia, Chicago, and New York generated the most requests—a tribute to the service, given the rich medical library resources in those cities. The College became an educational institution.

The College extended its educational activities to the public. At a time when cultural taboos kept cancer hidden, the CCSNA had formed a "cancer campaign committee" in 1912 to educate the public through articles in *Ladies Home Journal*, *McClure's*, and *Colliers*. The College collaborated with the American Society for the Control of Cancer (founded 1913, now the American Cancer Society) on spreading the message of early detection and advances in treatment. Films for the public covered a wide range of medical topics, although some, like child care and the regular medical checkup, were not directly related to surgery. The radio broadcasts to the general public by leading surgeons of the Clinical Congresses served a similar purpose. Martin held an expansive view of the College's place in American medicine, and these activities helped bring the College to public attention and to identify it with medical progress in the public mind.

Foreign Travel

Although established for the reform of surgery in the United States and Canada, the idea of establishing ties with surgeons in the rest of the Americas had been considered as early 1914. At that time some correspondence was conducted with leading surgeons in South America and a visit by College officials considered for 1916. WWI interrupted these plans. By 1919, the College had reestablished contact with surgeons in Peru, Chile, Argentina, and Uruguay in an attempt to "enlist the interest of the surgical profession [there] in the American College of Surgeons."[60]

Consequently, in January 1920, the former President of the College William Mayo and Secretary Franklin Martin undertook a two-month tour of Panama, Peru, Chile, Argentina, and Uruguay.[61] The long voyage deepened the friendship between Martin and Mayo and allowed Martin to try his hand at writing a shipboard mystery. The group met with medical leaders, toured hospitals and medical schools, and departed with high praise for the standards of South American surgery. Welcomed as distinguished guests, the Past-President and Secretary of the seven-year-old College even met with the Presidents of several of the countries. Following up on this visit, Francis P Corrigan, a young Fellow, made an official trip to Ecuador, Bolivia, Peru, and Chile at the end of the year. (Figure 3.3)

In early 1923, accompanied by Thomas J Watkins, a Governor of the College, Martin led a larger delegation that included wives and children to South America. The two month cruise on the chartered SS *Vandyck* passed pleasantly and allowed Martin to attend the laying of the cornerstone for the Gorgas Memorial Institute of Tropical Medicine in Panama. Martin had served during WWI with William Gorgas (1854–1920), Surgeon General of the Army and an expert in tropical disease. After Gorgas' death, Martin led the fund-raising for the memorial, an activity wholly separate from the College. But as we will see, activities like these, however valuable in linking North and South America's surgical communities (and gratifying to Martin's ego), would contribute to a growing uneasiness among some surgeons that the College

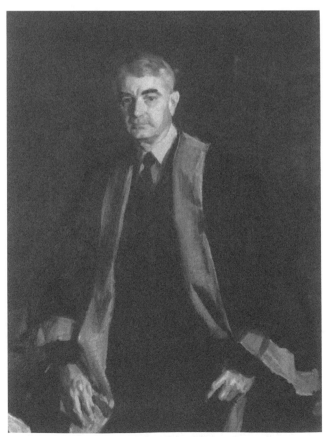

FIGURE 3.3 Dr. William J Mayo, ACS President, 1916–18.

had begun to stray from its original purpose and that Martin used it to raise funds for other activities.

The outreach effort itself succeeded—35 South American surgeons received fellowships at the 1920 Convocation in Montreal. Two years later, the Year Book would describe the College as "a society of surgeons of both North and South America."[62] By 1928, 242 Latin American surgeons had become Fellows, representing 17 countries. With the Depression, however, the number of new Fellows from Latin America declined. Between 1929 and 1935, only 14 received fellowships, eight of them before 1932.

Continuing their travels, William Mayo and Martin made a private visit to Australia and New Zealand in February and March of 1924. At the time, leading surgeons in Australia and New Zealand were considering establishing some form of association. Consequently, Mayo and Martin's talks on the formation of the American College of Surgeons found a receptive audience. Mayo's belief that, while the Royal Colleges had provided an example, a new country required a new approach resonated with his listeners.[63] After the visit, a number of prominent Australasian surgeons received "charter memberships" in the ACS.[64] The following year, several Australasian surgeons attended the annual meeting in New York City. On the way home, one member of the group, HB Devine, stayed with William Mayo in Rochester. The question of an Australian college came up. Devine received succinct advice from Mayo, "My boy, go home and found your own College," one adapted to Australasian conditions.[65] Devine later credited this with inspiring his efforts to organize what would become the Royal Australasian College of Surgeons.[66]

≋✤≋

The First Challenge

During the 1920s, Martin's expansive international and educational programs were matched by an expansion of the membership. From 1920 to 1929, the College awarded 6,183 fellowships. The character of the membership changed with this expansion. The proportion of Fellows from the South, West, and Northwest increased. As a result of this movement away from the larger cities, the proportion of Fellows representing a surgical specialty also decreased. The fellowship assumed a less urban and less academic character.[67]

By the early 1920s, elite surgeons, particularly in the Northeast, viewed these changes, which they saw as a devaluation of the fellowship, with mounting alarm. As the prominent Philadelphia surgeon WW Keene put it in a letter to Harvey Cushing, "to admit over 400 Fellows at one fell swoop is tending to cheapen the membership very seriously."[68]

In the spirit of quiet influence, despite his personal misgivings, Harvey Cushing reluctantly agreed to take the presidency of the College in 1922.[69] While conceding that Martin had created an important organization, Cushing thought the College needed "to be kept within bounds" to be respectable.[70] The influence of the President, however, was limited. Although an inner circle, including Charles Mayo, George Crile, and (behind the scenes) William Mayo, had some restraining effect, Martin had firm operational control of the College, particularly after the departure of Bowman. And Martin, many thought, needed an expanding membership to fund the College's ambitious programs.[71]

Even College insiders expressed disquiet about the expansion of the membership. By the mid-1920s, Crile and William Mayo had agreed that, in Mayo's words, "we have got to go on a quality basis instead of a quantity basis."[72] Both Charles Mayo and George Crile had recommended to Martin that the requirements for fellowship be raised. Charles Mayo believed that the written and oral exam of the American Board of Ophthalmic Examinations (founded in 1917), which for some years was based in College headquarters, offered the best model.[73] Martin, by now ten years out of active practice, took no action.

Consequently, despite internal pressure and the increasing importance to surgical practice of basic sciences like physiology and chemistry, fellowship requirements for surgeons remained essentially unchanged. True, diplomates of the new boards in Ophthalmology and Otolaryngology (1924) would be required to submit only 25 cases, but for all others, increasingly the majority of new members, the old standards applied. While the critics could agree that the fellowship should require a more rigorous exam, no consensus existed on what form that exam should take. Even Harvey Cushing believed that the "College should not fall into the errors of the Royal College by having too academic an exam."[74] Additionally, whatever the concerns about Martin's leadership, the College had a dual mandate—to identify the qualified surgeon (the focus of the critics) *and* to raise the level of surgical care throughout the continent, which necessarily required a focus on those *currently* in practice and which external critics largely ignored.

While Cushing and others of his generation tried to influence Martin, a younger generation of surgeons turned to direct confrontation. On June 12, 1924, two groups presented petitions to the Board of Regents—the Society of Clinical Surgery (SCS) and the Eclat Club. The Eclat Club represented a self-selected group of younger surgeons, all of whom had served in the Zone of Advance during WWI. They continued their association in the post-war years. By the mid-1920s both groups represented a rising generation of prominent surgeons.

At a meeting in Rochester, Minnesota that year, the SCS expressed support for the College goals, but recorded four "suggestions." To wit, the College should immediately reduce the number of Fellows; institute more rigorous tests of character, training, and "intelligence;" not reconsider those rejected for character flaws for at least three years; and stop "proselytizing" for members. In sum, all four suggestions spoke to concerns about the devaluation of the fellowship.[75]

The Eclat Club also praised the ideals of the College, but more openly criticized the College's policies and the Director General. The expanded membership included too many not "up to the original standard" as well as known fee splitters. Too much publicity attended the speakers at the public sessions of the Clinical Congresses and the sectional meetings. Neither provided much educational benefit, and the College should place more emphasis on encouraging clinical research. Higher standards not minimum standards should be set for hospitals. Financial statements should be issued annually. (This reflected a wider suspicion that Martin used his creations for personal financial gain. Mayo's committee had visited the same issue in 1917 and found the accounts in order.) The Regents needed to assume more responsibility from a dictatorial Director General, who ignored their advice. By taking action, the petitioners believed, the Regents would go a long way toward "reinstating itself in the confidence of its *original* members (emphasis added)."[76] The Eclat Club's petition received endorsements from the Interurban Surgical Society, the Milwaukee Surgical Society, and a number of other leading surgeons from around the country solicited by the petitioners. The petitioners hoped to show that they represented a broad-based coalition.

A tense discussion followed the presentation of the petitions to the Board of Regents at their June 12, 1924 meeting, much of which focused on the College's record in combating fee splitting. MacEachern and Craig (the assistant director of the standardization program) defended their efforts vigorously, while Judge Stephens explained the legal difficulties the College faced. Once the petitioners withdrew and after further discussion, the Regents gave Judge Stephens the task of replying to the petitioners in what would be a defense of the "middle way" the College had taken between egalitarianism and exclusivity.[77]

Stephens, in his lawyerly reply, distinguished between "questions of fact" and "questions of policy."[78] For the former, which included financial accountability, publicity, and arbitrariness, he provided brief answers. A respected accounting firm prepared the financial statements. Any interested Fellow could review them. (Unmentioned by Stephens, they would need to travel to Chicago to do so.) A committee supervised publicity at the Clinical Congresses. Stephens answered the charge of arbitrariness on the part of the Director General by pointing to the bylaws. The Regents served as a board of directors and its Executive Committee met frequently. Both acted to restrain the chief executive.

In answering the "questions of policy," Stephens continued his defense of the status quo particularly on the contentious issue of membership and fee splitting. Artfully re-framing the question as a choice between two extremes, Stephens argued that too large a membership would merely replicate the AMA's Section on Surgery, while too small a membership would duplicate the existing specialty societies. (In fact, the 7,465 fellowships awarded represented only about five percent of North American physicians.)[79] Further, as Stephens correctly noted, beyond a vague suggestion that the medical schools conduct some form of exam, the petitioners had offered no practical solutions. Even had they done so, Stephens pointed out that no organization would delegate responsibility for determining its own membership. With regard to fee splitting, Stephens, as he had at the meeting in June, explained the difficulty of proving the case and the risks of suits for defamation. Stephens' carefully worded reply forestalled any further action by the College's critics for another decade, but it proved to be a Pyrrhic victory.

Had the College, under Martin's leadership, paid closer attention to its critics and seriously considered revising the standard for fellowship, it might have maintained a position equivalent to that of the Royal Colleges as both a professional organization and a certifying body. Loyal Davis, whose work with the College had begun during this period and who remained a close associate of Martin, stated that by the 1920s the College's Regents had at least tacitly decided to defer the question of examination to others.[80] While the minutes for this period are incomplete, there are several reasons to reconsider this. First, at that time, only two boards had been established and the American Board of Surgery did not yet exist. Second, as we will see in chapter 6, the first impulse of at least some of the founders of the American Board of Surgery was to attempt to work through the College. When rebuffed, they went around the College. Finally, the Regents then argued that a board was unnecessary; there already was a certifying body in surgery—the College. In any event, no significant changes occurred, which would lead to a second confrontation a decade later.

REFERENCES

1. Crile, G. W., *Diary: The Third Battle of Chicago.* October 23, 1917, George W. Crile Papers (MSS 2806), Container 35, Folder 112, Manuscript Collections, Western Reserve Historical Society, Cleveland, OH. Davis, L. (1960). *Fellowship of Surgeons: A History of the American College of Surgeons* (pp. 188–9). Springfield, IL: Charles C. Thomas.
2. Ibid., pp. 487–8.
3. Crile, G. W., *Diary: The Third Battle of Chicago.* George W. Crile Papers (MSS 2806), Container 35, Folder 112, Manuscript Collections, Western Reserve Historical Society, Cleveland, OH.
4. Ibid.
5. Crile, G. W., *Diary: Franklin Martin.* October 24, 1917, George W. Crile Papers (MSS 2806), Container 35, Folder 112, Manuscript Collections, Western Reserve Historical Society, Cleveland, OH.
6. Martin, F. H. (1934). *Fifty Years of Medicine and Surgery: An Autobiographical Sketch* (pp. 331–2). Chicago: The Surgical Publishing Company.
7. Martin, F. H., *Letter to W J Mayo.* November 1, 1917, W. J. Mayo Papers, Box 1, Folder ACS 1913–1918, Mayo Historical Unit, Mayo Clinic, Rochester, MN.
8. Martin, F. H., *Letter to W J Mayo.* November 2, 1917, W. J. Mayo Papers, Box 1, Folder ACS 1913–1918, Mayo Historical Unit, Mayo Clinic, Rochester, MN.
9. American College of Surgeons. (1917) The by-laws. In *Year Book of the American College of Surgeons* (pp. 12–13). Chicago: American College of Surgeons.
10. Ibid.
11. Davis, L. (1960). *Fellowship of Surgeons: A History of the American College of Surgeons* (p. 235). Springfield, IL: Charles C. Thomas.
12. Martin, F. H., *Diary: August 31, 1920 to June 12, 1921.* September 8, 1921, Franklin Martin Diary, Archives of the American College of Surgeons, Chicago.
13. Martin, F. H., *Diary: August 31, 1920 to June 12, 1921.* November 3, 1920, Franklin Martin Diary, Archives of the American College of Surgeons, Chicago.
14. Bowman, J. G., *Letter to F H Martin.* December 1, 1932, Eleanor Grimm Papers, Archives of the American College of Surgeons, Chicago.
15. Stephens, H. M., *Letter to the Board of Regents.* May 27, 1921, C. H. Mayo Papers, Box 60, Folder 062, Mayo Historical Unit, Mayo Clinic, Rochester, MN.
16. American College of Surgeons. (1922). *Year Book of the American College of Surgeons: 1922* (p. 70). Chicago: American College of Surgeons.
17. American College of Surgeons. (1925, October 27). *Board of Regents: Minutes October 27, 1925.* Complete Minute Book 3. Archives of the American College of Surgeons, Chicago.
18. Martin, F. H. & MacEachern, M. T. (1925) Presentation of the official report of hospital standardization for the year 1924. *Bulletin of the American College of Surgeons, 9*(1), 9.
19. MacEachern, M. T. (n.d.). Hospital standardization. In *Year Book of the American College of Surgeons: 1927* (p. 49). Chicago: American College of Surgeons.
20. Crile, G. W. (1926). The American College of Surgeons. *Surgery, Gynecology, and Obstetrics, 43*, 262.
21. Ibid., p. 263.
22. Martin, F. H. & MacEachern, M. T. (1925) Presentation of the official report of hospital standardization for the year 1924. *Bulletin of the American College of Surgeons, 9*(1), 15–16.

23. American College of Surgeons. (1927, October 4). *Board of Regents: Minutes October 4, 1927*. Complete Minute Book 4. Archives of the American College of Surgeons, Chicago.

24. American College of Surgeons. (1929, October 15). *Board of Regents: Minutes October 15, 1929*. Complete Minute Book 4. Archives of the American College of Surgeons, Chicago.

25. American College of Surgeons. (1925, October 27). *Board of Regents: Minutes October 27, 1925*. Complete Minute Book 3. Archives of the American College of Surgeons, Chicago.

26. American College of Surgeons. (1929, October 15). *Board of Regents: Minutes October 15, 1929*. Complete Minute Book 4. Archives of the American College of Surgeons, Chicago.

27. Stewart, G. D. (1929). Ourselves–the college: Address of the retiring President. *Surgery, Gynecology, and Obstetrics, 48*, 144.

28. American College of Surgeons. (1925, October 27). *Board of Regents: Minutes October 27, 1925*. Complete Minute Book 3. Archives of the American College of Surgeons, Chicago.

29. Ibid.

30. Barnett, L. E. (1928). A history of the American College of Surgeons. *Journal of the College of Surgeons of Australasia, 1*, 30.

31. American College of Surgeons. (1924, June 12). *Board of Regents: Minutes June 12, 1924*. Complete Minute Book 3. Archives of the American College of Surgeons, Chicago.

32. Martin, F. H., *Letter to W J Mayo*. November 1, 1917, W. J. Mayo Papers, Box 1, Folder American College of Surgeons, Mayo Historical Unit, Mayo Clinic, Rochester, MN.

33. American College of Surgeons. (1924, June 12). *Board of Regents: Minutes June 12, 1924*. Complete Minute Book 3. Archives of the American College of Surgeons, Chicago.

34. See Rodwin, M. A. (1992). The organized American medical profession's response to financial conflicts of interest: 1890–1992. *The Milbank Quarterly, 70*(4), 703–741.

35. American College of Surgeons. (1929, October 15). *Board of Regents: Minutes October 15, 1929*. Complete Minute Book 4. Archives of the American College of Surgeons, Chicago.

36. American College of Surgeons. (1925, October 27). *Board of Regents: Minutes October 27, 1925*. Complete Minute Book 3. Archives of the American College of Surgeons, Chicago.

37. Ibid.

38. American College of Surgeons. (1927, October 4). *Board of Regents: Minutes October 4, 1927*. Complete Minute Book 4. Archives of the American College of Surgeons, Chicago.

39. American College of Surgeons. (1929, October 15). *Board of Regents: Minutes October 15, 1929*. Complete Minute Book 4. Archives of the American College of Surgeons, Chicago.

40. American College of Surgeons. (1925). *Year Book of the American College of Surgeons: 1925* (pp. 17–18). Chicago: American College of Surgeons.

41. American College of Surgeons. (1927). Judiciary committee report for 1926. In *Year Book of the American College of Surgeons* (p. 42). Chicago: American College of Surgeons.

42. Anonymous. (1924). Judiciary and advisory committee. *Surgery, Gynecology, and Obstetrics, 39*, 127.

43. Anonymous. (1922). Summary of group meetings of state and provincial sections of the Clinical Congress of the American College of Surgeons, 1920–1922. *Surgery, Gynecology, and Obstetrics, 35*, 248.

44. American College of Surgeons. (1919, October 23). *Board of Regents: Minutes October 23, 1919*. Complete Minute Book 1. Archives of the American College of Surgeons, Chicago.

45. Martin, F. H., *Diary: August 31, 1920 to June 12, 1921*. Franklin Martin Diary, Archives of the American College of Surgeons, Chicago.

46. American College of Surgeons. (1921, October 25). *Sectional meeting minutes: October 25, 1921*, Complete Minute Book 2, Archives of the American College of Surgeons, Chicago.

47. Grimm, E. K., *Letter to F H Martin*. January 13, 1931, Folder EKG–FHM Letters, Archives of the American College of Surgeons, Chicago.

48. American College of Surgeons. (1923, October 24). *Proceedings State and Provincial Committee Meeting*, p. 15. Complete Minute Book 2, Archives of the American College of Surgeons, Chicago.

49. Marchand, R. (1985). *Advertising the American Dream: Making Way for Modernity, 1920–1940* (pp. 10–4). Berkeley, CA: University of California Press.

50. American College of Surgeons. (1923). *Year Book of the American College of Surgeons: 1923* (p. 45). Chicago: American College of Surgeons.

51. American College of Surgeons. (1929). *Year Book of the American College of Surgeons: 1929* (p. 27). Chicago: American College of Surgeons.

52. Besley, F. A. (1933). Industrial medicine and traumatic surgery: Report of the board and list of approved medical services in industry. *Bulletin of the American College of Surgeons, 17*(4), 12.

53. Ibid.

54. Ibid.

55. Ibid., p. 13.

56. American College of Surgeons. (1933, October 10). *Board of Regents: Minutes October 10, 1933*. Complete Minute Book 9. Archives of the American College of Surgeons, Chicago.

57. Anonymous. (1930). Report of the board of medical motion picture films. *Surgery, Gynecology, and Obstetrics, 50*, 357–8.

58. Anonymous. (1921). Department of literary research. *Surgery, Gynecology, and Obstetrics, 33*, 320.

59. Walker, S. F. (1929). The correlation of the record department and medical library in the hospital. *Bulletin of the American College of Surgeons, 13*(4), 56.

60. American College of Surgeons. (1921). *Year Book of the American College of Surgeons* (p. 7). Chicago: American College of Surgeons.

61. Martin, F. H. (1922). *South America From a Surgeon's Point of View*. New York, NY: Fleming H. Revell.

62. American College of Surgeons. (n.d.). *Year Book of the American College of Surgeons: 1922* (p. 1). Chicago: American College of Surgeons.

63. Smith, J. O. (1971). The history of the Royal Australasian College of Surgeons. *Australian and New Zealand Journal of Surgery, 41*(1), 3.

64. Martin, F. H. (1925). Report of the director general. In *Year Book of the American College of Surgeons* (p. 78). Chicago: American College of Surgeons.

65. Smith, J. O. (1971). The history of the Royal Australasian College of Surgeons. *Australian and New Zealand Journal of Surgery, 41*(1), 4.

66. Ibid.

67. Kernahan, P. (2010). *Franklin Martin and the standardization of American surgery 1890–1940* (p. 159; Doctoral dissertation, University of Minnesota). Available from CIC Institutions. (Publication No. AAT 3422569).

68. Keen, W. W., *Letter to H Cushing*. November 1, 1921, Harvey Williams Cushing Papers. Microfilm. 1921, Manuscripts and Archives, Yale University Library, New Haven, CT.

69. Bliss, M. (2005). *Harvey Cushing: A Life in Surgery* (p. 384–5). Oxford, UK: Oxford University Press.

70. Cushing, H., *Letter to W W Keen*. November 2, 1921, Harvey Williams Cushing Papers. Microfilm, Reel 2 Box 2 Folder 35, Manuscripts and Archives, Yale University Library, New Haven, CT.

71. Jones, D. F., *Letter to H Cushing*. January 12, 1922, Harvey Williams Cushing Papers. Microfilm. Manuscripts and Archives, Yale University Library, New Haven, CT.

72. Mayo, W. J., *Letter to G W Crile*. July 4, 1924, W. J. Mayo Papers, Box 1, Folder American College of Surgeons 1913–18, Mayo Historical Unit, Mayo Clinic, Rochester, MN.

73. Mayo, C. H., *Letter to F H Martin*. June 28, 1924, C. H. Mayo Papers, Box 2, Folder 51, Mayo Historical Unit, Mayo Clinic, Rochester, MN.

74. Cushing, H., *Letter to F H Martin*. September 20, 1920, Harvey Williams Cushing Papers. Microfilm. Reel 2 Box 2 Folder 34 1920, Manuscripts and Archives, Yale University Library, New Haven, CT.

75. *Untitled*. n.d., C. H. Mayo Papers, Box 59, Folder 51, Mayo Historical Unit, Mayo Clinic, Rochester, MN.

76. *To the regents of the American College of Surgeons*. n.d., C. H. Mayo Papers, Box 59, Folder 51, Mayo Historical Unit, Mayo Clinic, Rochester, MN.

77. American College of Surgeons. (1924, June 12). *Board of Regents: Minutes June 12, 1924*. Complete Minute Book 3. Archives of the American College of Surgeons, Chicago.

78. Stephens, H. M., *Statement by the Board of Regents of the American College of Surgeons*. June 1924, 9–10, C. H. Mayo Papers, Box 2, Folder 51, Mayo Historical Unit, Mayo Clinic, Rochester, MN.

79. Kernahan, P. (2010). *Franklin Martin and the standardization of American surgery 1890–1940* (p. 176); Doctoral dissertation, University of Minnesota). Available from CIC Institutions. (Publication No. AAT 3422569).

80. Davis, L. (1960). *Fellowship of Surgeons: A History of the American College of Surgeons* (p. 234). Springfield, IL: Charles C. Thomas.

CHAPTER 4
The Last Years
of the Martin Era,
1930–1934

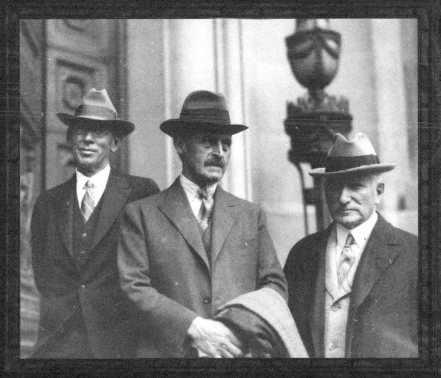

Dr Allen B Kanavel, Lord Dawson of Penn, Dr Franklin H Martin,
October 1, 1930 at ACS Headquarters

By early September 1929, the Dow Jones Industrial Average had reached an all-time high in a six-year bull market. America's leading economist, Yale's Irving Fisher, famously announced that stocks had reached "a permanently high plateau."[1] Small wonder, then, that when the Regents discussed the College's finances at their October 15, 1929 meeting, Bentley Squier asked whether Illinois law allowed non-profit organizations to purchase stocks.[2] Treasurer Besley replied that it did not. Even if it had, the sense of the meeting conveyed financial conservatism on the part of the Regents. Squier's timing had been unfortunate, if understandable. Nine days later the stock market crashed, and in the ensuing months the nation and the world would enter what came to be called the Great Depression.

The financial crisis would put strains on the College, but its greatest challenges would come from within the medical profession. A rising generation of full-time academic surgeons, personified by Evarts Graham of Washington University St. Louis, would attack Martin's management of the College. Conflict between the American Medical Association (AMA) and the American College of Surgeons (ACS), after a period of détente in the 1920s, would flare again over the health insurance question. Martin, now in his seventies, would suffer a serious stroke in 1930, recover, and continue as an increasingly controversial Director General.

❦

College Affairs

A charismatic individual, Martin had the ability to inspire loyalty and dedication from his subordinates. In general his management style was to give the College staff a fair degree of freedom to carry out their jobs, while remaining firmly in control of the direction of the College. Malcolm MacEachern, for example, ran the hospital standardization program with little direct interference from Martin and rapidly established himself as a leading figure in hospital management. Similarly, Marion Farrow, secretary to the Regents, and Martin's secretary Eleanor Grimm had considerable authority in the day-to-day operations of the College. Martin also offered relatively generous salaries to the staff and established a retirement annuity plan. (At the time, only about 15 percent of the nation's workforce had pension plans.)[3] Under Martin's management, hard work and loyalty would be rewarded and reciprocated.

These arrangements would be tested in April 1930 when the 73-year-old Martin suffered a severe left hemispheric stroke that resulted in amnesia, aphasia, and right hemiplegia. Hospitalized initially at Passavant Hospital and then convalescing at a local country club under the care of neurosurgeon and confidant Loyal Davis, Martin made a slow but progressive recovery in the ensuing months. By mid-June he could walk with assistance and had regained some speech and use of the right hand.[4] By late July, he resumed some College business. By October, any residual deficit was undetectable to the uninformed observer.[5] Nonetheless, the stroke had been hidden from the membership, reflecting a sense of vulnerability in the close identification of the College with its Director General. Significantly, no action was taken on a succession plan, despite JMT Finney's attempts to bring this issue to the College's inner circle.[6]

As a testament to Martin's organizational skills, however, his incapacity had caused no interruption in the routine tasks of the College. In the interim, George Crile, as Chairman of the Board of Regents, stepped in to provide overall direction and the actual management fell to the Executive Committee and to the College's staff. At the

Regents' meeting that October, Martin paid a handsome tribute to "my family" and "this marvelous organization" that had carried on in his absence.[7]

Financially, the College weathered the early years of the Depression relatively well. The conservatively managed endowment, having stood at $735,132 in 1928, reached a peak of $857,000 in 1932 before declining to $838,448 by 1936, as some municipalities and Latin American countries defaulted on their bonds. With some satisfaction, George Crile observed to the Regents on at least two occasions that the College's endowment had fared better than Harvard's.[8]

Still, the Depression had an impact on the membership. Besley, as Treasurer, reported to the Regents in 1932 that he was "receiving some very pathetic letters" from Fellows unable to pay their dues.[9] In keeping with the College's practice of referring issues concerning the Fellows to the Regents, many of these individual cases would be reviewed at Board meetings. The Board acted generously by excusing many of the hard-pressed Fellows from dues and dropping any debts owed the College. At the same time, membership growth slowed to about 5 percent to 10 percent per year during the Depression.

The Depression also affected the College staff. The number of office staff, which had reached 37 by 1930, was reduced to 26 in late 1931. The remaining employees had salaries reduced by 10 percent. Martin took a similar reduction. His distribution of small Christmas gifts continued. Staff morale and esprit de corps remained strong.[10]

Despite these medical and economic exigencies, the College carried on with its core functions. Sectional meetings were held, although with reduced frequency. The standing committees of the College continued their work. Hospital standardization inspections continued and remained the most demanding of the College's many activities. A handful of field representatives (between three and six in any given year) carried out the arduous work. By 1935, the surveyors had conducted more than 34,000 inspections, encompassing 3,565 individual hospitals.[11] Of those hospitals 2,523 had been approved.

For the largest hospitals (100 or more beds) the approval rate reached 92 percent by 1926 and 95 percent by the 1935 survey. Surveys of hospitals of 50–99 beds began in 1922 with an initial approval rate of 41 percent. By 1935, that rate had risen to 68 percent. Surveys of 25–49 bed hospitals began in 1924. These hospitals, many proprietary and rural or western, had the lowest approval rates—16 percent on the initial survey and 27 percent at the time of the 1935 survey. Interestingly, the Depression, which posed significant hardships for hospitals, resulted in no fall in the approval rates for any size of hospital. For medium-sized hospitals during this time, the rate of increase in approvals slowed but did not reverse. Even the smallest hospitals showed continued improvement during the Depression years, with approvals rising from 18 percent in 1930 to 31 percent in 1937.

The annual Hospital Standardization Conferences provided a venue for hospital administrators, nursing supervisors, physicians, and officials of the College and the American Hospital Association to meet and exchange ideas. The programs covered the full range of hospital activities from the organization of the medical staff to the laboratories, laundry, and medical records. Increasingly, the College used the accumulated data for what would now be called outcomes research—formalized in 1934 when a Hospital Research and Information Department was created within the hospital standardization program. In 1935, Malcolm MacEachern distilled his years of experience with hospital standardization into the 900 pages of *Hospital Organization and Management*, the first comprehensive textbook of hospital administration.[12]

The Changing World of the Surgical Elite

At its founding, the College had been part of a wider world of medical reform. Much of that reform, epitomized by Abraham Flexner's famous and muckraking report in 1910, concentrated on undergraduate medical education. Understandably at the time, given the condition of the medical schools, graduate education and specialty training received little attention. The College itself necessarily focused on the surgeons already in practice and the hospitals in which they worked. Identifying competent surgeons and improving the quality of care provided by those surgeons and their hospitals was the great goal of the standardization project. Under these circumstances the College essentially deferred the question of the education of surgeons to the medical schools, suggesting that they consider a supplemental degree for surgeons. This undoubtedly reflected the influence of the Mayo brothers as part of the College's inner circle. The Mayo Clinic's trainee fellows would, from 1915 onward, be enrolled as graduate students in the University of Minnesota and receive either the MS or the PhD degree at the completion of their training.[13] This "graduate school model," also adopted at the University of Pennsylvania, offered one solution to identifying the well-trained and qualified new surgeon.

The dominant model would, however, become the surgical residency pioneered by William Halsted at Johns Hopkins. At the same time, Abraham Flexner at the Rockefeller Foundation championed—and selectively funded—the full-time faculty system. Reformers like Flexner saw this as a way of freeing the medical schools' clinical faculty from the demands and distractions of private practice. So freed, the clinical faculty could devote itself to research and teaching. Not without a great deal of controversy (and a warning from the eminent William Osler that such a system risked producing "clinical prigs"), a number of leading medical schools adopted the full-time system. By the early 1930s, the combination of the Halsted residency and the full-time system had created a powerful new force in American surgery—the full-time teachers of surgery.

These full-time teachers would find their spokesman in Evarts A Graham of Washington University. The son of a prominent Chicago surgeon, Graham received an undergraduate degree from Princeton and then graduated from Rush Medical College in 1907. There he and his contemporary Dallas Phemister, who would become the first full-time chief at the University of Chicago, had trained under Martin's nemesis, Arthur Dean Bevan. Graham's early career included a brief and unhappy two years in Mason City, Iowa, where he hoped to help create a clinic modeled on that of the Mayos. The fee splitting and medical politics proved too much for him. His biographer, C Barber Mueller, attributes much of Graham's antipathy toward surgeons in private practice to those years.[14] For Graham, the true surgeon was the "composer" who created new knowledge in "temples of learning." Private practitioners were, at best, "merely surgical artists," and the number of cases performed—the standard that the College used—a "false standard."[15] (Figure 4.1)

By contrast, Franklin Martin had an abiding aversion to those he considered "academic *littérateurs*,"[16] perhaps reflecting his sensitivity to his sketchy educational background. He had founded *Surgery, Gynecology, and Obstetrics* in 1905 as a journal by and for practical surgeons, among whose number he included his close allies Crile and the Mayo brothers. Together, they remained firmly in control of the College's affairs. In addition, several of the relatively younger men most active in the management of

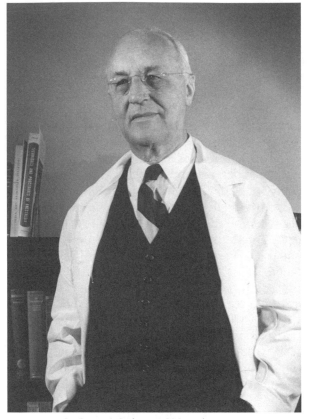

FIGURE 4.1 Dr. Evarts A Graham, ACS President, 1940–41, circa 1951.

the College, notably Frederic Besley, Allen Kanavel, and Loyal Davis, all of Northwestern University, combined, in the traditional manner, private practices with their academic work. Consequently, the College had been slow to recognize a significant new constituency competing for the leadership of American surgery.

Graham's long association with the College began when he became a Fellow in 1914. As Graham's post-war reputation grew at Washington University in St. Louis, Martin invited him to speak on thoracic surgery at the 1923 and 1926 Clinical Congresses. Graham subsequently declined an invitation from Martin to serve on the credentials committee for Missouri in 1925, but he and Martin did meet again briefly later that year. In 1932, Graham chaired the organizing committee for that year's Clinical Congress in St. Louis. That Congress marked the start of Graham's involvement in College leadership.

It was an inauspicious beginning for someone already concerned about the direction of the College and who believed that the discontent reflected by the Eclat Club's protest eight years earlier had only increased.[17] By custom, the chair of the organizing committee became the Second Vice President of the College the following year. Graham, unfortunately, learned of this from the front page of his morning paper on the last day of the conference.[18] His annoyance at this arbitrary action led to a long conversation with Crile about his generation's criticisms of the College and another with Martin and Squier. Learning that the Second Vice President had no power did nothing to appease Graham. In response Martin assured Graham that as Vice President he could attend the Regents' meetings and speak if he wished.[19]

An exchange of letters between Graham and Martin followed. The letters reveal two men talking past each other. To Graham's charge that a younger generation lacked representation, Martin could supply a list of younger men who held university appointments and had served as Regents in the past decade.[20] On the other hand, Graham, with some justice, could claim that they were not representative of the full-time teachers "who now hold the most important chairs of surgery."[21] Martin's emollient praise of Graham did nothing to soften the latter's stiff replies. His unexpected appearance in the Blue Book as First Vice President seemed to confirm his concerns about Martin's arbitrary management.[22]

While there had certainly been, as Martin argued, turnover in the Board of Regents, there was also a remarkable stability in its membership. Four of the then 16 members—Martin, Charles Mayo, JMT Finney, and George Crile—had served continuously since 1913. Two others, William Haggard of Tennessee and Robert McKechnie of Vancouver, were on the Board between 1913 and 1921. Allen Kanavel and Robert Greenough of Boston were members since 1921. In addition, the character of the Board had changed. In 1913, 12 of the Regents had been members of the American Surgical Association. By 1933, that number dropped to nine, of whom four (Crile, Greenough, Finney, and Kanavel) were inactive senior members of the older society.

During the summer of 1932, Graham prepared for the October meeting of the Board of Regents. He would use the opportunity Martin had given him to present his case to the Board. To strengthen his hand, he wrote to 20 surgeons who he felt represented his generation of leading surgeons.[23] Of these, the majority were full-time heads of university departments. He included two representatives of "large private clinics," Frank Lahey of the Lahey Clinic and E Starr Judd of the Mayo Clinic, in the belief that this made the group more representative.[24] Of the 20, all but four were Fellows of the College. With varying degrees of vehemence, most of his correspondents thought as he did.

Protest and Response

Invited to speak at the end of the meeting on October 10, 1933, Graham presented his case in measured and dispassionate terms.[25] He informed the Regents that his remarks were based on the responses he had received to his letter. He began with the general approval of the hospital standardization program and the scientific work of the College's various committees. He discussed the sense of alienation from the College and the belief that a small clique controlled the College. He went on to deplore the attention still given to John B Murphy ("ludicrous") who remained, 20 years after his death, a controversial figure, one who Graham and his correspondents believed did not represent the best in American surgery. Inadequate financial reports, lack of recognition of recent achievements in American surgery, lax membership policies, and a failure to address fee splitting completed the indictment. He concluded by reminding the Regents that the teachers of surgery would shape the views of the next generation of surgeons toward the College.

Graham's remarks came as the last item at the end of a long meeting during the Clinical Congress in Chicago. The Regents had already discussed controversial reports on health insurance (see next section) and surgical education (see chapter 6). Given this and the nature of Graham's charges, the response became testy at times. Besley, particularly, seemed stung by the criticism of the College's finances. "For your information, Doctor," he told Graham, detailed financial statements had "been published every year," were presented at meetings and "open to inspection by anyone."[26] Charles Mayo defended his old friend, John B Murphy. Martin argued that of 4,500 applicants only 2,000 were accepted at the state level and of those only 600 finally accepted. "It is a shifting process that is intricate, reliable, and mighty effective."[27]

Toward the end of the discussion, Chairman Crile diplomatically provided the soft answer. He began by empathizing with Graham about the unpleasantness of having to present criticism "from various of your colleagues" and that doing so demonstrated Graham's concern for the College.[28] Having depersonalized the debate, he went on to gently defend the College's actions. On fee splitting, he discussed the difficulties of proof and pointed out that only the ACS had taken action. Liability concerns meant that the names of expelled Fellows could not be published, which gave the erroneous impression of inertia. The initial large intake of Fellows had been necessary to gain momentum and to raise an endowment. Early on, the Regents had recognized that harmony and efficiency dictated a small inner circle, but everything was discussed before the full Board. Any in the inner group, all of whom had once been elected, would step aside, he concluded, if they thought it would improve the College.[29]

A few days after the meeting, Graham prepared a generally even-handed summary for his correspondents. Before circulating it, he sent a copy to JMT Finney, the College's first President. He told Finney that, although he had acted with the best of intentions, he felt his reception to have been "exceedingly cold."[30] Despite the disappointing response, Graham remained optimistic about the College. "My first experience at a meeting of the Board of Regents," he told Finney "convinced me of the enormous potentialities of the organization."[31] Finney declared himself "heartily in sympathy" with Graham's position, but cautioned that as long as Martin remained in charge little could be done.[32] Unfortunately, he went on, private talks with Crile and the Mayos had accomplished nothing and now Squier and Haggard seemed to be joining the inner circle. Finney concluded by expressing his own sense of powerlessness and his willingness to let Graham make his sympathies known. Graham then sent copies of his report to his correspondents and to Martin and Crile. To the latter two he also sent cover letters urging action.[33]

The inner circle itself remained divided on how to respond to the protest. Crile and Charlie Mayo experienced the growing frustration and anger first hand during the Society of Clinical Surgery's annual banquet a few weeks later. Several of Graham's correspondents, including Elliott Cutler of Peter Bent Brigham Hospital, already incensed that the Regents had not allowed him to present his report on education in October, attacked the College. Even the imperturbable Allen Whipple apparently lost his temper with Crile, and Elliott Cutler had to separate them.[34] Mayo stopped in Chicago to warn Martin that he had become a lightning rod for the disaffected.[35] The meeting brought home to Mayo and Crile the bitterness of the critics and the seriousness of the situation facing the College leadership.[36] As the year drew to a close, both increasingly favored compromise, as did Allen Kanavel. Recognizing that Graham "will probably be the strongest man in surgery ten years from now" he advised Martin to meet the critics at more than half way.[37]

On the other hand, Besley and William Mayo showed little inclination to compromise. Besley remained angry over the criticism of the College's financial management,[38] perhaps in part because he was finding the role of treasurer during a major depression increasingly thankless. For Mayo, the attack represented another front in a long campaign against the College by two groups—one from the East Coast centered in Boston and the other a Chicago group under the influence of Bevan.[39] The latter included Graham and Phemister—an opinion shared by Loyal Davis, a Martin loyalist, and reflected in *Fellowship of Surgeons*.[40] In Mayo's opinion, finding that they could not destroy the College, its enemies now wished to take it over. "Let 'em holler" and ignore them, he advised Martin.[41]

After considerable discussion, the Executive Committee prepared an official response to Graham, which Martin sent out on December 5, 1933. As with the Eclat Club, the 10 page reply, drawn up by Besley with the aid of Bowman Crowell and Marion Farrow,[42] consisted of a point-by-point refutation of the charges, some selective omissions, and a few concessions.[43] The primacy of the Board of Regents over the Director General in matters of policy was asserted. The minutes of the meetings were "open to all Fellows." The complaint about the age of the leadership was elided by giving the age *at election* (average 51) rather than the *current* age (61) of the Regents. The report provided a summary financial statement and confirmed that, with the death of Martin and his wife,

Martin's publishing interests would be left to the College. The books were open to any Fellow who wished to see them (in Chicago). Efforts to combat fee splitting were detailed.

Perhaps most importantly, the letter stressed the importance the College attached to improving surgery at the community level. In defending the fellowship, the letter noted that the College was not a restrictive society, but one that consisted "of men and women who have proven that they are safe surgeons from the standpoint of service to the patient."[44] The use of the inclusive phrase "men and women," uncommon in American medicine at the time, was probably not accidental. (Despite some of the critics' rhetorical claims about the size of the College, its membership represented slightly less than 8 percent of North American physicians.)[45] The report concluded with a list of names demonstrating that, far from ignoring contemporary achievements, 15 of the complainants had participated in Clinical Congresses. Martin sent it on to Graham with the hope that it would "satisfy some mistaken ideas" about the management of the College.[46]

The report did nothing to mollify Graham as he told Martin in late December.[47] To his mind, the central complaint, the underrepresentation of his generation of surgical leaders, had not been addressed. In addition, his request for a meeting between members of his group and a committee of the Regents had been completely ignored.

As the tumultuous year ended, Martin's allies became increasingly concerned about his health. His stroke in 1930 remained in their minds as did a recent attack of abdominal pain that had hospitalized him. Martin regarded the College as "his baby" and took criticism of it personally. He poured out his frustrations in a long and defensive letter to Charlie Mayo on New Year's Day 1934.[48] Calling his critics "rats" and "unworthy self-seekers," he vowed never to voluntarily surrender the organization to them.

When Martin and his wife left for their winter stay at the Biltmore Hotel in Phoenix, Besley, Loyal Davis, and Charlie Mayo decided to shield the absent Martin as much as possible.[49] The College staff had felt the crisis intensely, and the decision by his friends to protect Martin left them isolated. In the first of many such journeys over the next six years, on January 24, 1934, Crile made a morale-boosting visit to headquarters. Crile's vigorous defense of the College's policies, the good done the public by its programs, and the loyalty of its Fellows struck the right note. Eleanor Grimm quickly telegraphed and then wrote to the Martins the same day. "We were almost gleeful."[50]

Graham and his confidants also considered their options as the New Year began. Cutler led no mass resignation as once threatened. The only significant task was removing "the old crowd" and here, he felt, the critics had time on their side.[51] Graham too recognized that "nothing very radical" could happen in Martin's lifetime, and he decided to let the matter temporarily drop. A handwritten personal letter from Crile during the crisis and his earlier correspondence with JMT Finney had convinced him that he had influential support among the Regents.[52] Continued pressure on Martin, Graham believed, might jeopardize that support.[53]

≈⋘ ✶ ⋙≈

Accommodation and Conciliation

With tempers cooling, Martin extended a conciliatory invitation to 14 of the critics to a meeting of the Board of Regents on June 10, 1934. In doing so, he hoped to show how the College conducted its business.[54] Of those invited, Evarts Graham (Washington University); Samuel Harvey (Yale), who would soon become a Regent; Alton Ochsner

(Tulane); Dallas Phemister (Chicago); and Erwin Schmidt (Milwaukee) attended. As the last item of the day, Crile opened the floor to comments from the guests encouraging them not to "have the slightest hesitation … to tell us [how] we can improve our College."[55]

The visitors maintained the cordial tone. Ochsner stated that the meeting had given him a much more tolerant view of the Board of Regents. Phemister praised the College's efforts in continuing education through the Clinical Congresses and in hospital standardization. His main criticism was that the College needed to limit its activities "to surgery among the surgical profession"[56] and do for surgical education what it had done for what would now be called continuing education and the hospitals. The most critical, Harvey thought the organization too centralized. Graham emphasized that his criticisms came from a desire to strengthen the College. He repeated his calls for greater representation on the Board.

Kanavel, replying for the Regents, began by saying that he thought the visitors' remarks "have been made in the kindliest of spirit." (Figure 4.2) He felt that much of the criticism from Fellows came from ignorance, despite the *Bulletin of the American College of Surgeons* and the Blue Book, of the College's activities. Developing this theme, he stressed that the first priority of the College was elevating the standard of surgery in the community in the absence of any legal authority to prevent any licensed physician from operating. He pointed out that while the College had already begun a study of graduate surgical education, "Our problem is to bring to the man in Jonesville as competent a service as he could possibly get in that community, and to elevate the standard of the men there."

The conflict between Graham and Martin was both generational and, in some respects, as Peter Olch and C Barber Mueller have observed, a town-gown dispute.[57] More broadly, it illustrated the College's overlapping and competing constituencies: the prominent urban surgeon; the surgeon of the large private clinic; the surgeon in "Jonesville;" and Evarts Graham's constituency—the full-time teachers of surgery, to say nothing of the attempt to represent both general and specialty surgery. The conflict also raised the question of the public role of the College: Was it to confine its efforts to the improvement of surgery or did it have a larger role in organized medicine and public policy? Whoever had direction of the College in the future would need to balance these competing interests.

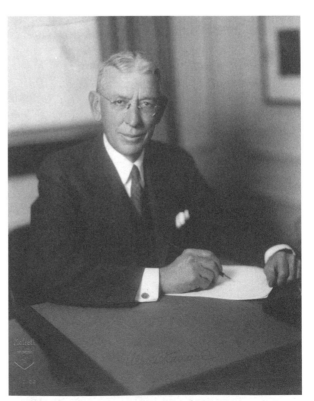

FIGURE 4.2 Dr. Allen B Kanavel, editor of *SGO*; ACS President, 1931–32.

The Insurance Question

While this debate raged among the leadership of surgery, the College and the AMA clashed again. Under Martin, the College's relationship with the AMA had never been an easy one. As Director General he played a prominent public role and by doing so challenged the AMA's determination to be the sole representative of organized medicine. After a period of relative quiescence in the 1920s, tensions flared again in the 1930s over the health insurance question.

Concerns about the expense and availability of medical care—particularly for people of modest means—had begun in the 1920s as costs increased with the growth of hospitals, technology, and specialization. In 1927, the Milbank Foundation sponsored the Committee on the Costs of Medical Care (CCMC) to study the pressing issues of medical economics and the delivery of care. In 1932, the committee's majority recommended (1) that medical services be provided through group practices; (2) insurance coverage for medical costs and lost wages; (3) a greater emphasis on prevention and public health; (4) coordination of health care through community and state agencies; and (5) improved education for all health care providers. The AMA swiftly condemned the report, and its representatives on the CCMC issued a minority report defending solo, fee-for-service practice as the only acceptable model for health care delivery.

The Depression—with 25 percent unemployment and many of the employed enduring reduced wages, salaries, or hours—exacerbated these concerns over the costs of care. The growing numbers of indigent patients threatened to overwhelm local charitable resources. With reduced hours and wages, even the employed had more difficulty paying for care. Physician incomes, particularly in rural areas and for general practitioners, suffered accordingly as did the finances of many hospitals. As a result, small experiments in hospital insurance and prepaid care began to occur around the country. The AMA, dominated by the more prosperous element of private practitioners, resolutely opposed all insurance schemes as "socialized medicine."[58] The College, more aware through the standardization program of the problems hospitals faced, demonstrated a greater interest and, so Crile later claimed, a greater sophistication in the insurance question—a view shared by some historians.[59] Always interested in matters of national importance, Martin organized a symposium on medical economics at the 1929 Clinical Congress.

When the Roosevelt administration took office in March 1933, Martin took three actions that would place the College at odds with the larger medical organization. First, through Judge Stephens, now an assistant attorney general, he arranged meetings with prominent New Dealers, including the new Secretary of Labor, Frances Perkins. The officials, frustrated with what they saw as AMA obstructionism, received Martin with enthusiasm, partly because of the College's work on industrial medicine. Martin understood Secretary Perkins to say that unless the profession did something for the poor and laboring classes, "a federal program was to be considered."[60] Second, Dr. MN Newquist, the College staffer most involved with industrial medicine standardization, was assigned to Washington, DC, to cooperate with the Federal Civil Works Administration.[61] Third, after speaking with Robert Greenough, a Regent from Boston who had an interest in socioeconomic matters, Martin asked the Regents to appoint a new committee, the Medical Service Board (MSB).

The Regents immediately directed the new board to study the problem of providing adequate medical services at a cost the community could afford. Greenough (and Martin) appeared to regard this as a logical extension of existing College programs. (Figure 4.3)

As Greenough told William Mayo, the five major activities of the College—certification of specialists; hospital certification; services within hospitals, including trauma, fracture and cancer care; post-graduate education; and public education—all involved "the great questions of Medical Economics."[62]

Greenough circulated a preliminary draft report to the committee members during the fall of 1933. The committee held its first meeting on October 9, 1933 and reported to the Board of Regents the following day. Granting that economic conditions required changes in the delivery of health services, the committee, after a prolonged almost line-by-line discussion of the draft, adopted a cautious call for evolution rather than revolution.[63] The report identified five groups that experienced difficulty obtaining adequate medical care—the indigent in communities lacking the resources to care for them; the "ignorant and credulous"

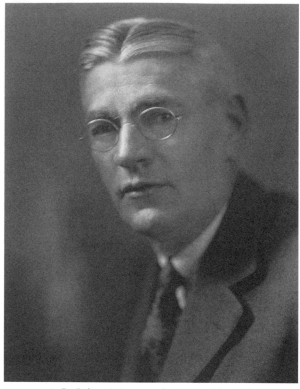

FIGURE 4.3 Dr. Robert B Greenough, ACS President, 1934–35.

who trusted unorthodox practitioners; those in remote districts who lacked access to care and where a physician would need to be subsidized; those of "moderate means" who could not meet the costs of serious illness; and those unable to find an adequately trained and up-to-date physician, particularly in smaller communities far from large medical centers.

The solutions proposed followed from the statement of the problem. For the indigent, the community must accept responsibility; for the credulous, better protection through strengthened medical practice acts; for the frontier, ethical oversight to insure that the contracted physician placed the patient first; for the moderate earner, some form of insurance without a commercial intermediary; and for those unfortunate in their choice of physicians, more stringent licensing, better qualification and certification of specialists, and cooperation between the ACS and other organizations to provide post-graduate education, particularly in the physician's locality. As Greenough had told Mayo, all this represented an extension of the College's existing work. The Regents greeted the report enthusiastically.

Martin, as he had so often in his career, had broader ambitions and enthusiasms. Clearly, he saw a leading role for the College in shaping any federal initiative and settling the insurance question. Comparing the insurance issue to hospital standardization, which the AMA had also avoided, Martin told the Regents:

> This will have to be done by an organization that has the nerve to put it through and not pussy-foot too much...let us guide this and accept all the aid that we can get, but let us keep it in the College of Surgeons or I am not interested in it.[64]

Martin graciously allowed that members of the American College of Physicians (ACP) and the AMA could join as individuals, but that only "a jam" would result if they had to report back to their organization as representatives.[65] Inspired by Martin, the Regents voted to continue the MSB. By doing so, as Martin pointed out, the Regents helped insure that if anything developed in Washington, DC, the College would be consulted. The report subsequently appeared in the *Bulletin of the American College of Surgeons* in June 1934.

In this final report, the College endorsed the idea of voluntary prepayment plans for hospital and medical services for those of moderate means. Given different conditions and insurance laws in different parts of the country, the report encouraged continued local experimentation. Six general organizing principles were established. First, the plans must be free of commercial promotion—beyond clerical costs and reserves, all other funds should be available to subscribers. Second, medical and hospital administrators must supervise the plan, albeit with citizen consultation. Third, subscribers were to have free choice of physician and hospital. Fourth, physician compensation would be based on a fee-for-service model. Fifth, any plan must conform to existing codes of ethics. Finally, participating medical groups would be responsible for the quality of care.

The report included a second section on standards for industrial medical contracts— with the understanding that prepayment schemes would eliminate the need for contract practice. (The AMA regarded any form of contracted, industrial practice as unacceptable. The College saw it as inescapable and that it therefore required regulation.) Significantly, a third section on surgical fees, which condemned commercialism (manifested by newspaper publicity and exorbitant charges for operations), was never published.[66]

In 1934, the endorsement of prepayment put the College on a collision course with the AMA as well as some of its own Fellows. Unfortunately, the MSB report, picked up by the leading newspapers, appeared in the *Bulletin of the American College of Surgeons* on the day that the AMA began its annual meeting.[67] The Regents had been aware of the possibility of misinterpretation of their action but had voted, given the interest in the insurance question by Fellows, eight to four to proceed with publication.[68]

The AMA leadership chose to see this as a deliberate affront. On June 12, the House of Delegates responded with a resolution that claimed for the AMA the sole right to speak for the medical profession. The press quickly seized on a story that appeared to show a division between the country's two major medical organizations.[69] Newspaper coverage tended to be less favorable to the AMA's position.[70]

Reading the resolution, the delegates seem to have been upset in equal parts by the presumptuousness of the Regents in speaking on such matters, the fact that the report had received much favorable press coverage, and that it had recommended that prepayment be "restricted to so-called 'approved hospitals.'"[71] The Regents as members of the AMA were to be called by the Trustees and the Judicial Committee "to explain the reasons for their action and to justify the attempt by this small group…to legislate for all the medical profession of this country."[72] In other words, as Hugh Cabot, a medical reformer and surgeon at the Mayo Clinic, observed, the AMA resolution represented a clear attempt to intimidate any medical organization that spoke out on socio-economic matters.[73]

The delegates' actions probably had as much to do with a professional demarcation dispute as with voluntary health insurance. At that same meeting, the AMA began its slow movement toward accepting voluntary insurance.[74] On the recommendation of the Trustees, the delegates approved a position paper establishing 10 principles for assessing voluntary health insurance plans. But it was a very small first step. The collaboration between physicians and administrators that the ACS recommendations envisioned was completely absent. For the AMA, any plan that did not give complete control and freedom to the medical profession and that did not allow the individual practitioner to do as he or she saw fit would be unacceptable.[75]

Meanwhile, the AMA leadership followed up on the resolution condemning the Regents. In the event that the latter read neither the newspapers nor the *Journal of the American Medical Association*, Olin West, secretary of the AMA, helpfully sent them a copy of the resolution together with the Trustees' demand for an explanation.[76] But as the executive board of an autonomous organization, the Regents felt under no obligation to explain their actions to anyone other than their own membership.

A group of Fellows in Indiana demanded just such an explanation. (The Regents considered Indiana a long-standing "problem" for its antipathy to the College, probably over the fee splitting campaign.)[77] Indicating their support for the AMA resolution, they wanted to know why the College did not stick to scientific and surgical matters. As opposed to the "undemocratic College," the Indiana Fellows argued that the AMA was the only "democratic" and legitimate policy voice of the medical profession.[78]

When the Regents next met on Tuesday, October 16, 1934, Crile kept the AMA letter for last. Feelings ran high. As Crile said in introducing the subject, "We cannot allow other people to tell us what we may or may not do concerning our own job."[79] Martin in particular opposed any meeting, official or unofficial, with the AMA. His remarks reflected a lifetime of conflict and mutual antagonism with that organization:

> You are going to get us into difficulty when you do that. They have invited us repeatedly and it has always been an insult. Why do we have to deal with them at all? ... I have had experience with these people. There is no help in them. Give them a lee-way, and that is all they want. Let us invite them and then you will be sorry; I will tell you that.[80]

Crile wisely postponed any decision until Friday morning, the last day of the Congress.

After further discussion that Friday, the Regents decided to reply to the Indiana Fellows and the AMA in the same fashion. Kanavel, noted for his tact, drafted the letters that went out over Crile's signature as Chairman of the Board. For the Indiana Fellows, the letter traced the history of the MSB as a response to questions from Fellows about the ethics of prepayment plans. The College, the Regents explained, had a duty, as the representative of 11,000 surgeons and their hospitals, to be part of the solution to the problem of adequate medical care for the "moderate income group." Finally, as an international organization, the College represented not only American but also Canadian Fellows confronting the same problem.[81]

The letter to the AMA simply stated that a careful reading of the report would indicate that the College stood ready to cooperate with other organizations on a solution to the insurance problem and reminded the AMA of the international character of the ACS. Canadian Fellows, the letter patiently pointed out, were not represented by the AMA.[82] The letter refrained from any comment or discussion of the AMA's own set of principles and can certainly be read as an implied criticism of AMA inaction.[83] Asked later by West how the Trustees were to use this letter, Crile replied that "the Board of Regents will be very glad to have you use the letter of October 19, 1934, in any way you may choose."[84] Even conciliation had its limits.

For the profession, Robert Greenough gave the clearest statement of the College's position in his inaugural address as President at the Clinical Congress in October of 1934.[85] Although not endorsing compulsory insurance, Greenough presented a strong argument for prepaid health care. While acknowledging the tendency of voluntary systems to become compulsory, he drew a distinction between two extremes—Russia with complete socialization and Britain where, under National Health Insurance, the medical profession retained control. This was a distinction sometimes lost in the debate. Nonetheless, he did not endorse any single national scheme for the United States—in so diverse a country, no single national plan could be everywhere satisfactory.

The answer, he argued, would be found in local experimentation in which the medical profession must take the lead.[86] For the indigent, the community must provide reimbursement for care rather than rely on the charity of financially strained physicians and hospitals. For the wealthy, no support was necessary. For the vast middle of American economic life, the more prosperous could afford premiums for prepaid care. For the less prosperous, the community would be required to subsidize premiums. However arranged, such plans needed to be "free from the intervention of commercial organizations."[87] Significantly, the question of qualification of specialists, national certification, and graduate instruction of specialists received equal attention. Compared with the AMA's dogged characterization of any insurance scheme as "socialized medicine" and opposition to any constraints on an individual physician's independence, Greenough's address was radical indeed.

While the two medical organizations feuded, the new administration in Washington had begun considering Social Security legislation. In June 1934, Roosevelt appointed a Committee on Economic Security (CES) to study the social insurance question and make policy recommendations. Members of the CES technical staff, a prominent group of New Dealers, many with ties to the Milbank Foundation and the CCMC, advocated a compulsory health insurance provision within Social Security.[88] In response, Secretary of Labor Perkins appointed a Medical Advisory Council of 12 prominent physicians to the technical subcommittee on health insurance. Advisory Council members included Harvey Cushing; Walter Bierring, president of the AMA; George Crile and Robert Greenough for the ACS; and George H Piersol, vice president of the ACP. Franklin Martin, through his Washington contacts, had first suggested the appointment of the leaders of the three major medical organizations—the AMA, the ACS, and the ACP. Accepted by the CES staff, the recommendation, as Martin intended, gave the AMA representation without the power of nomination.[89]

That accomplished, Martin continued lobbying the administration to the consternation of the AMA. He remained in communication with the executive director of the CES, Edwin Witte, a prominent New Dealer and former University of Wisconsin economist, who regarded Martin as an influential ally.[90] Martin also wrote to Roosevelt—whom he knew from his Washington service during WWI when FDR ("the Boy" as Martin knew him) was Assistant Secretary of the Navy—advocating that a federal department of health be established.[91] Roosevelt demurred on the grounds that this would mean adding Departments of Education, Housing etc.[92]

These activities did not escape the notice of the AMA, where they caused considerable alarm. Olin West, AMA secretary, shared that organization's concerns about Martin's influence in Washington with Harvey Cushing. As West informed Cushing, he had confidential information that Martin's visits to Washington had left the impression that America's surgeons favored some form of health insurance.[93] The fact that two of the advisory committee members, Greenough and Crile, might "have been tarred by the FH Martin brush" proved a source of added concern.[94]

Indeed, during the advisory council's deliberations, Crile spoke strongly in favor of importing Saskatchewan's system of municipally subsidized doctors to the United States and in support of the benefits of health insurance in general. For the committee as a whole, however, concerns about the possible malign effects of government intervention outweighed any perceived benefits. Despite offers of compromise by the advocates of compulsory insurance on the committee staff, the advisory committee itself rejected any form of state insurance.[95] What role the advisory committee played in the administration's final decision not to include health insurance as part of Social Security remains a matter of debate among historians. So too does the importance of the connection between FDR and Cushing through the marriage of Cushing's daughter to FDR's son. It seems likely that even before the final meeting of the committee in late January 1935, the administration had already decided—in the face of opposition from the AMA, the anticipated difficulty of passing any Social Security legislation, and the absence of a significant political constituency in favor—not to include health insurance in the bill sent to Congress.[96]

With this, the health insurance question would, for the next three decades, be addressed largely through the private sector. In September 1934, the American Hospital Association, with the endorsement of the ACS, had given its support to prepayment plans.[97] Similar endorsements of group hospitalization came from the Duke Endowment, the Commonwealth Fund, and the Julius Rosenwald Fund. These would form the conceptual basis of the Blue Cross program, just as hospitalization programs like Baylor University's would provide the practical model. But as JT Richardson noted in his 1945 review of the development of group hospitalization:

> The support of the group hospitalization movement by the American College of Surgeons was very important. This organization had long been active in helping to secure higher standards for hospitals in the United States.[98]

It was not until 1942 that the AMA unequivocally accepted and approved voluntary group hospitalization plans.[99]

REFERENCES

1. Fisher sees stocks permanently high. (1929, October 16). *New York Times (1923–Current file)*, p. 8. Retrieved November 11, 2011 from ProQuest Historical Newspapers: The New York Times (1851–2007). Document ID: 96000134.

2. American College of Surgeons. (1929, October 15). *Board of Regents: Minutes October 15, 1929*. Complete Minute Book 4. Archives of the American College of Surgeons, Chicago.

3. Badger, A. J. (1989). *The New Deal: The Depression Years, 1933–1940* (p. 229). New York, NY: Farrar, Straus & Giroux.

4. Grimm, E. K., *Letter to G W Crile*. June 16, 1930, George W. Crile Papers, Container 49, Folder 181, Manuscript Collections, Western Reserve Historical Society, Cleveland, OH.

5. Crile, G. M., *Letter to G W Crile, Jr.* October 16, 1930, George W. Crile Papers (MSS 2806), Container 50, Folder 183, Manuscript Collections, Western Reserve Historical Society, Cleveland, OH.

6. Finney, J. M. T., *Letter to W J Mayo*. February 2, 1931, W. J. Mayo Papers, Box 2, Folder "American College of Surgeons, 1930–33," Mayo Historical Unit, Mayo Clinic, Rochester, MN.

7. American College of Surgeons. (1930, October 14). *Board of Regents: Minutes October 14, 1930*. Complete Minute Book 7. Archives of the American College of Surgeons, Chicago.

8. American College of Surgeons. (1932, October 18). *Board of Regents: Minutes October 18, 1932*. Complete Minute Book 8. Archives of the American College of Surgeons, Chicago. American College of Surgeons. (1933, October 10). *Board of Regents: Minutes October 10, 1933*. Complete Minute Book 9. Archives of the American College of Surgeons, Chicago.

9. American College of Surgeons. (1931, October 13). *Board of Regents: Minutes October 13, 1931*. Complete Minute Book 8. Archives of the American College of Surgeons, Chicago.

10. American College of Surgeons. (1932, October 18). *Board of Regents: Minutes October 18, 1932*. Complete Minute Book 8. Archives of the American College of Surgeons, Chicago.

11. Tenth annual hospital standardization report. (1935). *Bulletin of the American College of Surgeons, 20*(3), 5–20.

12. MacEachern, M. T. (1935). *Hospital Organization and Management*. Chicago: Physicians' Record Co.

13. Gunn, J. L. (2003). The first adequate graduate school of medicine in America: A brief history of the University of Minnesota–Mayo Graduate School of Medicine. *Minnesota Medicine, 86*(9), 63–8.

14. Mueller, C. B. (2002). *Evarts A. Graham: The Life and Times of the Surgical Spirit of St. Louis* (p. 33). Hamilton, ON: BC Decker.

15. Graham, E. A. (1925). What is surgery? *Southern Medical Journal, 18*(12), 864–7.

16. Martin, F. H. (1934). *Fifty Years of Medicine and Surgery: An Autobiographical Sketch* (pp. 286–7). Chicago: The Surgical Publishing Company.

17. Graham, E. A., *Letter to J M T Finney*. October 23, 1933, Evarts A. Graham Papers, FC 3, Box 9, Folder 60, Washington University School of Medicine, St. Louis, MO.

18. Ibid.
    Mueller, C. B. (2002). *Evarts A. Graham: The Life and Times of the Surgical Spirit of St. Louis* (p. 216). Hamilton, ON: BC Decker.

19. Graham, E. A., *Letter to J M T Finney*. October 23, 1933, Evarts A. Graham Papers, FC 3, Box 10, Folder 63, Washington University School of Medicine, St. Louis, MO.
20. Martin, F. H., *Letter to Evarts Graham*. October 24, 1932, Evarts A. Graham Papers, FC 3, Box 10, Folder 63, Washington University School of Medicine, St. Louis, MO.
21. Graham, E. A., *Letter to F H Martin*. November 4, 1932, Evarts A. Graham Papers, FC 3, Box 10, Folder 63, Washington University School of Medicine, St. Louis, MO.
22. Graham, E. A., *Letter to J M T Finney*. October 23, 1933, Evarts A. Graham Papers, FC 3, Box 9, Folder 60, Washington University School of Medicine, St. Louis, MO.
23. Graham, E. A., *Letter to 20 Surgeons*. July 14, 1933, Evarts A. Graham Papers, FC 3, Box 9, Folder 60, Washington University School of Medicine, St. Louis, MO.
24. Graham, E. A., *Letter to Dear___*. October 14, 1933, Evarts A. Graham Papers, FC 3, Box 9, Folder 60, Washington University School of Medicine, St. Louis, MO.
25. American College of Surgeons. (1933, October 10). *Board of Regents: Minutes October 10, 1933*. Complete Minute Book 9. Archives of the American College of Surgeons, Chicago.
26. Ibid.
27. Ibid.
28. Ibid.
29. Ibid.
   American College of Surgeons. (1932, October 18). *Board of Regents: Minutes October 18, 1932*. Complete Minute Book 8. Archives of the American College of Surgeons, Chicago.
30. Graham, E. A., *Letter to J M T Finney*. October 23, 1933, Evarts A. Graham Papers, FC 3, Box 9, Folder 60, Washington University School of Medicine, St. Louis, MO.
31. Ibid.
32. Finney, J. M. T., *Letter to Graham*. October 31, 1933, Evarts A. Graham Papers, FC 3, Box 9, Folder 60, Washington University School of Medicine, St. Louis, MO.
33. Graham, E. A., *Letter to F H Martin*. November 8, 1933, C. H. Mayo Papers, Box 2, Folder 19, Mayo Historical Unit, Mayo Clinic, Rochester, MN.
   Graham, E. A., *Letter to George Crile*. November 8, 1933, C. H. Mayo Papers, Box 2, Folder 19, Mayo Historical Unit, Mayo Clinic, Rochester, MN.
34. Cutler, E. C., *Letter to E A Graham*. November 6, 1933, Elliott C. Cutler Papers (H MS c170), Box 9, Folder 1, Harvard Medical Library, Francis A. Countway Library of Medicine, Boston, MA.
35. Mayo, C. H., *Letter to George Crile*. November 8, 1933, C. H. Mayo Papers, Box 2, Folder 19, Mayo Historical Unit, Mayo Clinic, Rochester, MN.
36. Mayo, C. H., *Letter to Frederic Besley*. November 16, 1933, C. H. Mayo Papers, Box 2, Folder 19, Mayo Historical Unit, Mayo Clinic, Rochester, MN.
   Mayo, C. H., *Letter to George Crile*. Mayo, November 8, 1933, C. H. Mayo Papers, Box 2, Folder 19, Mayo Historical Unit, Mayo Clinic, Rochester, MN..
37. Kanavel, A., *Letter to F H Martin*. Quoted in Davis, L. (1960). *Fellowship of Surgeons: A History of the American College of Surgeons* (p. 299). Springfield, IL: Charles C. Thomas.
38. Besley, F. A., *Letter to C H Mayo*. November 22, 1933, C. H. Mayo Papers, Box 2, Folder 19, Mayo Historical Unit, Mayo Clinic, Rochester, MN.
39. Mayo, W. J., *Letter to F H Martin*. January 9, 1934, W. J. Mayo Papers, Box 2, Folder 6, Mayo Historical Unit, Mayo Clinic, Rochester, MN.
40. Davis, L. (1960). *Fellowship of Surgeons: A History of the American College of Surgeons* (p. 366). Springfield, IL: Charles C. Thomas.
41. Mayo, W. J. *Letter to F H Martin*. January 9, 1934, W. J. Mayo Papers, Box 2, Folder 6, Mayo Historical Unit, Mayo Clinic, Rochester, MN.

42. Besley, F. A., *Letter to C H Mayo*. December 29, 1933, C. H. Mayo Papers, Box 2, Folder 12, Mayo Historical Unit, Mayo Clinic, Rochester, MN.
43. *Untitled*. (1933). Evarts A. Graham Papers FC 3 Box 9 Folder 60, Becker Medical Library, Washington University.
44. Ibid., p. 7.
45. American Medical Association. (1940). Comparative statement on the number of physicians in the United States, Dependencies and Canada In *AMA Directory* (p. 250). Chicago: American Medical Association.
   American College of Surgeons. (1935) The by-laws. In *Year Book of the American College of Surgeons: 1935* (pp. 194–8). Chicago: American College of Surgeons.
46. Martin, F. H., *Letter to E A Graham*. December 4, 1933, Evarts A. Graham Papers, FC 3, Box 10, Folder 63, Becker Medical Library, Washington University, St. Louis, MO.
47. Graham, E. A., *Letter to F H Martin*. December 21, 1933, Evarts A. Graham Papers, FC 3, Box 9, Folder 60, Washington University School of Medicine. St. Louis, MO.
48. Martin, F. H., *Letter to C H Mayo*. January 1, 1934, C. H. Mayo Papers, Box 2, Folder 12, Mayo Historical Unit, Mayo Clinic, Rochester, MN.
49. Mayo, C. H., *Letter to F A Besley*. January 10, 1934, C. H. Mayo Papers, Box 2, Folder 12, Mayo Historical Unit, Mayo Clinic, Rochester, MN.
   Besley, F. A., *Letter to C H Mayo*. January 17, 1934, C. H. Mayo Papers, Box 2, Folder 12, Mayo Historical Unit, Mayo Clinic, Rochester, MN.
50. Grimm, E. K., *Letter to FHM*. January 24, 1934, Eleanor Grimm Correspondence, Archives of the American College of Surgeons, Chicago.
51. Cutler, E. C., *Letter to E A Graham*. January 2, 1934, Elliott C. Cutler Papers (HMS c170), Box 9, Folder 1, Harvard Medical Library, Francis A. Countway Library of Medicine, Boston, MA.
   Cutler, E. C., *Letter to E A Graham*. November 6, 1933.
52. Crile, G. W., *Note to E A Graham*. n.d., Evarts A. Graham Papers, FC 3, Box 8, Folder 55, Washington University School of Medicine, St. Louis, MO.
53. Graham, E. A., *Letter to F A Coller*. February 24, 1934, Evarts A. Graham Papers, FC 3, Box 9, Folder 60, Washington University School of Medicine, St. Louis, MO.
54. Martin, F. H., *Letter to C H Mayo*. May 5, 1934, C. H. Mayo Papers, Box 2, Folder 12, Mayo Historical Unit, Mayo Clinic, Rochester, MN.
55. American College of Surgeons. (1934, June 10). *Board of Regents: Minutes June 10, 1934*. Complete Minute Book 9. Archives of the American College of Surgeons, Chicago.
56. Ibid.
57. Olch, P. D. (1972). Evarts A. Graham, the American College of Surgeons, and the American Board of Surgery. *Journal of the History of Medicine and Allied Sciences, 27*(3), 247–261.
   Mueller, C. B. (2002). *Evarts A. Graham: The Life and Times of the Surgical Spirit of St. Louis* (p. 33). Hamilton, ON: BC Decker.
58. A complete review of the debates over health insurance is beyond the scope of this book. Relevant works include: Hirshfield, D. S. (1970). *The Lost Reform: The Campaign for Compulsory Health Insurance in the United States from 1932–1943*. Cambridge, MA: Harvard University Press.
   Engel, J. (2002). *Doctors and Reformers: Discussion and Debate over Health Policy, 1925–1950*. Columbia, SC: University of South Carolina Press.
59. American College of Surgeons. (1935, April 6). *Executive committee: Minutes April 6, 1935*. Complete Minute Book 10, Archives of the American College of Surgeons, Chicago.
   Fox, D. M. (1986). *Health Policies, Health Politics: The British and American Experience, 1911–1965* (p. 85). Princeton, NJ: Princeton University Press.

60. American College of Surgeons. (1933, October 10). *Board of Regents: Minutes October 10, 1933.* Complete Minute Book 9. Archives of the American College of Surgeons, Chicago.

61. Martin, F. H., *Letter to F Perkins.* July 19, 1933, Papers of Franklin D. Roosevelt, Folder PPF 2373, Franklin D. Roosevelt Library, Hyde Park, NY. Hopkins, H. L., *Letter to M H McIntyre.* March 2, 1934, Papers of Franklin D. Roosevelt, Folder PPF 2373, Franklin D. Roosevelt Library, Hyde Park, NY.

62. Greenough, R. B., *Letter to W J Mayo.* August 23, 1933, W. J. Mayo Papers, Box 2, Folder 5, Mayo Historical Unit, Mayo Clinic, Rochester, MN.

63. Greenough, R. B. (1933, October 9). Report of the medical service board. Mayo, CH MHU 0618 SG3 S 2 Box 2 Folder 18.

64. American College of Surgeons. (1934, June 10). *Board of Regents: Minutes June 10, 1934.* Complete Minute Book 9. Archives of the American College of Surgeons, Chicago.

65. Ibid.

66. Medical Service Board. (1934, October 17). *Medical Service Board: Section III, Report of the sub-committee on surgical fees.* Complete Minute Book 10: Medical Service Board, Archives of the American College of Surgeons, Chicago.

67. *American College of Surgeons.* (1934). Principles of prepayment plans for medical and hospital service. *Bulletin of the American College of Surgeons, 18*(3).
Surgeons' group drafts health insurance rules: Provides medical care on partial payments. (1934, June 11). *Chicago Daily Tribune (1923–1963),* p.9. Retrieved November 11, 2011 from ProQuest Historical Newspapers: Chicago Tribune (1849–1987). Document ID: 439498652.
Surgeons back health insurance; Vote to lead national movement: Regents adopt program for system of voluntary prepayments for hospitalization and medical care to aid persons of moderate means. (1934, June 11). *New York Times (1923–Current file),* p. 1. Retrieved November 11, 2011 from ProQuest Historical Newspapers: The New York Times (1851–2007). Document ID: 94539799.

68. American College of Surgeons. (1934, October 16). *Board of Regents: Minutes October 16, 1934.* Complete Minute Book 10. Archives of the American College of Surgeons, Chicago.

69. Ator, J. (1934, June 12). Doctors urged to fight Legion hospital plan: Political bloc called way to beat project. *Chicago Daily Tribune (1923–1963),* p. 9. Retrieved November 11, 2011 from ProQuest Historical Newspapers: Chicago Tribune (1849–1987). Document ID: 439500932.
Ator, J. (1934, June 13). Medical group spurns move for 'New Deal': Health insurance proposal draws attack. *Chicago Daily Tribune (1923–1963),* p. 10. Retrieved November 11, 2011 from ProQuest Historical Newspapers: Chicago Tribune (1849–1987). Document ID: 439503682.
Laurence, W. L. (1934, June 12). Doctors resent health insurance: Resolution opposing stand of surgeons offered as medical association meets. *New York Times (1923–Current file),* p. 24. Retrieved November 11, 2011 from ProQuest Historical Newspapers: The New York Times (1851–2007). Document ID: 95048180.
Doctors condemn health insurance: American association 'rebukes' surgeons for advocating socialized medicine. (1934, June 13). *New York Times (1923–Current file),* p. 27. Retrieved November 11, 2011, from ProQuest Historical Newspapers: The New York Times (1851–2007). Document ID: 93631176.

70. Brenner, A. (1934, July 15). The 'health insurance' issue stirs doctors to new debate. *New York Times (1923–Current file)*, p. XX3. Retrieved November 11, 2011 from ProQuest Historical Newspapers: The New York Times (1851–2007). Document ID: 94551864.

71. American Medical Association, "Resolution of the House of Delegates", June 12, 1934. *Board of Regents: Minutes October 16, 1934*. Complete Minute Book 9, Archives of the American College of Surgeons, Chicago.

72. Ibid.

73. Cabot, H. (1935). *The Doctor's Bill* (p. 235). New York, NY: Columbia University Press.

74. Burrow, J. G. (1963). *AMA: Voice of American Medicine* (pp. 235–7). Baltimore, MD: Johns Hopkins University Press.
See also Richardson, J. T. (1945). The origin and development of group hospitalization in the United States, 1890–1940. *The University of Missouri Studies, 20*(3), 82–84. Richards dates the shift to a year later, 1935.

75. Editorial: The Cleveland Session. [Editorial]. (1934). *JAMA 102*(25), 2106.

76. West, O., *Letter to George Crile and Regents*. October 12, 1934, Board of Regents Minutes October 19, 1934, Archives of the American College of Surgeons, Chicago.

77. American College of Surgeons. (1933, October 17). *Executive Committee: Minutes October 17, 1933*. Complete Minute Book 9, Archives of the American College of Surgeons, Chicago.

78. Indiana Fellows, *Letter to the Board of Regents*. n.d., Medical Service Board File, Archives of the American College of Surgeons, Chicago.

79. American College of Surgeons. *Board of Regents: Minutes October 16, 1934*. Complete Minute Book 9, Archives of the American College of Surgeons, Chicago.

80. Ibid.

81. Crile, G. W., *Letter to Indiana Fellows*. October 19, 1934, Medical Service Board File, Archives of the American College of Surgeons, Chicago.

82. Crile, G. W., *Letter to Olin West*. October 19, 1934, Medical Service Board File, Archives of the American College of Surgeons, Chicago.

83. Davis, L. (1960). *Fellowship of Surgeons: A History of the American College of Surgeons* (pp. 312–3). Springfield, IL: Charles C. Thomas. Rosemary Stevens attributes this to the ACS' greater familiarity with hospitals and their financial plight during the Depression.
Stevens, R. A. (1998). *American Medicine and the Public Interest: A History of Specialization* (2nd ed.; p. 191). Berkeley, CA: Johns Hopkins University Press.

84. West, O., *Letter to G W Crile*. March 22, 1935, Board of Regents Minutes March 22, 1935, Archives of the American College of Surgeons, Chicago. Crile, G. W., *Letter to Olin West*. April 6, 1935, Medical Service Board File, Archives of the American College of Surgeons, Chicago.

85. Greenough, R. B. (1935). Efficient surgical service for the whole community. *Surgery, Gynecology, and Obstetrics, 60*, 432–40.

86. Ibid., p. 437.

87. Ibid.

88. Hirshfield, D. S. (1970). *The Lost Reform: The Campaign for Compulsory Health Insurance in the United States from 1932–1943*. Cambridge, MA: Harvard University Press.
Witte, E. E. (1962). *The Development of the Social Security Act: A memorandum on the history of the Committee on Economic Security and drafting and legislative history of the Social Security Act*. Madison, WI: University of Wisconsin Press.
Derickson, A. (2005). *Health Security for All: Dreams of Universal Health Care in America*. Baltimore, MD: Johns Hopkins University Press.

Fox, D. M. (1986). *Health Policies, Health Politics: The British and American Experience, 1911–1965.* Princeton, NJ: Princeton University Press. Starr, P. (1982). *The Social Transformation of American Medicine.* New York, NY: Basic Books.

89. Witte, E. E. (1962). *The Development of the Social Security Act: A memorandum on the history of the Committee on Economic Security and drafting and legislative history of the Social Security Act* (p. 176). Madison, WI: University of Wisconsin Press.

90. Ibid., p. 184, n. 95.

91. Martin, F. H., *Letter to F D Roosevelt.* August 17, 1934, Papers of Franklin D. Roosevelt, Folder PPF 1449, Franklin D. Roosevelt Library, Hyde Park, NY.

92. Roosevelt, F. D., *Letter to F H Martin.* August 20, 1934, Papers of Franklin D. Roosevelt, Folder PPF 1449, Hyde Park, NY.

93. West, O., *Letter to H Cushing.* October 31, 1934, Harvey Williams Cushing Papers. Microfilm. Manuscripts and Archives, Yale University Library, New Haven, CT.

94. Cushing, H., *Letter to O West.* November 9, 1934, Harvey Williams Cushing Papers. Microfilm, Manuscripts and Archives, Yale University Library, New Haven, CT.

95. Medical Advisory Council. (n.d.). Minutes of the meetings of the Medical Advisory Council. *Social Security Online.* Retrieved October 27, 2011 from http://www.ssa.gov/history/reports/ces/ces7intro.html

96. Derickson, A. (2005). *Health Security for All: Dreams of Universal Health Care in America* (p. 69). Baltimore, MD: Johns Hopkins University Press. Bliss, M. (2005). *Harvey Cushing: A Life in Surgery.* Oxford, UK: Oxford University Press.
Kooljman, J. (1999). Soon or later on: Franklin D. Roosevelt and national health insurance, 1933–1945. *Presidential Studies Quarterly, 29*(2), 336–350.

97. Convention upholds group hospital plan: Surgeons approve monthly payments by individuals to cover care when needed. (1934, September 28). *New York Times (1923–current file)*, p. 25. Retrieved November 11, 2011 from ProQuest Historical Newspapers: The New York Times (1851–2007). Document ID: 93643236.

98. Richardson, J. T. (1945). The origin and development of group hospitalization in the United States, 1890–1940. *The University of Missouri Studies, 20*(3), 24.

99. Ibid., p. 84.

CHAPTER 5
The End of the
Martin Era

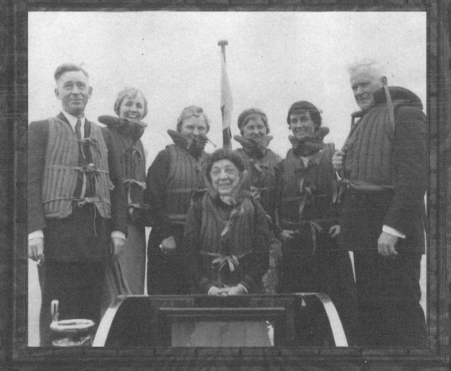

Dr. Martin, Cuba, 1930s

For Martin the health insurance debate would represent his last act on the national stage and the last battle with his old institutional enemy. Within surgery, the détente between Martin and his critics collapsed after an unfortunate newspaper interview during the 1934 Congress in Boston. As a result, Martin and the College at last confronted the question of his retirement and succession. Martin's death in March 1935 would disrupt these plans and begin a 15 year interregnum without an executive director.

The Boston Debacle

The controversy over Martin's leadership reignited during the 1934 Clinical Congress in Boston. Momentarily left unguarded by Eleanor Grimm and hurrying between meetings, Martin gave a brief and impromptu interview to a persistent reporter from the *Boston Herald*. The next day a banner headline proclaimed "If Taken Sick in Boston, Would Fly West, Says Surgeon."[1] Whatever Martin actually said, in the published article he unfavorably compared surgery and surgeons in Boston and Europe to their counterparts in the West at some length. "The West," said Martin according to the newspaper, "is so far ahead of the East as far as surgical progress is concerned that there is simply no comparison." A large photograph of Martin accompanied the article.

Martin learned of the article as he arrived in New York City on his return journey from the Congress. He immediately contacted Robert Greenough and Frederic Cotton, his close Boston allies, and Arthur W Allen, the chair of the local arrangements committee, and disavowed the remarks. In a letter to the editor of the *Boston Herald,* Martin made the disavowal public, although the reporter stood by his story. (Figure 5.1) Allen, Cotton, and Greenough, aided by Crile, did their best to diffuse the situation and within a week Greenough informed Martin that "the medical profession is assured that the impression

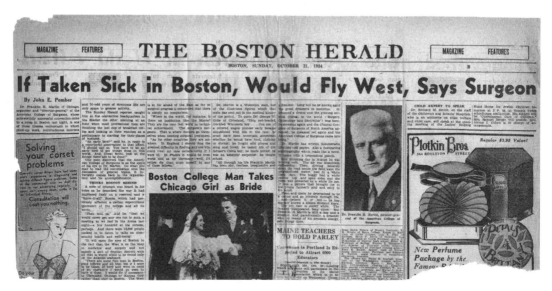

FIGURE 5.1 The headline that helped precipitate Martin's decision to resign as Director General.

given by the newspaper article is erroneous."[2] The College's Executive Committee decided that the best course was to make no official reply and to let the controversy fade.

But as JMT Finney warned Will Mayo, the angry reaction of many East Coast Fellows reflected far deeper frustrations with Martin and the College.[3] Beyond threats of mass resignations, two incidents capture the level of antagonism towards the Director General. A well-respected Boston surgeon sent an angry note to Charlie Mayo with "worthless" scrawled across a clipping of Martin's letter to the *Herald's* editor.[4] A caricature of Martin sent to Elliott Cutler, one of Evarts Graham's correspondents and chair of surgery at Harvard and Peter Bent Brigham, combined regional, academic, and generational prejudice. In the sketch, a rustic Martin claims "there ain't no surgery east of Oshkosh."[5] Small wonder that Finney advised Mayo that only Martin's immediate resignation would save the College in the East.[6]

The mass resignations did not occur and that year's meeting of the Society of Clinical Surgery passed peaceably.[7] For the first time, however, Martin began to seriously, if reluctantly, consider retirement. On October 31, Crile met Martin at College headquarters. In a letter of November 2, 1934, Crile summarized his understanding of the meeting. Both he and Martin would step down and either Allen Kanavel or former Army Surgeon General Merritte Weber Ireland would become Director General.[8]

By then, however, Martin's attitude had hardened and he denied that this plan was anything more than something that could be considered "at our leisure" at the June Executive Committee meeting.[9] He increasingly saw the whole Boston controversy as having been engineered to discredit him, a view he expressed forcibly to Robert Greenough and Will Mayo.[10] "Your Director General," he told Mayo, "would never resign from the Director Generalship of the College while this whispering gallery is being continued against his reputation."[11]

In his reply, Martin's old friend, now making his own transition from the leadership of the Mayo Clinic, performed a signal service for the College. While his letter began "hurrah for the old scrapper" Mayo offered Martin a face-saving way out. Martin should ignore his enemies and, as Mayo had done, gracefully relieve himself of the burden of day-to-day management while mentoring his successor. Mayo assured Martin that this meant not retirement but "a position of responsibility in which I can aid in helping those who are to continue, to prepare for their duties." He also gave his guarantee that the College would provide both Martin and his wife with a secure income for life.[12] Martin took Mayo's counsel to heart.[13]

As he did that of Allen Kanavel with whom he corresponded and then visited in Pasadena for four days in December. Together they laid out a plan that followed Mayo's experience. Martin would assume the position of honorary Director General while the selection of a new Director General began. In the interim the Board of Regents would take on greater administrative oversight with Crile as Chairman and Kanavel as Vice-Chairman. Pending the selection of a new Director General, an Administrative Board, composed of department heads and the secretaries Eleanor Grimm and MT Farrow, would supervise day-to-day activities and report to the chairman.

The members of this new Administrative Board who met on December 29, 1934, somewhat distracted by the holidays, were unprepared for the surprise they were about to get. Present were Drs. Martin, MacEachern, Crowell, Newquist, and Williamson; and Mr. Ballou, Mrs. Farrow, and Miss Grimm. Miss Grimm recorded the bombshell in the minutes: "Dr. Martin stated that he had an important matter which he wished to bring up: His proposed retirement from the Director Generalship of the College immediately following the Clinical Congress in San Francisco in October, 1935."[14] Martin said that he wanted the inner administrative group (Dr. Newquist and Dr. Williamson, not in the "inner" group, had been excused before the announcement) to know about his retirement before the Board of Regents was notified. He then distributed the letters announcing his retirement that would be sent to Crile and the other Regents after the meeting.[15]

Given the lack of an obvious successor and pending the appointment of one, Martin went on to say that the current administrative group was to meet weekly. One member of the group should be chosen as chairman each week. The group should have someone record the minutes of meetings to send to the Chairman of the Board of Regents and the President of the College, so they would know what was taking place at College headquarters. Any matter that dealt with fundamental principles or matters of policy should be referred to the Director General or to the Board of Regents, as had been done in the past. To make sure that his instructions were carried out, he specified that "a list of those who were present should be given and absences recorded, with reasons for absence."[16] Martin was making certain that the staff would hold the meetings, attend them, and conduct the business of the College. The dutifully recorded minutes document that the staff indeed met weekly for the next 15 years as Martin had intended. The Administrative Board's meetings dutifully continued until 1950, when MacEachern was named Director of the College.

Martin assured them that the Board of Regents "has the greatest confidence in the inner group" gathered around the table. He admonished them to hold his decision in confidence. Clearly this was a shock to them; they were members of his family, and they knew that the College would not be the same without its leader.[17] Yet, they had been working together for a long time, had handled many difficult problems, and knew that they would be able to keep the College functioning normally. Martin's style had been to let them run their own shops. They had managed well and were confident that they would maintain the same high level of performance in his absence. With these administrative arrangements in hand, Martin officially informed Crile and the Regents in writing of his intention to resign as Director General after the San Francisco Clinical Congress in October 1935.

≈✳≈

Martin in Phoenix

Martin attended the weekly Administrative Board meeting on January 4, after which he went to Phoenix for his now customary winter vacation, where he stayed in a cottage at the Biltmore with his wife Isabelle. He corresponded regularly with Miss Grimm by handwritten notes on Biltmore stationery and she responded with formal, typewritten letters. He asked her to send copies of his books, *The Joy of Living* and *Digest of the Proceedings of the Council of National Defense during the World War,* which he called the "war book," to various people he had met in Phoenix. He requested some blank checks, which she sent, and asked her to get his umbrella and raincoat from a closet in their home and send them to him. Mrs. Martin sent Miss Grimm income tax information, presumably for Mr. Ballou, who handled the finances of the Martins and the Surgical Publishing Company. Franklin and Isabelle enjoyed their vacation in Phoenix, socializing, exercising, and tending to the mundane activities of daily living. He made plans for the Clinical Congress in San Francisco in October and for another meeting in Los Angeles, which he and Miss Grimm were to attend in March. On Martin's suggestion, Miss Grimm would take a vacation in Phoenix before they left for Los Angeles.[18] He remained actively involved with the health insurance question and in regular communication with Greenough on this issue. He also, according to Loyal Davis, had several telephone conversations with President Roosevelt, the last a heated one on February 25.[19]

On February 26, while dictating to a stenographer in the Biltmore lobby, Martin suddenly developed pain behind the sternum that radiated into the neck and down the left arm. Leaving his work, he went to his cottage on the Biltmore grounds to rest. He experienced some initial improvement but after 30 minutes he had another episode that was so severe he almost collapsed and was too weak to call for help. He was seen by his doctor at 7:00 pm that evening. He continued to have episodes of pain and at 2:00 am on February 27, he was awakened from sleep by severe chest pain. The diagnosis was "coronary embolism"—Franklin Martin was having a severe heart attack. His physician initially treated him in his cottage at the Biltmore—a decision fully within the standard of care at the time.

On the morning of February 28 Martin's condition deteriorated. During the afternoon he developed atrial fibrillation, an abnormal heart rhythm, and was at times disoriented. Martin initially resisted all efforts at care and attention and refused to be placed in an oxygen tent, but after capitulating, his condition improved. The fortunate presence of Loyal and Edith Davis in Phoenix proved a source of support for Isabelle Martin, as would the presence of Allen Kanavel and Eleanor Grimm who would both arrive shortly.

On March 1 Allen Kanavel arrived in Phoenix and on March 2 wrote to George Crile describing Martin's illness.[20] Kanavel believed that Martin's intense worry and concern over the insurance issue had precipitated the heart attack. In advice recapitulating the decision at the time of Martin's stroke, Kanavel recommended to Crile that Martin, in the event of a recovery, be shielded as much as possible from business affairs and reassured that the College would not succumb to the domination of the AMA. He added that Mrs. Martin, supported by the Martins' many friends, was holding up under the strain. On March 2 Eleanor Grimm arrived and Kanavel returned to Pasadena the following evening.

Martin was taken to the hospital on March 3. Dr. Robert S Flynn of Phoenix made a record of his illness, stating that Martin was 77 years old and had suffered a coronary thrombosis five days earlier.[21] His past history revealed that he had diabetes and had been taking insulin twice daily for many years. Previously, he had a stroke with hemiplegia on his right side and difficulty in speech. These symptoms had resolved completely. His blood pressure had been above 160 for several years (normal 120), but there was no shortness of breath on exertion, pain or discomfort, or anything suggesting angina (chest pain) or coronary artery disease.

Martin had been feeling well, Dr. Flynn wrote, since arriving in Arizona in January. He was walking three miles daily and had even danced without untoward symptoms. But Dr. Flynn observed that he had failed considerably since his last visit to Arizona a year earlier and was forgetful and somewhat unstable emotionally. These observations may throw some light on the Boston episode and Martin's response to the subsequent criticism.

On admission to the hospital, Martin was disoriented and confused. On the morning of March 7, his condition deteriorated further and he died at 5:15 pm.[22] An autopsy on March 8 confirmed that he had died of a heart attack.[23] Isabelle Martin, Eleanor Grimm, and Loyal Davis accompanied the body to the station for the journey back to Chicago. In a fitting tribute to Martin and his life's work, a procession of local Fellows and nurses followed behind.[24]

The body was transported back to Chicago for the funeral on Tuesday, March 12, in the Murphy Memorial Hall on Erie Street.[25] The pallbearers were close personal and professional friends who had worked with him for many years, including Mr. AD Ballou, Dr. Frederick Besley, Dr. William Cubbins, Dr. Loyal Davis, Dr. Allen Kanavel, and Dr.

Sumner Koch.[26] After the service the body was cremated, and on March 18, 1935, his ashes placed in a grave in the Hollister lot, belonging to Isabelle's family, in Graceland Cemetery. About 12 of his friends, relatives, and associates—including the ever loyal Miss Grimm—were present to pay their last respects and to support Isabelle. [27]

In a testament to his stature, reports of Martin's death appeared in newspapers throughout the country and the world. Both the *Times* of London and the *Argus* of Melbourne, Australia printed obituaries.[28] Hundreds of telegrams, letters, and cards expressing sympathy to Isabelle Martin and the College flowed in from Martin's personal friends and professional associates. They extolled his charisma and his expertise in founding and leading the College. Obituaries appeared in Australian, British, Canadian, and Latin American medical journals—a recognition of the international reputation of Martin and the College he had founded. But the Martin era had ended.

≈⋙ ✻ ⋘≈

The Martin Years in Retrospect

Franklin Martin had been an outstanding leader and organizer. As a leader, Martin set clear expectations for the College staff. Each week he convened a meeting of the Administrative Board, composed of selected members of the staff, which took place even when he was traveling. The manager of the Clinical Congress, AD Ballou, was present and often the advertising man for the journal, *Surgery, Gynecology, and Obstetrics*. A number of minor officials of the College were also invited. Martin encouraged attendees to think freely at these meetings and to criticize one another, describing them as family gatherings. Today's executives try to put teamwork into practice in their organizations, but Martin created a team and integrated teamwork into the culture of the College administration almost a century ago, a practice that has persisted through the tenures of most of the Directors of the College.

Having established policy, Martin delegated well. He once told the Regents he gave the staff free rein to lead their departments as they saw fit. If they failed, he said, they did not remain at the College. With great pride he told the Fellows and Governors at their meeting in October, 1934, that women also attend the staff meetings. He said that they are so talented, if they were men, they would be paid salaries of $25,000–$50,000 per year. Reflecting the era in which he lived, while he recognized their merit and had the power to pay these women more money, he did not do so.[29]

Martin was also adept at engaging young men as his associates and then mentoring them. His decision to hire Kanavel as associate editor of the *Surgery, Gynecology, and Obstetrics* and to have Crowell and MacEachern as associate directors served him and the College extremely well. From the early 1930s, he brought Dr. Newquist along by assigning him a gradually increasing portfolio of activities, beginning with taking over the duties of Mr. Walter E Carr, who managed the College's mortgages and insurance but had become incapacitated. Six months later he assigned Newquist as an understudy to Dr. MacEachern, doing hospital surveys, and shortly thereafter put him in charge of the industrial certification program. He had an easy way with his employees and colleagues. He believed in thorough discussion and was open to both criticism and new ideas. His letters to his secretary, Eleanor Grimm, were formal, yet friendly and complimentary. He engendered the respect of those with whom he worked, and most were in awe of him. He had positioned the College as the leading specialty organization in the country, with a mission to elevate the standards of surgery. Franklin Martin had been the ideal founder and leader of the American College of Surgeons.

He left the College in good condition with a satisfactory endowment and many active programs. Associate Director Malcolm MacEachern, already establishing an international reputation for his expertise in hospital administration, had managed and steadily improved the hospital standardization program. By 1935 there were 3,538 hospitals in the program, and 2,480 were on the approved list. Martin's *SGO* became the official journal for the College. Its readers learned about both the latest developments in surgery and the activities of the College, including information about where its meetings were to be held, the meeting programs, and information about hotels and how to access them. The annual Clinical Congress attracted thousands of surgeons. New operations and modifications of old ones were described and actually performed so that the attendees could learn how to do them. Five well-attended sectional meetings brought continuing education and the College's program to physicians and the public each year.

Since their inception, MacEachern estimated in 1935 that the College had held more than 200 sectional meetings and congresses, and that more than one million citizens had participated in the public meetings. By 1935 these meetings followed a well-established pattern. On the first day, operative clinics were held in the approved hospitals in the host city. Two major scientific sessions, one on the evening of the first day and the other on the afternoon of the second day complemented the operative clinics. Speakers were experts in surgery and many of them leaders in the College. Medical motion pictures were shown daily from 12:30 pm to 2:30 pm Fellows participated in elections for various state offices for the ensuing year and in discussions of College activities. Sessions for hospital administrators, consisting of papers, roundtable discussions, and demonstrations dealing with administrative, medical, and economic problems were held. The average attendance at these sessions ranged from 800 to 1,000. As with all of Martin's projects, the emphasis was on the practical and the practicing surgeon.

Under Martin the College reflected an American tradition of volunteerism and mutual association. Before television and government involvement in the lives of citizens, many advances in the United States were made through community involvement. Citizens met with one another, formally or informally, discussed problems in their communities, suggested solutions, and often implemented them, leading to improvement of their communities. Franklin Martin understood that communities must be involved to improve hospitals and to improve the quality of surgery and surgeons. Consequently the sectional meetings included public meetings.

These community meetings, held in the evening on the last day of each sectional meeting, were a remarkable marketing tool. They were designed to inform the public about common diseases and conditions through presentations by famous surgeons such as the Mayo brothers or George Crile. The work of the College, especially its hospital standardization program and its commitment to ethical, competent surgical practice, was highlighted. The notion that members of the community should choose Fellows of the College as their surgeons was implied, if not expressly stated. This, of course, resonated with the fellowship and stimulated surgeons throughout the country to apply for fellowship.

Reporters were invited to attend the meetings and interview participants. This resulted in extensive coverage of the meetings in the local and national press. The College also arranged lectures to community groups, local radio broadcasts, and talks before high school and junior college students. The community health meeting was held as the closing session of each sectional meeting, drawing audiences ranging from 2,000 to 12,000, depending on the size of the city and the venue. In Los Angeles alone, representatives of the College had spoken at 32 high schools and to 272,000 students at the request of the Los Angeles School Board. For both the profession and the public, these meetings identified the College with medical progress and its standardization of hospitals and surgeons with surgical quality. In the absence of a legislative mandate, publicity was the College's only tool, one that Martin used effectively.

The College was a good medical citizen, responding helpfully when the government sought assistance whether in war or peace—by overseeing medical mobilization or sharing its work on industrial medicine with the Department of Labor. Martin had actively involved the College in the insurance question. It cooperated with the American Medical Association (AMA) on matters of mutual interest, even though the relationship was sometimes strained by competing agendas and by Martin's distrust of its leadership. The College respected and supported the development of surgical specialties, and invited the participation of the American College of Physicians in the hospital standardization program. Under Martin, the College had a significant voice in organized medicine and medical politics.

So Martin left as his legacy an active, prominent, and important organization. But his death also left unresolved the question of who could lead the College into the future. Any hopes for an orderly transition had been disrupted. Would the Regents be able to find a new Martin to guide the College into its fourth decade?

≈ ✳ ≈

Beginning the Next Era

On the day of Martin's funeral, Board Chairman George Crile brought the Executive Committee together for a special meeting.[9] Doctors Crile, Greenough, Abell, Besley, Kanavel, and Squier were present. In contrast to their usual loquaciousness, the discussions at the meeting were stilted and truncated, symptomatic of their shock and grief over the death of their beloved colleague. Isabelle Martin came to the meeting. The Martins had no children and in many ways the College was their child, one that they had supported and nurtured. The leaders of the College were their closest friends, and now in her grief and sadness she turned to them. She gracefully conveyed her appreciation for the "cordial and sympathetic relations" between the College and Dr. Martin. The committee was moved by her comments and quickly decided to give her Martin's salary for the entire month of March. They also made tentative plans to memorialize Martin's life in a lecture at the Clinical Congress in October. As a more practical matter the arrangement between the College and Martin's *SGO* needed to be clarified. Members of the committee knew that Martin had planned to transfer ownership of the *SGO* to the College upon his death, so Crile appointed himself, Greenough, and Squier as a subcommittee to work out the details with Mrs. Martin.

The Committee then turned to fill some voids created by his death. They appointed J Bentley Squier, the prominent urologist at Columbia University in New York, to fill Martin's seat on the Board of Regents. They gave Mrs. Marion Farrow, Executive Secretary of the College, the authority to sign checks, and appointed Miss Eleanor Grimm, Martin's secretary and the person who held the College together, as Secretary to the Board of Regents and the Executive Committee. (Figure 5.2)

Before his death, Martin and the staff introduced items for discussion at meetings of the Executive Committee and the Board of Regents without a formal agenda. As a result, discussions often became prolonged and sometimes unfocused and inconclusive as the Regents thought through the issues and developed their attitudes about them. This inefficiency had been a source of irritation to the Regents. They now directed staff to draw up an agenda before meetings of the Executive Committee and the Board of Regents. Members would at last have the opportunity to think about the issues on the agenda and prepare themselves for the meetings.

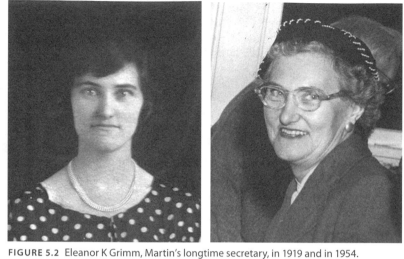

FIGURE 5.2 Eleanor K Grimm, Martin's longtime secretary, in 1919 and in 1954.

Another vexing matter was their concern about the legal liability associated with expelling Fellows from the College for various problems, particularly fee splitting. The bylaws were imprecise about the process for expulsion, and the Regents had not developed clear policies that were followed consistently. Accordingly, the Executive Committee directed Miss Grimm to request from the College's lawyer a change in the bylaws that would protect the College from liability when a Fellow was expelled.

The immediacy of Martin's death and the funeral service earlier in the day made a discussion of his successor seem inappropriate, and they avoided it. This would require a great deal of thought and discussion. Mindful that a regular meeting of the Board was scheduled in less than a month, they decided that Crile, as Chairman of the Board of Regents, should manage the affairs of the College temporarily and that given the uncertainty of the future, they would meet more frequently, probably monthly. Crile, always faithful and available, said he would do whatever was best for the College. [30]

A Fateful Decision

The Executive Committee met again in Cleveland at the Statler Hotel on April 6, a month after Martin died. They went over the agenda for the Board of Regents meeting, which was to follow immediately. Crile, in his home town, opened the Board meeting by stating, "The first question is one of policy and conduct of the organization, whether a Director General or the Executive Committee and the Board of Regents shall have charge of the conduct of the organization."[31] Crile left no time for discussion, and the wording of the "first question" made it clear that Crile and those he had consulted saw only two options. The fact that he did not propose discussing the process for selecting a new Director General, the normal course of action for an organization that had lost its chief executive, meant that Crile already had decided that the College should not select a leader to replace Martin, but he did not tip his hand yet.

The Regents then went into executive session to discuss the succession issue.[32] Martin had led the founding of the College, he nourished it and ran it; it was "his baby."

In many respects, he was the College. The central question for Crile and his colleagues was how to preserve and extend this legacy. Could another individual take over from the founder and shepherd the organization without altering it, when altering it might negate much of what it was in the process of accomplishing? The leaders wanted the College to stay the same, to stay on its mission, to have the same feel, to do the same good. A new appointee would inevitably make changes that would make them uncomfortable. The recent challenge from Evarts Graham and his group served as a reminder of the potential for disruption.

Within the framework of this conservatism, the Regents believed that it would be impossible to find anyone who could adequately replace Martin. Another Martin could not be appointed because another Martin did not exist. Before Martin's death, John Ireland, the former Army Surgeon General, and Allen Kanavel had been mentioned as possible candidates for the Director Generalship. Ireland, however, was 68 and Kanavel, having moved from Chicago to California, had no interest in the position. Besides his personal circumstances, Kanavel firmly believed that his appointment would be resented by many as a continuation of rule by the "Chicago crowd."[33] In the weeks after Martin's death, Hugh Young of Johns Hopkins and Elliott Cutler of Peter Bent Brigham lobbied to have Robert U Patterson, the retiring Army Surgeon General, considered for the position. Patterson was a respected administrator regarded as competent and neutral, and as a urologist, his appointment would have emphasized that the College represented all surgical specialties. The Regents, however, believed that there was no need for a rapid decision because the present members of the administrative group in Chicago were functioning very efficiently. Nothing would go seriously wrong, they apparently felt, while this group carried on the work of the College.

The members of the administrative group then returned to the meeting as the executive session ended. Crile told them that, because Dr. Martin had such unusual talents and administrative abilities, it would be very difficult to replace him at this time. He then asked those attending the meeting whether they wanted to have the responsibilities of the Board of Regents delegated to the office of a director general or whether the Board of Regents and the Executive Committee themselves should take the responsibility. While all present agreed that it would be impossible to replace Dr. Martin, opinions were divided on the question of succession. Several attendees expressed concern that too much central control was inadvisable. Others felt that a large measure of central control was advisable. All at least agreed that nothing should be done in haste. Some believed that in due course, another leader would be necessary, whereas others thought that the Board of Regents and the Executive Committee should meet more frequently and manage the organization through the administrative group. The latter view prevailed. The College would not seek another director general.[34]

The decision not to replace their chief executive officer was understandable but unusual. The organization had approximately 11,500 Fellows, an endowment of $868,000, and ran the program that was primarily responsible for the quality of health care delivered in the 3,538 hospitals in its standardization program. Its CEO frequently had to manage conflicts with the government, the AMA, and groups of Fellows in several states who were critical of College policy and leadership. Many Fellows, including some prominent surgical leaders, wanted Martin out; his decision to retire shortly before he died resulted in part from the criticism he was under. Not all was well with the Fellows; discontent over College policy existed in all parts of the country. Any other organization of this size and scope that lost its leader would have replaced him.

A new leader would have had a mandate to make peace with the disaffected Fellows, grow the organization, and renew its quest for surgical care of the highest quality. Instead, members of the Board chose to run the College themselves, using a staff team that would keep the gears turning, but, with the possible exception of Malcolm MacEachern, had no expertise, experience, or reputation in leadership or in developing a vision for the future. Members of the Board were comforted by the fact that George Crile would bring the issues to them for decision making, but they knew he would be in Chicago only one day each month, not enough contact time even to manage the staff well, let alone work through complex issues. As the liaison between the College staff and Crile and subsequent chairs of the Board of Regents, Eleanor Grimm would, in many ways, act as the de facto chief administrative officer in the coming years.

The Board wanted to run the College. They chose to perform the duties of the chief executive officer in addition to their governance tasks. Experts in organizational structure and management would have predicted that the College would not make progress under this arrangement. The typical separation of duties between a board and the chief executive is clear and simple: the board governs and the executive manages. Perhaps the Regents' desire to both govern and manage arose from the penchant of surgeons to be in control, which at the time was essential in the operating room and on the wards. As if to put an exclamation point on the decision not to replace Martin, the Executive Committee met two months later and removed all references to the Director General from the bylaws. [35]

Whatever the reasons, the Regent's decision not to replace Martin would profoundly affect the College for the remainder of its first hundred years. In one immediate consequence, the College adopted a more conciliatory approach to the AMA. On April 6, Crile wrote to Walter Bierring, the AMA's president, indicating the College's willingness to hold an informal meeting on the contentious insurance question.[36] He added, however, the proviso that he made the offer without compromising the ACS's independence. Also, Martin had left many in Washington, DC with the impression that the ACS favored compulsory health insurance, and this had been a particular source of vexation for the AMA leadership. Crile's letter to FDR on July 17, 1935, clearly and unequivocally corrected this "misapprehension."[37] With Martin's death and in the absence of a successor, on socioeconomic matters, the AMA would now speak for the entire profession.

Fifteen years later, after World War II, a different Board of Regents—confronted with a looming financial deficit, the possibility of a federal health insurance program, major changes in the paradigm of surgical education, and new surgical approaches based on scientific discovery—sought a Director to lead it out of trouble and into uncharted waters. Ironically, given that two former Army surgeons general had been proposed once as successors to Martin, the Regents would chose a military surgeon. Although the College was never without a Director thereafter, the Board often slipped into managing. The implied power of the executive to manage on one hand and the occasional desire of the Board of Regents to manage certain operations of the College on the other, and the manner in which each exercised their authority, would create serious problems on several occasions.

REFERENCES

1. Pember, J. F. (1934, October 21). If taken sick in Boston, would fly west, says surgeon. *Boston Herald* [Sunday edition], sec. B, p. 1.
2. Greenough, R. B., *Letter to F H Martin*. October 28, 1934, Martin Papers, Franklin H. Martin Letters, Archives of the American College of Surgeons, Chicago.
3. Finney, J. M. T., *Letter to W J Mayo*. October 31, 1934, W. J. Mayo Papers, Box 2, Folder 6, Mayo Historical Unit, Mayo Clinic, Rochester, MN.
4. Jones, D. F., *Note to C H Mayo*. October 21, 1934, C. H. Mayo Papers, Box 2, Folder 12, Mayo Historical Unit, Mayo Clinic, Rochester, MN.
5. *Untitled Caricature*. (1934, October 22). Elliott C. Cutler Papers (H MS c170), Box 9, Folder 1, Harvard Medical Library, Francis A. Countway Library of Medicine, Boston, MA.
6. Finney, J. M. T., *Letter to W J Mayo*. October 31, 1934, Mayo Historical Unit, Mayo Clinic, Rochester, MN.
   Finney, J. M. T., *Letter to W J Mayo*. November 20, 1934, W. J. Mayo Papers, Box 2, Folder 6, Mayo Historical Unit, Mayo Clinic, Rochester, MN.
7. Greenough, R. B., *Letter to F H Martin*. Martin Papers, Franklin H Martin Letters, Archives of the American College of Surgeons, Chicago.
8. Crile, G. W., *Letter to F H Martin*. November 2, 1934, Martin Papers, Franklin H Martin Letters, Archives of the American College of Surgeons, Chicago.
9. Martin, F. H., *Telegram to G W Crile*. November 3, 1934, Martin Papers, Franklin H. Martin Letters, Archives of the American College of Surgeons, Chicago.
10. Martin, F. H., *Letter to R B Greenough*. October 30, 1934, Martin Papers, Franklin H. Martin Letters, Archives of the American College of Surgeons, Chicago.
    Martin, F. H., *Letter to W J Mayo*. November 27, 1934, W. J. Mayo Papers, Box 2, Folder 6, Mayo Historical Unit, Mayo Clinic, Rochester, MN.
11. Ibid.
12. Mayo, W. J., *Letter to F H Martin*. November 28, 1934, W. J. Mayo Papers, Box 2, Folder 6, Mayo Historical Unit, Mayo Clinic, Rochester, MN.
13. Martin, F. H., *Letter to W J Mayo*. November 30, 1934, W. J. Mayo Papers, Box 2, Folder 6, Mayo Historical Unit, Mayo Clinic, Rochester, MN.
14. American College of Surgeons. *Abstracted Minutes. Administrative Board.* Archives of the American College of Surgeons, Chicago.
15. Ibid.
16 Ibid.
17. Ibid.
18. Martin, F., *Letter from Franklin Martin to Eleanor Grimm*. undated, Archives of the American College of Surgeons, Chicago.
19. Davis, L. (1960). *Fellowship of Surgeons: A History of the American College of Surgeons* (p. 316). Springfield, IL: Charles C. Thomas.
20. Kanavel, A. B., *Letter to G W Crile*. March 2, 1935, George W. Crile Papers (MSS 2806) Western Reserve Historical Society, Cleveland, OH.
21. Flynn, R., *Dr. Franklin Martin. His last illness.*, in *FH and IH Martin Papers*, Archives of the American College of Surgeons, Chicago.
22. Flynn, R., *Dr. Franklin Martin. His last illness.*, in *FH and IH Martin Papers*, Archives of the American College of Surgeons, Chicago.
23. Mills, H., *Franklin H Martin. Report of Autopsy*, in *FH and IH Martin Papers*. 1935, Archives of the American College of Surgeons, Chicago.

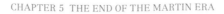
24. Palmer, E. P., *Letter to W J Mayo*. March 9, 1935, W. J. Mayo Papers, Box 2, Folder 6, Mayo Historical Unit, Mayo Clinic, Rochester, MN.

25. Rotary Club of Chicago sustains double loss during past week. (1935, March 17). *The Gyrator*, Chicago.

26. *Active pallbearers*. In FH and IH Martin Papers, Archives of the American College of Surgeons, Chicago.

27. *Letter from Eleanor Grimm to Charles Nicola*. (1935, March 22). Archives of the American College of Surgeons, Chicago.

28. Dr. Franklin H. Martin: An eminent American surgeon. (1935, March 9). *The Times* (London, UK), 17.
   Dr. Franklin Martin. (1935, April 10). *The Argus* (Melbourne, AUS), 6.

29. American College of Surgeons. (1934, October 18) *Minutes of the meeting of Governors and Fellows of October 18, 1934*. Archives of the American College of Surgeons: Chicago.

30. American College of Surgeons. (1935, March 12). *Minutes of the meeting of the Executive Committee of March 12, 1935*. Archives of the American College of Surgeons, Chicago.

31. American College of Surgeons. (1935, April 6). *Minutes of the meeting of the Executive Committee of April 6, 1935*. Archives of the American College of Surgeons, Chicago.

32. American College of Surgeons. (1934, June 10). *Board of Regents: Minutes June 10, 1934*. Complete Minute Book 9. Archives of the American College of Surgeons, Chicago.

33. Kanavel, A. B., Letter to C H Mayo. May 11, 1935, W. J. Mayo Papers, Box 2, Folder "American College of Surgeons, 1934–1939," Mayo Historical Unit, Mayo Clinic, Rochester, MN.

34. American College of Surgeons. (1935, April 6). *Minutes of the meeting of the Board of Regents of April 6, 1935*. Archives of the American College of Surgeons, Chicago.

35. American College of Surgeons. (1935, May 29). *Minutes of the meeting of the Board of Regents of May 29, 1935*. Archives of the American College of Surgeons, Chicago.

36. Crile, G. W., *Letter to Walter L. Bierring*. April 6, 1935, Medical Service Board File, Archives of the American College of Surgeons, Chicago.

37. Crile, G. W., *Letter to F D Roosevelt*. July 17, 1935, Papers of Franklin D. Roosevelt, Folder PPF 2373, Franklin D. Roosevelt Library, Hyde Park, NY.

CHAPTER 6
The Board Is Created

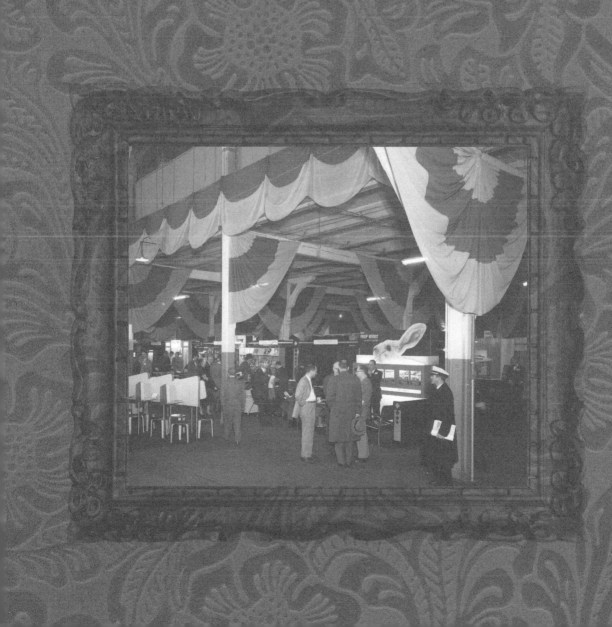

Nothing concerned the College leadership more during its first 100 years than the formation of the American Board of Surgery (ABS) in 1937 and the cachet it bestowed on surgeons through its certification process. The College's role as the only arbiter of the competence of surgeons was now challenged, stinging its leadership.

⁓ ✣ ⁓

Specialization, Training, and Certification

Board certification was not new. The American Board of Ophthalmology was founded in 1916, followed by the American Board of Otolaryngology in 1924. By the end of 1941, 15 certifying boards had been established. The boards set standards for education and training, which had to be met for admission into their examinations. Usually, the boards required a written exam that covered the knowledge necessary to practice the specialty, followed by an oral examination on management of patients by the eminent members of the board. Successful candidates were, and are, awarded a certificate; hence, the term "board certified." Certification was an outgrowth of specialization, a movement as old as the profession, which gained momentum in the late 1800s. Some physicians who were affiliated with medical schools and those who practiced in large cities studied and even conducted research in a limited area of their practices. As physicians became more proficient, the public recognized their expertise as specialists, and their practices grew accordingly. In medical schools, groups of specialists pushed for designation as departments or divisions, bringing them more prestige and authority, a practice that continues today.

Technology and the desire of specialists to master its use were, and still are, a driving force behind specialization. Ophthalmology is a typical example. The ophthalmoscope, invented by the Viennese scientist von Helmholtz in 1851, allowed budding ophthalmologists to view the back of the eye, the retina, and begin to understand diseases of the eye more fully. They also noted findings associated with other diseases such as diabetes, adding to the number of clues used for diagnosis. Elucidation of the complex optical characteristics of the eye spawned devices and practices for prescribing lenses to correct visual impairment. The physician who owned and used the instruments attracted patients who had eye problems; soon he was a specialist in ophthalmology.

Ophthalmologists joined together to learn from one another as the American Ophthalmological Society, founded in 1864. Soon, departments and chairs of ophthalmology were established at leading medical schools. The American Academy of Ophthalmology and Otolaryngology was first organized as one of many regional specialty societies and grew into a national organization at the turn of the century. It was not until 1979 that it split into separate organizations representing each of the two specialties. Standards for residency training in ophthalmology and for admission to the board examination process were established by cooperating committees of the American Medical Association (AMA) and the two leading ophthalmologic specialty societies, with each of these organizations appointing members of the board. The pattern of interest in an organ or organs and their diseases, the resulting specialization, and introduction of the specialty into medical schools, was repeated until 1991, when the last of the current 24 primary certifying boards was established.

Internships, developed by many hospitals in the 1880s, became increasingly popular. By 1914, 75-80 percent of medical school graduates were opting for internships.[1] They served as the clinical experience after medical school, which often was devoid of adequate facilities and patients. Depending on the hospital and its attending physicians, internships tended to be weighted toward medicine or surgery, leading to subsequent specialization. The internship was established as a fundamental, permanent segment of medical education during World War I. At that time, the Council on Medical Education of the AMA, which accredited medical schools, began to inspect hospitals for accreditation of their internships. In 1919, the Council published its first "Essentials for Approved Internships" and a year later changed its name to the Council on Medical Education and Hospitals, reflecting its control over the hospitals that sponsored internships.[2]

Dr. William S. Halsted established the prototype of the surgical residency, derived from German medical clinics, at the Johns Hopkins University in 1889. The resident was given increasing responsibility as he moved up the ladder, and the department chairman decided when his training was complete. But cuts were made annually at the levels of assistant resident and senior resident, and only one survived to be appointed "resident"—or as we call him or her today, "chief resident." This "pyramid" system had many variations as residencies were developed at hospitals associated with elite medical schools, but the central features were the progressive responsibility and the fact that only one individual experienced the entire program.

This system was not designed to populate the country with well-trained surgeons. Although some residents who were dropped from pyramidal systems were able to obtain adequate training elsewhere, others entered the practice of surgery, often with less than optimal training. Because the "surviving" resident eventually functioned as a junior faculty member, the pyramidal systems' best products stayed on as academic surgeons, many of whom made extraordinary contributions to their fields. During the latter half of the 20th century, the pyramidal system was replaced by a structured five-year program that all residents completed if their performance was satisfactory.

As early as 1919, Dr. William J Mayo advocated three years of surgical training for fellowship in the College, even though many surgeons were admitted with far less.[3] The public gradually became aware of internships and residencies, and correctly surmised that specialists were better equipped to solve their medical or surgical problem than was the general practitioner. Successful general practitioners referred certain cases to specialists, usually because they were not trained to handle them or did not have the time to devote to them. The unethical practice of fee splitting rewarded general practitioners for not handling the cases themselves, and in a perverse way encouraged specialization. Finally, the better hospitals, easily identified by the public, actively recruited and were proud to have the widest possible array of specialists on their staffs.

During the 1920s and 1930s, graduates of medical schools increasingly sought an internship and one to three or more years of specialty training at a university or a public or large community hospital, but the programs were unregulated and varied markedly in quality. Residencies were valuable resources; residents had access to patients and received on the job training, and hospitals had the services of physicians to supplement and extend the care given by its medical staff. Residents usually were assigned patients who were unable to pay a private physician, thereby enabling the hospital to provide a much needed service for those patients and the community.

Although residencies proliferated after World War I, especially in hospitals affiliated with medical schools, by 1939 there were only 1,791 positions, in all residencies of three years or longer, for the approximately 5,400 medical school graduates.[4] Medical educators were concerned that there were no standards or guidelines to ensure that residents obtained the best possible training and that when they completed their training, patients would be safe under their care. Most specialists were being produced by methods of training inferior to the long, structured residencies of some medical schools. As more specialty organizations discussed the possibility of creating a certifying board, the lack of standards for training became a major issue.

By 1928, the AMA had established essential standards for approved internships and residencies, but it was in the 1930s that the College, the AMA, and the American Surgical Association (ASA), despite the tensions that existed among them, made great progress toward establishing the framework for graduate medical education in surgery. Since then, that framework has enabled the surgical community to replicate and regulate itself, and thereby meet its obligations to the public as a profession. The framework included the Advisory Board for Medical Specialties, the ABS, and the Joint Council of the AMA and the ACS, which eventually became the current Residency Review Committee (RRC) for Surgery, the body that sets the standards for residency programs. Currently, there are RRCs for 27 of the specialties in medicine.

≈✳≈

Creation of the Advisory Board for Medical Specialties

The lack of standardization of graduate medical education was a frequent topic of discussion at medical meetings, including the AMA meeting in Milwaukee in 1933, when its Council on Medical Education and Hospitals was asked to "devise a plan and procedure for the certification of specialists in all branches of medicine and surgery."[5] At the same meeting the Council was authorized to "formulate standards of administration" for specialty examining boards along the lines of those of the four existing boards (Ophthalmology, Otolaryngology, Obstetrics and Gynecology, and Dermatology and Syphilology) "and officially recognize new boards meeting these standards.[6] This bold move gave the AMA self-designated authority to set standards for the certifying boards and determine what other specialty boards would be added to the original four, a grand endeavor that structured the profession of medicine throughout the 20th century and beyond. A prime mover in this action of the AMA was the Chairman of the Reference Committee on Medical Education, Dr. Irvin Abell of Louisville, a Regent of the ACS. (Figure 6.1)

The AMA Council on Medical Education and Hospitals chose to carry out its charge by convening the leadership of the existing specialty boards (Ophthalmology, Otolaryngology, Obstetrics and Gynecology, and Dermatology and Syphilology) along with representatives of the National Board of Medical Examiners, the Association of American Hospitals (AHA), the Association of American Medical Colleges (AAMC), the Federation of State Medical Boards, and several specialty sections of the AMA. They discussed the need for a coordinating board of the organizations interested in graduate training in the medical and surgical specialties and in the recognition of specialists. Not surprisingly, they also believed that they were the "interested" organizations.

The group resolved that the examination and certification of specialists should be carried out by national certifying boards that would represent the specialty societies, and that an advisory board should be formed to counsel and advise those boards in existence and those to be formed in the future. The advisory board, formally organized later in 1933 as the Advisory Board for Medical Specialties (later to be called the American Board of Medical Specialties), consisted of two representatives from each of the organizations that participated in the meeting. They declared that the purpose of the Advisory Board was to "furnish an opportunity for the discussion of problems common to the various specialty examining boards in medicine and surgery, to act in an advisory capacity to these boards, and to coordinate their work as far as possible." The board also was "authorized to stimulate improvement in postgraduate medical education."[6]

Thus did the existing boards and the other organizations that formed the Advisory Board declare and implement their intent to control the examination and certification of physicians and surgeons and, by virtue of the requirements to sit for examinations, the training of specialists. The Advisory Board still controls these elements of certification.

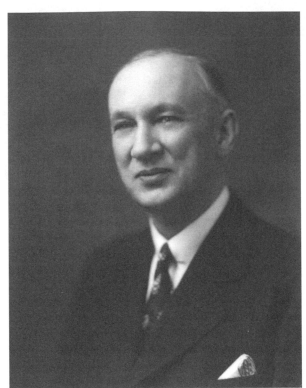

FIGURE 6.1 Dr. Irvin Abell, ACS President, 1946–47.

The Board of Regents, knowing that the ACS was not represented in the AMA initiative, realizing that an insufficient number of surgeons was receiving good training, and reacting to the growing criticism for accepting to membership surgeons with inadequate training, appointed a Committee on Graduate Training in Surgery at its meeting on October 19, 1934, chaired by Dr. Samuel C Harvey, chairman of surgery at Yale and a protégé of Cushing. The Regents expressed the view that the College should take active leadership to improve training, so the committee was charged with determining the best possible ways to train surgeons.[7]

Planting the Seeds for the American Board of Surgery

At the annual meeting of the prestigious, senior surgical organization, the ASA, in June 1935, president Edward Archibald, chairman of the department of surgery at McGill University in Montreal, severely criticized the College for its low standards of training for admission, which were a medical degree, an internship, and two years as a surgical assistant. He believed that training should include a long apprenticeship with a master surgeon and an examination.

After Archibald's address, the Association held a symposium on graduate medical education. Drs. Elliott C Cutler of Harvard, George J Heuer of Cornell Medical College, and Allen O Whipple of Columbia University, critics of the College, had prepared talks on education for the 1934 Clinical Congress of the College, but because they had been critical of the College and its leaders, they were denied access to the floor to present them. Having then been invited to present them at the ASA meeting, a distinct honor, they spoke on undergraduate and graduate medical education, stressing the need to provide more opportunities for surgical education and to improve residency programs.[8] (A few hours later, at the scientific session of the ASA annual meeting, Whipple described his pancreatic resection for cancer, known thereafter and currently as the famous Whipple procedure.[9])

The brilliant and brash chairman of surgery at Washington University in St. Louis, Evarts Graham, commented that Archibald's talk and the education symposium were "only a continuation of the discussion that has been going on for many years among those of us who are teachers of surgery. Yet nothing has come of it in regard to the most important matter of establishing proper standards of qualification of those permitted to practice surgery."[8] At Graham's suggestion, Archibald appointed a committee to study the matter and to report at the 1936 meeting of the ASA. The committee consisted of Drs. Archibald, Whipple, Arthur W Elting, Thomas M Joyce, Thomas G Orr, and, as chairman, Evarts Graham, who was determined to improve the quality of surgery.

≈ ✳ ≈

Graham Goes into Action

Graham's agenda was to propose an independent certifying board. George Crile, Chairman of the Board of Regents of the College at the time, had attended the ASA meeting and knew that this meant trouble for the College, which had been the sole arbiter of surgical qualifications. He met with Graham and urged him to use the College as the certifying authority, but Graham, convinced that the College would not change until the old guard was gone, rejected his proposal.[8,10] Graham was defying one of the most illustrious men in surgery; Crile had founded the Cleveland Clinic, performed thousands of operations, been president of every important surgical society, and served on the Board of Regents of the College from its founding.

Graham's committee decided that other surgical organizations should be consulted, and this resulted in a meeting on October 23, 1935, between representatives of the College, the AMA, and the ASA. Graham read a resolution from his committee that proposed a Joint National Committee to pursue a program to "consider the elevation of standards of the practice of surgery and to increase the hospital facilities for the training of young surgeons."[11] The National Committee would be comprised of 24 members, six each from the ACS, the AMA, and the ASA; and two each from the Southern Surgical Association (SSA), the Western Surgical Association, the New England Surgical Society, and the Pacific Coast Surgical Society. These regional societies, which had memberships restricted to well-trained surgeons recommended by peers, held annual meetings for fellowship and the presentation of papers by members. These continue to the current day.

The College representatives, not fully understanding Graham's plan that these representatives would eventually become directors of the ABS, resisted the creation of the Joint National Committee, contending that it was not necessary because the College had always promoted high standards and would continue to do so. Dr. J Stewart Rodman, representing the AMA, spilled the beans, explaining that the proposal was actually for a certifying board, which would be under the authority of the Advisory Board for Medical Specialties and would certify individual surgeons. In the ensuing heated discussion, the College representatives argued that the proposed board would duplicate what the College did. Members of the group assuaged the College representatives by acknowledging the fine work of the College in elevating surgical standards through its hospital standardization program.

Finally, the College representatives conceded and reluctantly agreed that there was a separate need to examine and certify individual surgeons. They also read the handwriting on the wall: the certifying board would be formed with them or without them, and they had a better opportunity to influence the direction of surgery by going along with the board's formation. From that time forward they publicly supported the establishment of the board. Everyone at the meeting realized that the proposed board would not be successful without the support of all the surgical organizations, and they formally approved Graham's resolution.[11]

The Board of Regents met a few days later. Concerned about the rapidly moving events, they asked Dr. Samuel Harvey, Chairman of the Committee on Graduate Training in Surgery they had appointed in 1934, to report on the best methods to train surgeons.[12] He reviewed the initiative of the ASA to elevate the standards of training in surgery as well as notes from the meetings of Graham's committee. Harvey said that Graham's resolution had stimulated the College committee to meet, although only Abell, Kanavel, Munroe, and Chairman Harvey were present. (Figure 6-2)

The committee reviewed the current methods of training and rejected the preceptor concept, in which a young man would work under a senior partner in an informal training arrangement. A second method of training was for an individual to enter general practice and gain experience in surgery until he became expert. The committee rejected this as well. The third method was through a visiting staff appointment to a hospital, where some surgeons on the staff were willing to teach and the young man would learn from them and gain experience. This was the most common method of learning surgery at the time, but the committee rejected it as inadequate, while recognizing that it would have to be accepted until a better system was in place. Harvey said the fourth method is the so-called resident system, chiefly in hospitals associated with medical schools. It essentially prolongs the internship over several years, he said, allowing the student to obtain a concentrated experience. He pointed out that these residencies were very limited in number.

The committee recommended this as the preferable method of training. They recommended that hospitals with the proper personnel, facilities, and organization should offer these residencies and that minimum standards be established for this type of training. The committee also agreed that residents

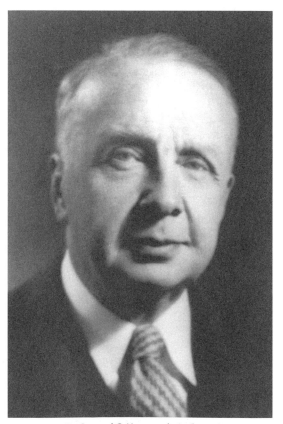

FIGURE 6.2 Dr. Samuel C. Harvey, chair, Committee on Graduate Training in Surgery.

needed to be taught special knowledge pertinent to surgery, including the fundamental sciences of anatomy, physiology, and pathology.

Harvey then discussed how minimum standards might be set and implemented, dismissing use of the licensing authority of state medical boards because of their heterogeneity and because their efforts to raise standards were met by opposition from the profession. He said that federal licensure was not legally possible. He pointed out that some specialties had created examining boards, which had been developing according to minimum standards laid down by the Advisory Board of Medical Specialties.

Finally, he reported that his committee believed it was highly probable that a board for certification of surgeons would be organized in the near future and he recommended that the College cooperate in its formation. He said that the committee recognized that the requirements of a board might not mesh well with the requirements for fellowship in the College, and recommended that the College restudy the requirements for admission to fellowship.

So, after careful consideration, the members of this committee, Harvey, Abell, Munroe, Kanavel, and all Regents of the College, favored creation of the board, even though they understood that control of the standards for residency training would be given over to the board and the Advisory Board of Medical Specialties. They then delivered the final blow: the College should rethink its admission criteria, meaning that it should require board certification for admission. An important element of the College's scrutiny of candidates and control of the surgical profession should be given away to a board founded by dissidents.

Allen Kanavel, the retired head of surgery at Northwestern University, who was adept at getting things done behind the scenes, suggested to the Administrative Board of the College (senior College staff) at a meeting in January 1936 that MacEachern and Crowell, the associate directors of the College, should develop a tentative plan for training surgeons.[13] He envisioned that the College's hospital standardization program could be used to standardize the training of surgeons. Through this, the College could gain control of graduate surgical education and thereby minimize the influence of the new board.

The fast train of events leading to the formation of the American Board of Surgery, engineered by the College's critic Evarts Graham, was beginning to leave the College in the dust. Martin's death and the decision not to appoint a successor were compromising the ability of the College to head off what it saw as competition. Malcolm MacEachern, who understood the strategy, got to work quickly.

≋ ✳ ≋

The Joint National Committee Acts

In February 1936, the Joint National Committee met again.[14] They elected officers, who were Graham as chairman, Allen O Whipple as vice chairman, and J Stewart Rodman as secretary. They selected a new name for the committee that was long and telling: The National Committee Appointed to Improve the Graduate Teaching of Surgery and the Qualifying Standards of Those Desiring to Specialize in Surgery. They intended to improve graduate education in surgery by setting the standards that would qualify an individual to be a surgical specialist. Graham then appointed two subcommittees. Subcommittee A was to focus on the organization of the ABS, and Subcommittee B was to develop a plan for increasing the opportunities for training in surgery.

Subcommittee A decided that the board should consist of 13 members who would serve six year terms, three each from the ACS, the ASA, and the Surgical Section of the AMA, and one each from the New England Surgical Society, the Pacific Coast Surgical Association, the Southern Surgical Association, and the Western Surgical Association. They agreed that the proposal to establish the American Board of Surgery should be submitted for approval to the Advisory Board for the Medical Specialties, thereby putting the new board in the company of the other certifying boards and subjecting it to the standards of the Advisory Board, later to become the American Board of Medical Specialties (ABMS).

Subcommittee A also decided that two groups of surgeons desiring certification would be formed: A Founders Group consisting of members of the above surgical organizations represented on the board and all full and associate professors of medical schools who had restricted their practices to surgery for 15 years. They would not need to take an examination. All others would be certified by examination. Members of the latter group would be eligible for examination after an internship and five years of postgraduate study. Clearly, the average community surgeon who was not on a medical school faculty or had not been eligible for membership in one of the elite surgical organizations was discriminated against in this arrangement, but Graham and his allies were trying to garner the support of the surgical elite in their efforts establish the board, and the strategy worked, because there was little opposition. If a new organization grants its credential to an individual without examination, the grantee is not likely to be critical of the organization.

Perhaps the most important decision of Subcommittee A was to set requirements that candidates had to meet to sit for the examinations, for in so doing they mandated the type and length of training required for surgical specialists. The subcommittee specified that candidates hold the MD degree, have completed an internship, and have completed a residency of not less than three years if taken in a graduate school of medicine or under a sponsorship accredited by the ABS, plus an additional two years of surgical study or practice of surgery. The training was to include anatomy, physiology, pathology, and the other basic sciences as well as sufficient operative experience.

A written exam would cover the basic sciences and the principles and practice of surgery, and, if the candidate passed the written exam (Part I), he would be admitted to Part II, which consisted of two days of examinations in clinical and operative surgery. Later, the training requirements were revised by the National Committee to include five years of graduate study beyond the internship year. Although many modifications have been made in the structure and educational content of the surgical residency, the basic requirement of five years of training, required today, was established by the board's founders.

Subcommittee B, charged with increasing the opportunities for surgical training, acknowledged that expanding hospital residencies could not be accomplished without the cooperation of the two organizations that accredited hospitals and hospital training programs—the ACS and the Council on Medical Education and Hospitals of the AMA. The subcommittee recommended that these two organizations form a council "to organize and carry out a program for the training of surgeons in properly qualified hospitals, setting up such standards as will meet the requirements of the qualifying board in surgery now being established."[15] To help the Council along they suggested that the training include education in the basic sciences and pathology, that there be a ward service managed by a director responsible for resident education, that the resident perform procedures under supervision and guidance of the director and his staff, and that the training include follow-up clinics, conferences, and autopsies. Not leaving much for the new Council to determine, the subcommittee also suggested "careful and competent surveys … to ascertain that this [meeting their requirements] is being done."[15] Finally, they specified that the surveys could be carried out only by surgeons who were certified by the American Board of Surgery.

The full Joint National Committee approved both subcommittee reports on February 16, 1936, and Graham took the proposed plan to create the board to the Executive Committee of the Advisory Board for Medical Specialties, which was meeting the same evening in the same hotel, the Palmer House in Chicago. They informally approved it, and Graham then sent the plan to the member organizations for their approval.

The Executive Committee Cogitates

The Executive Committee of the Board of Regents met on March 29, 1936, and discussed the report of the National Committee. Crile agreed that the multiple ways in which physicians and surgeons were trained was a problem. He said that there was no general plan nor was there anyone or any organization in charge. Crile was also concerned about the future of potential Fellows of the College after their five years of medical school and internship. He believed that it would be beneficial to them if there were facilities to give them additional training in surgery and ethics until they were eligible for fellowship.

While seeming to agree with the recommendations of the Graduate Training in Surgery Committee that the College should restudy its requirements for fellowship, Crile stated that "certification by the specialty boards cannot be accepted by the College in lieu of its requirements for fellowship. A man may pass a good examination, but in actual practice he may have faults or deficiencies which make him ineligible for fellowship in the College."[14] The thread through the ensuing discussion was the Regents' insistence that fellowship in the College was contingent on an evaluation of the ethics of the candidate. They also believed that candidates for fellowship should come from the junior candidate group, who had been mentored and were known by the state and provincial credentials committees that could steer them along the proper course professionally and ethically. The consensus was that the College should continue to set its own standards, but that the regulation of surgical training and board certification were worthy additions to the system of professional development in surgery.

Samuel Harvey then turned the discussion to the problem of providing facilities in which young men could obtain the training they had agreed was necessary. MacEachern pointed out that there were not enough opportunities for training to meet the demand. He thought that in five years there would be ample facilities for training, but of the 114 hospitals on the list of institutions that were satisfactory for residency training, there were about 327 slots for graduate training in surgery. The Executive Committee decided that the College should identify the current qualified, nonacademic, non-teaching hospitals, and develop graduate training in surgery in them. MacEachern, who had already been working on this, was told to bring a final plan to the Regents.

Harvey reiterated the conclusion of the Joint National Committee that only a joint council of the Council on Medical Education and Hospitals of the AMA and the ACS would be able to develop the needed training opportunities for surgeons. Regent J Bentley Squier, the prominent urologist from Columbia University, said that the College should proceed rapidly to supply facilities for graduate training; George Muller and the others agreed. Harvey said that the College had to decide whether it would cooperate in formation of the council with the AMA. The problem for the Regents here was that this was engineered by Graham on behalf of the fledgling board, and that the standards to be developed by the new council were to meet the requirements of the board. Crile repeated that the standards for fellowship should be those of the College, and then reluctantly agreed that the College should participate in formation of a council with the AMA.[15]

Tightening the Rules

At the Regents' meeting in May 1936, the agenda revolved around issues created by the criticism of the College and the threats created by the proposed ABS. Their actions were meant to deflect some of the criticism and to align the College with the requirements of the board, an interesting development in that the board, not even operational, was already elevating the standards of surgery.

The Regents tightened up the training requirement for applicants for fellowship. They decided that all applicants for fellowship whose qualifying medical degree was obtained after January 1, 1938, must have three years of hospital service in one or more hospitals approved by the College, of which two years shall have been spent training in surgery. This was a significant step because the previous bylaws stated, "The candidate shall give evidence that he has served at least one year as intern in a creditable hospital and two years as surgical assistant, or he shall give evidence of apprenticeship of equivalent value."[16]

The new certifying board would require that applicants restrict their practices to surgery, but the College had no similar hard and fast rule about this. Regent Irvin Abell had previously proposed to the Executive Committee of the Board of Regents that College applicants should spend a minimum of 75 percent of their time as a specialist in surgery, and that the College should not consider applicants from unrecognized schools.[17] The Regents then discussed this and changed Article 5 in the bylaws to specify that "the candidate's professional activity shall be restricted to the study, diagnosis, and operative work in general surgery or in special fields of surgery."[16] While moving the College closer to encompassing only surgical practitioners, the Regents maintained their conviction that small communities need surgeons who, because of economic or medical manpower issues, may need to do some general practice, by adding,

> The College desires to admit only those who are primarily specialists in surgery and the minimum proportion of specialization which is acceptable may vary according to the character and size of the community in which the candidate resides. Each case should be judged on its individual merits as to the professional ability, training and experience of the candidate, in the particular field of surgery in which he is engaged.[16]

At least for that time, the notion that the College could improve surgical standards by being an inclusive instead of an exclusive organization prevailed.

The discussion turned to the proposed ABS. Harvey reported that the member organizations of the new board were expected to give formal approval by late fall, and he expected the board to be functional in January 1937. Despite their concerns that the board would diminish the standing of the College, they supported its establishment and passed a resolution pledging cooperation and indicating that they would name three nominees to serve on the board when it was organized.[16]

≈ ✳ ≈

The Graduate Medical Education Quandary

MacEachern, who believed that the College should control graduate medical education through the hospitals on its approved list, presented a remarkable document that detailed standards for three- to five-year residency programs in hospitals, and a list of 116 hospitals that he thought should develop such programs, many of which became outstanding comprehensive medical centers, such as the University of Iowa Hospitals and the Massachusetts General Hospital.[18] The Regents thought that Dr. MacEachern's document was too specific for the time and accepted it in principle only. MacEachern, who was a font of ideas and a compulsive worker, often made proposals that the Regents were not ready for and this was one of them. He must have been very disappointed because the length and specificity of the plan had obviously taken a great deal of time and effort. At the moment, the Regents had other plans.

They then turned to the issue of forming a joint council with the AMA that would work to increase the facilities for graduate training in surgery. Howard Naffziger, the pioneering San Francisco neurosurgeon, pointed out that one third of the fellowship of the College was specialists, so they agreed that the Joint Council should deal not only with graduate training for general surgery, but with the specialties of surgery as well. They considered adding the Association of American Medical Colleges to the Council, as well as the Canadian Medical Association (because the College was a North American organization). But in the end, they voted to set up the Joint Council between the two organizations with the recommendation that other bodies be consulted, in particular, the Canadian Medical Association.[16]

MacEachern introduced a resolution that each junior candidate for fellowship be assigned an advisor or counselor to guide him to obtain adequate training in surgery, proper ethical relations, and all other issues that had a bearing on his professional career as a surgeon. The advisor or counselor stimulated the candidate to take advantage of advanced courses, to participate in scientific programs, to prepare articles for medical journals, and to use every available resource to develop himself as a competent surgeon. This was approved.[1]

MacEachern notified the AMA that the College agreed to form the Joint Council with them to set up residencies in general surgery and the surgical specialties. Subsequently, he had two meetings with officers of the Council on Medical Education and Hospitals who told him that they had no plans for developing more residencies in surgery, but they planned to survey hospitals that currently had residencies in various fields of medicine and surgery and the specialties. Many of these were residencies of one, two, or three years, but were not of the quality that the College wanted to develop.[19]

Later, Crile received a letter from Dr. Olin West, general manager of the AMA, stating that the AMA was rejecting the College's request to form a joint council to consider increasing the facilities for adequate training for surgeons.[20]

This created a huge problem for the ABS. The board required three years of training plus two in study or practice for eligibility to take the examinations, but there were not enough residency programs to produce surgeons who met the eligibility requirements, and the quality of many of the programs was suspect. The board had no system for setting the standards for residency programs or measuring their quality. The directors wanted to expand the number of programs and were counting on the College and the AMA to encourage qualified hospitals, especially those not affiliated with medical schools, to establish residencies. By calling for the creation of the Joint Council, they planned to use the expertise and influence of both the AMA and the College. The AMA had established standards and inspected hospitals for internships, and the College set standards and inspected them for approval in its standardization program. Together, they could develop a program for establishing standards and monitoring quality. They could use their considerable influence to push for more residency programs. This was not to be.

MacEachern, sensing that a rift between the organizations would stop or at least delay the improvement needed in graduate medical education, developed a session on graduate medical education and training for the 1937 Clinical Congress. In seeking approval of the Regents, he said that the object was to pool the information and opinions of the various interested institutions and organizations so that the greatest good would accrue. No fixed program or definite recommendations were to come from the program, but there would be frank discussions on all aspects of the subject, which is of interest now to the ACS, the ASA, the ABS, the AMA, as well as individual institutions and surgeons. Expressing his approval, Chairman Crile said that "the best means of building goodwill is by service rendered." He said, "It is the effort of the College to cooperate with every group that is engaged in a genuine worthwhile effort."[1]

Meanwhile, in 1937, the ABS was incorporated, with Graham as chairman, Whipple as vice chairman, and J Stewart Rodman as secretary-treasurer. By the end of the year, examinations had begun.[22] Graham's dream became a reality in less than two years, a testimony to his extraordinary leadership and drive. This was a seminal event in the development of surgery in the United States. Since its founding the board has set a high bar for vetting the young men and women who graduated from their surgical residencies, ensuring that the surgical workforce is competent to provide appropriate care. The support by all the certifying boards of their umbrella organization, which began as the Advisory Council for the Medical Specialties and is now known as the American Board of Medical Specialties, has led to standardization across all specialties of medicine, frequent improvements in the certification process, and a commitment to serve the public by advancing safe, competent medical care.

The vacuum left by the AMA's unwillingness to participate with the College in evaluating hospitals for residency programs had to be filled, and the Regents would need to decide if they wanted to fill it. They had MacEachern, who already had proposed standards and knew which hospitals could implement them. Up for grabs was the opportunity to set the standards for training surgical specialists and to regulate surgical residencies. The bold decisions of the Regents around this issue would improve the care of surgical patients immeasurably, alter the focus of the College, and expand its influence.

REFERENCES

1. Stevens, R., *American Medicine and the Public Interest. A History of Specialization.* Updated Edition ed. 1998, Los Angeles and Berkley: University of California Press.
2. Ludmerer, K.M., *Time to Heal. American Medical Education from the turn of the Century to the Era of Managed Care.* 1999, Oxford: Oxford University Press.
3. Stephenson, G.W., *The American College of Surgeons and Graduate Education in Surgery. A Chronicle of Surgical Advancement. Bulletin of the American College of Surgeons.* 1971, Chicago: American College of Surgeons.
4. Commission on Graduate Medical Education, *Graduate Medical Education. Report of the Commission on Graduate Medical Education.* 1940, Chicago: University of Chicago Press.
5. American Medical Association, Minutes of the House of Delegates 84th Annual Session, Milwaukee, June 12-15, 1933. 1933; Available from: *http://192.159.83.55:8080/ AMA_NDLS/jsp/vieweer2.jsp?doc.*
6. Titus, P., *The Advisory Board for Medical Specialties. Information Booklet.* 1935, Paul Titus: Pittsburgh.
7. *Minutes of the Adjourned Meeting of the Board of Regents of October 19, 1934.* 1934, Archives of the American College of Surgoens: Chicago.
8. Ravitch, M.M., *A Century of Surgery. The History of the American Surgical Association.* 1981, Philadelphia: J.B. Lippencott Co.
9. Whipple, A.O., Parsons, W.B., Mullins, C.R., *Treatment of carcinoma of the ampulla of Vater.* Annals of Surgery, 1935. **102**: p. 763-779.
10. Olch, P., *Evarts A. Graham, the American College of Surgeons, and the American Board of Surgery.* Journal of the History of Medicine and Allied Sciences, 1972. **27**: p. 247-261.
11. Griffen, W.O., Jr., *The American Board of Surgery---Then and Now.* 2004, Philadelphia: American Board of Surgery.
12. *Minutes of the meeting of the Board of Regents of October 29, 1935.* 1935, Archives of the American College of Surgeons: Chicago.
13. *Abstracted minutes of the Administrative Board,* Archives of the American College of Surgeons.
14. *Minutes of the meeting of the Executive Committee of the Board of Regents of March 29, 1936. Exhibits A and B.* 1936, Archives of the American College of Surgeons: Chicago.
15. *Minutes of the meeting of the Executive Committee of the Board of Regents. Exhibit C.* 1936, Archives of the American College of Surgeons: Chicago.
16. *Abstracted minutes of the meeting of the Board of Regents of May 9,10, 1936.* 1936, Archives of the American College of Surgeons: Chicago.
17. *Minutes of the meeting of the Executive Committee of February 8,1936.* 1936, Archives of the American College of Surgeons: Chicago.
18. *Minutes of the meeting of the Board of Regents of May 10, 1936, Exhibit A.* 1936, Archives of the American College of Surgeons: Chicago.
19. *Abstracted minutes of the meeting of the Board of Regents of October 18, 1936.* 1936, Archives of the American College of Surgeons Chicago.
20. *Minutes of the meeting of the Executive Committee of October 9, 1937.* 1937, Archives of the American College of Surgeons: Chicago.
21. *Minutes of the meeting of the Executive Committee of July 29, 1939.* 1939, Archives of the American College of Surgeons: Chicago.
22. Rodman, J.S., *History of the American Board of Surgery. 1937-1952.* 1956, Philadelphia: J.B. Lippincott Co.

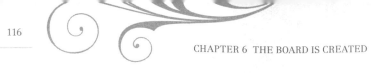

CHAPTER 7
Wrestling
with Diversity

Surgeons gather after opening ceremonies in the ballroom
of the Biltmore Hotel, Los Angeles, 1948

African Americans were excluded from the profession of medicine during our country's first century, when most of them were slaves. More than 200 years later, despite the recent lifting of restrictions and even some incentives, they remain underrepresented in the physician workforce and in the pool of applicants to medical schools. By 1847 there were approximately 40 medical schools in the country turning out thousands of white physicians, yet in that year David Jones Peck was the first African American to graduate from an American medical school, Rush Medical School in Chicago.[1] The first African American woman physician graduated from the New England Female Medical College (now Boston University School of Medicine) in 1864. Roscoe Giles (1890–1970), was the first African American admitted to Cornell Medical College (now Weill Medical College of Cornell University) and in 1938 he was the first certified by the American Board of Surgery.[2]

After the Civil War and the abolition of slavery, Jim Crow laws and white-directed segregation continued to leave African Americans with inadequate medical care. To avoid integrating existing facilities, whites supported the development of separate facilities and institutions for blacks. The notion that blacks should have their own hospitals and medical schools to train black physicians to care for blacks fit in with the prevailing attitudes of white supremacy. Accordingly, important African American medical institutions sprang up during the late 19th and the early 20th century, including the department of surgery at Howard University College of Medicine (1868), Meharry Medical College (1876), Harlem Hospital (1881), Provident Hospital in Chicago (1891) and in St. Louis (1894), Freedmen's Hospital in Washington, DC (1908), and the Tuskegee Veterans Administration Hospital in Alabama (1923). These and many other hospitals were built exclusively for African American physicians and patients, while African Americans were either denied admission or relegated to segregated wards and clinics in other hospitals. Racial separatism in hospital construction was sanctioned as late as 1946, when the Hill-Burton Act allowed the use of federal funds for construction of segregated hospitals. It was not halted until 1965, when the law that established Medicare and Medicaid effectively banned racial segregation in hospitals.

Membership in a medical society was a prerequisite for hospital medical staff privileges by the early 1900s. African Americans were excluded from membership in the American Medical Association (AMA) by its action to refuse to seat delegations from the National Medical Association, an African American organization, and the National Medical Society, an integrated Washington, DC organization that was formed because its African American members were refused admission to the all-white Medical Society of the District of Columbia. The seating of delegations was the route to membership in the AMA. Through this convoluted process of exclusion, African Americans were effectively kept off hospital medical staffs and therefore kept from giving adequate care to their African American patients. Southern blacks were excluded from membership in state and local medical societies, a prerequisite for AMA membership.[1]

Against this background, in 1913 early leaders formed the Founding Group of the College. Included was Dr. Daniel Hale Williams (1856–1931), the first African American to graduate from Northwestern University Medical School in 1883.[2] He practiced in Chicago for 10 years before serving as surgeon-in-chief at the renowned Freedmen's Hospital in Washington, DC.

Louis T Wright, MD, Candidate for Fellowship

Nothing that confronted the officers and Regents of the American College of Surgeons (ACS) was more reflective of the racial attitudes of the public in 1934 than the matter of Dr. Louis T Wright, an African American surgeon from New York City. (Figure 7.1)

Wright's father was an African American physician who died when Louis was four. By the time the boy was seven, his mother had married the man who would have the greatest influence on his life, encouraging him in his development and guiding him in his education. His stepfather was the respected Dr. William Fletcher Penn, the first African American physician to receive a medical degree from Yale.

Growing up in Atlanta during the turn of the century, the young Wright watched while white guards whipped Negroes working on chain gangs. He felt terror as he saw a black man lynched by a mob of whites. Wright was at the impressionable age of 15 during the Atlanta race riot in 1907. The Wrights' white neighbors, toting guns, were on the street in front of their house. Militia roamed the streets. Gunshots cracked in the distance. Dr. Penn, determined to protect his family, gave his son a loaded Winchester rifle and told him to shoot anyone who tried to enter their yard at the front of the house, while he defended the rear. Young Wright was terrified. The next day, a white auto mechanic rescued the family by driving them to a safe area of town. As an adult, Wright reflected on this act of kindness as the experience that led him to never judge an individual by the color of his skin. He believed that the terror of the racial injustices he experienced as a boy strengthened his character and made him fearless when faced with difficulty. This trait made life difficult for him during his personal and professional formation, but it served him and society well during his adulthood.[3]

Wright graduated from the tiny, historically black Clark College in Atlanta (now Clark Atlanta University). Encouraged by his stepfather, he applied and was admitted to Harvard Medical School, but the admissions office had mistaken the Clark College on his application for the more familiar Clark University down the road in Worcester, Massachusetts. When Wright arrived at Harvard they discovered their mistake and told him that he was not properly prepared to enter Harvard. In fact, he had not taken and passed the chemistry examination that Harvard required. To deal with his protest, they referred him to the venerable Dr. Otto Folin, professor of chemistry, who reiterated that he was not prepared for Harvard Medical School. Wright demanded to be admitted. Eventually the eminent chemist relented with the proviso that Wright must pass Folin's

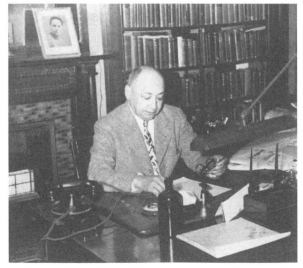

FIGURE 7.1 Dr. Louis T Wright, Chairman, Department of Surgery, Harlem Hospital. Published in "Louis Tompkins Wright, 1891-1952." Reprinted from Journal of National Medical Association, March, 1953, Vol. 45, No.2, p..130–148. Used with permission.

oral chemistry examination. He passed a very difficult exam and was admitted. (Neither Folin nor Wright knew that Folin would later become the father-in-law of a surgical icon and ultimately a President of the College, Dr. Jonathan Rhoads.) Wright put in a strong academic performance as a student, which entitled him to an annual scholarship.

During his third year, Wright was assigned to a black physician in Boston for his obstetrics rotation rather than the standard rotation at Boston Lying-In Hospital; the hospital would not accept a black medical student on its wards. Wright was indignant, and demanded to be assigned to Boston Lying-In. He said that Harvard's catalogue specified Boston Lying-In for the obstetrics rotation; he had paid his tuition and should be assigned as stipulated in the catalogue. Harvard capitulated. Wright was developing his deep resolve to fight racial inequality, a characteristic that defined him throughout his adult life and career.[3] He cut classes for three weeks during his senior year to join a protest of *The Birth of a Nation*, considered by African Americans to be a racist film. Despite his abrasiveness and the problems he created for Harvard, Wright managed to remain in good standing and graduate fourth in his class.

His race was a major hurdle in finding an internship. After rejections by three hospitals because he was black, his stepfather advised him to apply to Freedmen's Hospital, Howard Medical School's teaching hospital in Washington, DC, where he was accepted. At Freedmen's he conducted research that contradicted the conventional wisdom that the Schick skin test for diphtheria immunity was unreliable in African Americans. Many believed that it was impossible to decipher changes in black skin in response to the inoculation of diphtheria toxin. The *Journal of Infectious Diseases* published his work, the first research publication ever from Freedmen's Hospital.

His training completed, Wright returned to Atlanta to practice with his stepfather and began to specialize in surgery. There he worked to start the Atlanta branch of the National Association for the Advancement of Colored People (NAACP) and pushed to advance education for African American students. Although he was pleased with his rapidly growing practice, he chafed at the racial prejudices held by southern whites. On several occasions he responded vociferously when he was denigrated by racial insults. Once, he threatened to choke a man who insulted him. He worried about the depth of his anger and was afraid that he would be provoked to violence. Finally, he decided that he had to leave the South.

The opportunity came with the outbreak of World War I in 1917. He joined the Army and was stationed at Camp Upton on Long Island, where he conducted the research that created the Army's method of smallpox inoculation. In 1918, he was sent to France as a battalion surgeon.

Returning from the war, he settled in New York City, where no African American physician had ever been appointed to the staff of a hospital. After six months of applications to medical staffs of New York hospitals, all of which were denied, he was finally asked to work as a volunteer in the outpatient department of Harlem Hospital by the superintendent, Dr. Cosmo O'Neal, who knew of Wright's work with diphtheria and smallpox. Most of the patients at Harlem Hospital were black, but the medical staff was white, and Wright's lowly appointment, which did not include privileges to admit patients, was the beginning of his lifelong battle to transform the hospital into an institution where skin color of a patient, doctor, nurse or other staff was irrelevant.

Wright was the first African American physician appointed to the medical staff of a New York City hospital. But things did not go smoothly. Four white members of the medical staff resigned on Wright's first day in the clinic. On pressure from the white physician community, Dr. O'Neal was removed from his position and moved to a minor position at Bellevue Hospital.

The Harlem community and its alderman agitated for more African American physicians, complaining about the poor medical care in the hospital and ascribing it to white doctors who cared only about their paying white patients. In 1921, seven more African American physicians were appointed to the outpatient department, but they too were denied hospital privileges. Wright encouraged the NAACP and the North Harlem Medical Society, an African American group of physicians, dentists, and pharmacists who practiced in Harlem, to hire an African American Columbia law school graduate to investigate Harlem Hospital. The lawyer's report documented cases of patient abuse and tension between white and African American physicians. Charges of abuse by Harlem residents and politicians spilled into the country's black newspapers. After the NAACP became involved, the mayor launched an investigation. Subsequently, he recommended conversion of the hospital to a black institution with an entirely black medical staff. Wright and others fended this off, asserting that the hospital and its medical staff should be open to people of both races.

A positive outcome of the investigation was the establishment of a black nursing school at the hospital. Throughout his career at Harlem Hospital, Wright taught nurses and guided the school as it became a major source of well-trained black nurses for the New York area. Soon Wright was promoted to Adjunct Assistant Visiting Surgeon.

In 1926 three African American medical school graduates applied for internships at Harlem Hospital. With high examination scores and Wright as their advocate, they were appointed. This led to the resignation of five white doctors, but the African American members of the medical staff were unrelenting in their insistence on equality. Gradually, white gentile physicians left and the majority of the remaining doctors were Jews. Wright was appointed to the surgical staff, and in 1929 he was named a New York City police surgeon. Dr. John Fox Connors, director of Harlem Hospital Department of Surgery, opposed Wright at first, but soon recognized his talents as surgeon, teacher, and investigator. They became friends, and Connors, who was admitted to fellowship in the prestigious American Surgical Association (ASA), became his advocate.

Working together, they recruited more black physicians to the staff. Tensions surfaced again and Wright and Connors were pitted against a faction led by Drs. Louis Friedman and Henry Pascal, who opposed more black staff appointments. Pascal was openly critical of black physicians.[4] Friedman and Pascal and others charged that Wright and Connors politicized the medical staff appointment process and were riding roughshod over their opponents. By 1929 the open warfare on the medical staff compromised the care of patients and the operation of the hospital. The Commissioner of Hospitals, William Schroeder, stepped in and took the extraordinary action of abolishing the Harlem Hospital Board and the hospital's entire medical staff.

In the reorganization, 23 white and 2 black doctors were fired and 12 additional black doctors were appointed at various levels of the medical staff. Wright was promoted to attending surgeon and given control of the internship. Schroeder's reorganization now put black and white physicians on an equal footing, a relationship that did not exist in any other hospital in the country. Wright's influence was now established and he used it to control Harlem Hospital for the rest of his life.[5]

The Regents Bite the Bullet

The College staff referred to Wright in letters and minutes of meetings as "Dr. Louis T. Wright (colored)." This was not unusual in medical circles. The designation "col." appeared after the names of all African American physicians in the AMA Directory. In the southern states and in Washington, DC, blacks were barred from membership in the constituent societies of the AMA, including state and local medical societies.

At their October 1934 meeting during the Clinical Congress, Martin asked the Regents to approve the list of initiates for admission to fellowship at the convocation later in the week. Because the candidates had been formally vetted by both the state and the central credentials committees, this was usually routine business, a "rubber stamp" with no questions or discussion. But this time Martin informed them that a "Negro" was on the list: Dr. Louis T Wright. He did not want them to approve the list without knowing that a black man was on it. Wright's application had been approved by the 30-man New York Committee on Credentials without a single dissenting vote. Martin told the Regents that some of the best men in New York City were present at the meeting and they discussed the issue thoroughly. Martin said, "Professionally, he is all right. He is apparently a gentleman in every way." But Martin then reminded the Regents of the trouble in 1913 when the College had admitted Dr. Daniel Hale Williams of Chicago in the Founding Group.[6]

Regent John E Jennings, a founder of the Brooklyn-Long Island Chapter of the College, was asked to comment. He said he knew Wright and his reputation. "He is one of the most brilliant surgeons of the city. His work has been striking. His chest work and his work on blood vessels has (sic) been outstanding. Among his own people (African Americans) Wright represents the highest ideals of the College." Jennings thought it would be a mistake to turn him down.[7]

There followed a long discussion about whether Wright was qualified and whether or not the College should accept African Americans. The Regents knew that they needed to face the issue and that their decision could set a precedent.

Hubert Royster, from North Carolina, said that in his region of the country surgeons consulted with Negroes and worked with them in schools and hospitals. He felt that Negroes should have their own hospitals. He focused on the fact that they were not members of the state medical societies, such membership giving evidence of competence and approval by peers. Crile, irritated, quickly pointed out that the College did not require membership in a local or state medical society, and added that College fellowship was available in Canada and in other countries that had no state societies. Royster retorted that if they had their own hospitals and their own societies they would progress faster because so few of them were eligible for racially mixed organizations.

Crile reiterated that the discussion was whether or not the College should admit Negroes. He pointed out that a Negro had been accepted previously (Daniel Hale Williams), but he was now dead. The Negro in question is white in color and appearance, he said. All of those who spoke, including Martin, JMT Finney, Charles Mayo, Royster, George Crile, and J Bentley Squier, said that if the Committee on Credentials in New York City approved him, he should be approved.

The conversation wandered, and Mayo asked how the College, acting on behalf of society, could do the most good for Negroes. He questioned whether the Regents should encourage blacks to begin their own advanced surgical society, or should be admitted to the American College of Surgeons. He said, "They are going to increase faster in population than white people. They have doubled it to this point, and in 50 years there will be millions of them. There are currently 14 million and in 50 years' time there will be 28 million" [his prediction was remarkably accurate]. Mayo questioned whether the millions of Negroes in the population would be better off if Negro surgeons had a society of their own, one that the College could help them start, or whether the Negro population would be better served by the few of them who could get into the College.

Finney, born in Natchez, Mississippi and professor of surgery at Johns Hopkins, said there were two issues: one was whether or not the College would want to take in Negroes, and that had been settled in the affirmative. The other was whether the College should help them start their own organization. He thought that the latter would be the best thing to do. If they had their own society, they could feel as if there was an opportunity for them to get ahead. Finally, the Regents voted to accept the list of initiates without making specific reference to Wright.[7] They did not establish a formal policy that the College should admit African Americans, although several of them tacitly assumed that the admission of Wright set that precedent.

∾—✱—∾

Louis T Wright, MD, FACS

Wright and his wife Corrine went to Boston for the convocation at which he was admitted to fellowship in the College. The Bay State Medical, Dental and Pharmaceutical Society held a grand banquet in his honor with distinguished speakers who celebrated his achievement.

The remainder of Wright's career vindicated the decision of the College to admit him. The NAACP elected Wright to the chairmanship of its board in 1934, a position he held until his death in 1952. He was the first black to hold the position. Wright published 100 scientific papers, many of which appeared in prestigious journals. He used the extensive Harlem Hospital experience with all varieties of trauma to develop new methods of diagnosis and treatment of trauma victims. He invented a brace used for the transport of patients with cervical injuries. Dr. Charles L Scudder, chairman of the College's Committee on Fractures, invited him to write a chapter on head injuries for his classic book, *The Treatment of Fractures*, making Wright the first African American to contribute to a major medical text.

At Harlem Hospital, he was appointed director of the department of surgery, and later chairman of the Harlem Hospital Board of Trustees. In 1945 he initiated and directed a 5-year residency in surgery. He mentored many budding black surgeons who became very successful, including Dr. Myra Logan, who in 1951 was the second black woman to achieve fellowship in the ACS and the first woman to perform an operation on the heart,[8] and Dr. Aubre de Lambert Maynard, Wright's successor as director of surgery at Harlem Hospital.

At the end of World War II Wright established the Harlem Hospital as a research center for aureomycin, one of the first antibiotics. He and his colleagues tested aureomycin in the treatment of a wide variety of surgical diseases and conditions, resulting in 30 publications. At the beginning of the use of chemotherapy as adjunct therapy for cancer he also investigated the effects of several chemotherapeutic agents.[4]

Throughout his life Wright opposed segregation in all of its forms, believing that it led to inferior treatment of blacks and destruction of their self-confidence. He believed in the simple principle that blacks should have "equal opportunity, no more, no less."

In 1930 the Julius Rosenwald Fund offered money for an all-black hospital in New York. Wright led the opposition, which was successful in preventing the building of the hospital, much to the consternation of many blacks, including black physicians, who thought the care of blacks was better in all-black than in segregated institutions, and that black physicians had more opportunity to use their education and training in all-black hospitals.[9]

In the context of Wright's distinguished career and the fact that our country has had a black President, the angst of the Regents over the decision to admit him to fellowship now seems trivial and disgraceful. But given the general views of American society at the time, theirs was a courageous and bold decision. The many indignities Wright suffered during his personal and professional formation were commonplace and culturally accepted by whites. The Regents' views reflected those of our society.

Fallout

As the Regents expected, news of Wright's election was not well received in the South or in Washington, DC. Two Fellows from Yazoo City, Mississippi resigned from the College in protest. Washington and Birmingham were on the schedule for sectional meetings, and Fellows from both cities asked for a ruling on the participation of black surgeons. They suggested that separate meetings should be held for black doctors in their cities, but this was ignored.[10]

At the February 9, 1935 meeting of the College staff, a letter from a southern surgeon, chairman of the local credentials committee of the College, was read:

> ...I have always been under the impression that the American College of Surgeons was made up of white surgeons entirely. I would like to have a letter from you stating why this has occurred, that a Negro surgeon is now a member of the American College of Surgeons. It will be necessary for me to explain to the local members the reason why this Negro was admitted to this organization. I would appreciate a letter from you, because I feel there must be some mistake. Assuring you that I am not prejudiced against the College and that a mistake has been made, I stand ready to lend my assistance to right same.[10]

This letter forced Franklin Martin to articulate, on behalf of the College, his feelings regarding fellowship for African American surgeons. He replied,

> The candidacy of the surgeon referred to was thoroughly investigated. The local credentials committee recommended him without a dissenting vote. The committee on history reviews favorably recommended his histories. The administrative officers of the College, including myself, were at some pains to make personal investigations in this case. The Board of Regents, at a meeting at which several members from the South were present, discussed the case at length and admitted him to fellowship in the College. This surgeon is one who has attained a considerable

degree of distinction in his profession, and his work has led him to be highly esteemed by the surgical profession, not only of his own scientific and practical organization with professional, ethical, and moral standards, and when in the opinion of its officers and committees a candidate attains those standards he is entitled to fellowship. It is not the opinion of the officers of the College, nor of its committees, that its standard has been lowered by the admission of this candidate.[10]

≈✻≈

One Is Sufficient?

The fact that a distinguished black surgeon was admitted to fellowship in the ACS did little, if anything, to correct the indignities visited on African American surgeons and physicians throughout the country. In 1937, Roscoe Giles, the first African American graduate of Cornell Medical School, was elected president of the National Medical Association, an organization of black physicians. A year later his successor appointed Giles to a "Goodwill Committee," tasked with convincing the AMA to remove the designation "col." from the AMA Directory. His colleague on the committee, Dr. Carl G Roberts, pointed out to the AMA trustees that he had lost his malpractice insurance and other black physicians had lost their credit ratings because of this designation. The AMA took no action.

After several meetings and various proposals by the AMA designed to placate the complainants, none of which were implemented, the AMA finally removed the "col." designation from the 1940 edition of the American Medical Directory. Nevertheless, their constituent state and local medical societies in the South continued to deny membership to black physicians.[2]

At the April 1940 meeting of the Board of Regents, Associate Director Bowman Crowell raised the question that has been before the Board before

> —that of candidates of the colored race. There are candidates, who from all professional standpoints are well qualified for fellowship in the College. This Board has not gone on record for or against. Any action of this Board has not been included in the minutes because the Board did not wish to go on record, making it impossible for these men to come into the College. All the sidestepping of the issue has been thrown on me. I have consulted with a number of these men, and they have been very decent about it. I have talked about it to them frankly and told them that the time was not ripe for their acceptance into the College...[6]

Regent William Darrach asked, "The College is not taking in any colored surgeons?" Crowell replied that Dr. Louis Wright from New York was taken in, which caused quite a disturbance in the South. He said criticism was being received from members of the College that colored surgeons were not being admitted. The hour was late and Board Chairman Abell told the group that they would discuss the issue at the next meeting.[6]

A Policy Is Established

That issue was not addressed until October 1940, when Associate Director Crowell told the Board that there were applications from 12 to 15 colored surgeons, seven of whom had at one time or another been recommended for fellowship by their respective credentials committees. Their applications had been held up by the central credentials committee, acting on instruction of the Board of Regents. Among them were Lt. Col. Roscoe Giles, chief of surgery at Ft. Huachuca, Arizona, who was the first black surgeon certified by the ABS; Aubre de Lambert Maynard, Wright's successor at Harlem Hospital; Peter Marshall Murray, a prominent New York surgeon; and Charles Drew, chairman of the department of surgery at Howard University.[2] Evarts Graham said, "These men were coming from excellent medical schools, receiving four years or more of extensive training and the College simply cannot refuse them admission because they are black."

Regent James Monroe Mason, of Birmingham, Alabama, read a letter he had sent to Dr. Crile in which Mason discussed how segregation had helped the Negro, citing

> the record of the Tuskegee Institute, where, over a long period of years, the wisest colored leaders have done wonderful work in the educational and industrial advancement of members of their race. They have been encouraged and taught to work for their own racial improvement, and never has there been an attempt to bring the Negro into social or scientific competition with his white neighbors.[11]

Mason said,

> It will be very deleterious with [sic] the College to give any particular recognition to these men. Recognition by the College is different from certification by a Board. The College fellowships work closely into the social relationship. It wouldn't be safe for the College to get mixed up in this subject. I don't think it would be a good thing.

Board Chairman Irvin Abell pointed out that on May 13, 1939, the following resolution had been unanimously carried: "being resolved that no applicant shall be granted fellowship in the ACS, whose admission would be injurious to the good order, peace, or interest of the college, or derogatory to its dignity, or inconsistent with its purposes."[12] Crile said he believed that the Regents understood that this resolution was germane to the issue, and that "it would be very unwise to change our point of view now and admit these men as Fellows." Mason said that the resolution should be formally reiterated at this time. Rudolph Matas, from New Orleans, said there would be a great protest in the South if there was any change in the present policy that blacks would not be admitted. Finney said that Fellows told him they would leave the College if Negroes were admitted. "It is not the way to help the Negro by putting him into the College." Regent Albert Singleton said he approved of Dr. Mason's statement in general.

> But, it is difficult to explain that we are trying to help them and yet denying them fellowship in the College. The problem is recognizing them socially. I don't think the United States of America is ready

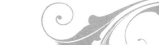

to acknowledge that the Negro is accepted socially. He is given scientific recognition, but we are not doing him an injustice by denying the social privileges, at least at this time.

Alton Ochsner said he was a transplanted Northerner and that he believed that the Negro was abused, but he was now convinced it would ruin the College in the South if the Negro were admitted. Crile moved that the Board reiterate the May 13, 1939, resolution. His motion passed. Crowell asked what he should tell applicants. Ending the discussion, Chairman Abell said, "You can tell them that for the present, the Board of Regents has decided not to admit any more Negro Fellows."[13] Thereafter, College staff used this statement, orally and in writing, in response to blacks who applied for fellowship and to Fellows who proposed them.

In May 1941, after Louis Wright and newly elected Regent Henry W Cave urged that black surgeons in New York be considered for fellowship, Miss Grimm summarized the College's experience with applications for fellowship from black surgeons and presented it to the Central Credentials Committee, chaired by Dr. Besley and composed of Dr. MacEachern, Dr. Crowell, Mrs. Farrow, and Miss Grimm, all College staff. She said that 24 applications had been received. Fellowship had been granted only to Daniel Hale Williams, a member of the Founding Group of the College, and Louis T Wright. The committee decided to not to bring this information to the Board of Regents because of the policy established by the Board and articulated by Dr. Abell.[14]

As the nation headed into World War II, the College's stance on the admission of African Americans was consistent with attitudes in other sectors of society. During the war, blacks were drafted in accordance with the Selective Service Act of 1940, which prohibited the selection and training of citizens because of race or color. Once they volunteered or were drafted, however, black soldiers were assigned to segregated units headed by white officers. They functioned in support roles, not in combat, until the Battle of the Bulge, when more combat troops were needed because of the large number of casualties. Blacks were then allowed to volunteer for combat as truck drivers, and 2,000 did so. As casualties depleted their segregated platoons, the survivors were integrated into white units, thus beginning the integration of the Army,[15] which was not formal policy until President Truman ordered an end to segregation in the Armed Forces in 1946.

On the home front, racism and segregation continued to be the norm during the war. For example, the Wright Aeronautical Corporation in Cincinnati transferred seven black workers into a shop that had been all-white, sparking a walkout of 450 employees.[15]

At the May, 1945, Regents' meeting, Crowell reported on an editorial in the

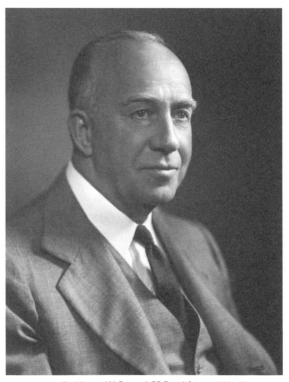

FIGURE 7.2 Dr. Henry W Cave, ACS President, 1950–51. Courtesy of the Connecticut State Medical Association.

Pittsburgh Courier by Dr. Louis T Wright that was very critical of the College for refusing to admit qualified African American surgeons.[16] Regent Henry Cave of New York said he was told that 100,000 people read the newspaper and the editorial created "quite a stir." He had talked with Dr. Wright, who was willing to let the matter go along and follow the process of evolution. He told Wright that two or three years earlier, the reason for deferring action was because, if the College took in Negroes, Fellows in the South would resign. Cave said that a committee should be appointed to study the subject. (Figure 7.2)

Mason thought that people in the South were being picked on by people in other sections of the country who were trying to break down social barriers in the South. He said white and black people were not ready to get along on social and professional lines and that if the College took any active steps to recognize Negroes it would be worse in the South than at any previous time. He said the so-called Negro question, including the political aspect of the Negro as a voter, "has gained much momentum under the guise of social justice and other propaganda promulgations." "There are 3,000 members of the College in the South and admission of Negroes could have serious consequences for the College."

Cave replied that he thought there was a great deal in what Dr. Mason said, but he moved that a committee study the subject; this motion was passed. The committee, called the Committee on the Relation of the Colored Surgeon to the American College of Surgeons, consisted of Drs. Cave (chair), Coller, and Ochsner.[17] Cave subsequently interviewed a group of black surgeons to understand their views and sent a questionnaire on the issue to several hundred Fellows.

Dr. George Thorne, a prominent black surgeon at Harlem Hospital, was turned down for fellowship. Public protests by Louis Wright and The New York Medical Society, which admitted blacks, were reported in *Time Magazine.* Editorials in New York papers attacked the College, and a New York assemblyman, who noted that the College was in violation of New York's anti-race-discrimination law, sponsored a resolution to investigate the College for racial discrimination.[18]

The College office received many requests for information from the press. *Time Magazine* quoted Malcolm MacEachern, the College's Associate Director: "It is strictly and entirely a matter of professional qualifications. If Dr. Thorne is properly qualified, he can be admitted." He added, "The College is studying the question of admitting Negroes and until the committee reports and the College acts, Dr. Thorne cannot get an application." Associate Director Bowman Crowell, always forthright and less politic, was quoted in the same article as saying that many Negroes meet the College's educational standards, but are barred because of their color.[19] The controversy, now widely reported, portrayed the College as anti-black and confused.

In June 1945 the Regents heard the results of his questionnaire from Dr. Cave: 201 Fellows replied that Negroes should be admitted if they meet the qualifications and 26, mostly from the South, were against their admission. In spite of a dramatic entreaty from Dr. Mason and a warning of resignations in the South from the respected Matas, conveyed by Ochsner, Cave moved that qualified Negroes be admitted. Mr. Vedder, the lawyer, advised that there be no formal vote, but that if this was the will of the Regents, they simply admit Negroes. This was their will, and four were initiated in 1945, ten in 1946, and by 1950 at least 40 had become Fellows,[20] including, in 1950, the first African American woman, Dr. Helen Octavia Dickens. Dickens, an obstetrician-gynecologist, was a graduate of the University of Illinois and practiced in Philadelphia, where she ended her career as a member of the faculty of the University of Pennsylvania. She was also the first African American woman to be admitted to fellowship in the American College of Obstetricians and Gynecologists. She died in 2001.[21]

In discussing a recommendation for posthumous fellowship of an individual, the College staff noted that in 1951, Dr. Charles R Drew, head of the department of surgery at Howard for 10 years from 1941 until his death, was fatally injured in an automobile accident prior to his interview with the committee on applicants. His name was included in the 1952 supplement to the Year Book only in the list of deceased Fellows with a note that he was granted posthumous fellowship.[22]

Typically, the Board closed ranks after making decisions on difficult issues, as exemplified by Regent James Monroe Mason, who said, "I am a member of the Board of Regents of this College and so long as I remain a Regent, I pledge you, I shall support the rules and regulations of the College."[23] This ended the debate for the College and closed a chapter that had reflected the shameful mind set of the American public.

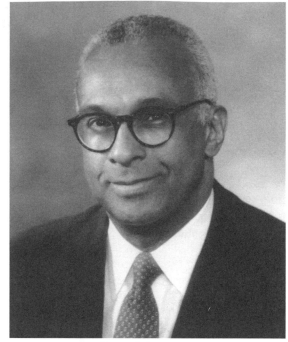

FIGURE 7.3 Dr. LaSalle D Leffall Jr, ACS President, 1995–96.

The Regents' struggle with the racial issue, spawned by Wright's candidacy for fellowship, eventually produced an impressive legacy for the College, organized medicine, and African Americans. In 1995, during the hundredth anniversary celebration of the National Medical Association, important positions were filled by black physicians, including Dr. LaSalle Leffall, (Figure 7.3) President-Elect of the American College of Surgeons; Dr. Gerald Thomson, president-elect of the American College of Physicians; Dr. Lonnie Bristow, president-elect of the American Medical Association; Dr. William G. Anderson, president of the American Osteopathic Association; and Dr. David Satcher, Director of the U.S. Center for Disease Control and Prevention. Satcher was later Surgeon General of the United States.[5]

During the 1990s, a committee of the Board of Governors pushed for more diversity, this time including women in the mix. They asked for a Governors' committee on diversity, but this was not approved until 2002, when the College created a committee on diversity issues, with the charge "to study the educational and professional needs of underrepresented surgeons and surgical trainees and the impact of its work on elimination of health disparities among diverse population groups."[24,25]

Dr. Claude Organ, the African American editor of *Archives of Surgery* and chairman of the department of surgery at University of California/Davis East Bay, had also chaired the department of surgery at Creighton University. He was elected Second Vice President of the College in 2001, and President in 2003–4. Dr. LD Britt, Brickhouse professor and chairman of the Department of Surgery at Eastern Virginia Medical School, became the third African American President of the College in 2010. He had the distinction of serving as a Regent and Chairman of the Board of Regents prior to his presidency.

As the College celebrates its Centennial, the issue of diversity remains, but it is clear that the College's leadership is no longer restricted by gender or race.

REFERENCES

1. Baker, R., Washington, HA, Olakanni, O, et al., *African American physicians and organized medicine, 1846-1968.* JAMA, 2008. **300**: p. 306-313.
2. Organ, C., Jr, Kosiba, MM,eds., ed. *A Century of Black Surgeons. The U.S.A. Experience.* Vol. 1. 1987, Transcript Press: Norman, OK. 298.
3. Hayden, R., *11 African American Doctors.* 1976, Frederick, Maryland: Twenty-First Century Books.
4. Maynard, A.D., *Surgeons to the Poor. The Harlem Hospital Story.* 1978, New York: Appleton-Century-Crofts.
5. Hayden, R., *"Mr. Harlem Hospital." Dr. Louis T. Wright. A Biography.* 2003, Littleton, MA: Tapestry Press.
6. *Minutes of the meeting of the Board of Regents of April 30, 1940.* 1940, Archives of the American College of Surgeons: Chicago.
7. *Minutes of the meeting of the Board of Regents of October 16, 1934.* 1934, Archive of the American College of Surgeons: Chicago.
8. *Death. Dr. Myra T. Logan.* J Nat Med Assn, 1977. **69**.
9. O'Shea, J., *Louis T. Wright and Henry W. Cave. How they paved the way for fellowships for black surgeons.* Bull Am Col Surg, 2005. **90**(10): p. 22-29.
10. *Abstracted Minutes. Administrative Board.*, Archives of the American College of Surgeons: Chicago.
11. Mason, J., *Letter from JM Mason to George Crile dated March 21, 1939.* 1939, Archives of the American College of Surgeons: Chicago.
12. *Minutes of the meeting of the Board of Regents of October 20, 1940.* 1940, Archives of the American College of Surgeons: Chicago.
13. *Minutes of the meeting of the Board of Regents of October 22, 1940.* 1940, Archives of the American Colllege of Surgeons: Chicago.
14. *Minutes of the Central Credentials Committee of January 22, 1941.* 1941, Archives of the American College of Surgeons: Chicago.
15. Ambrose, S., *D-Day. June 6, 1944: The Climactic Battle of World War II.* 1994, New York: Simon and Schuster.
16. *Minutes of the meeting of the Board of Regents of May 5, 1944. Exhibit D.* 1944, Archives of the American College of Surgeons: Chicago.
17. *Minutes of the Board of Regents meeting of May 5, 1944.* 1944, Archives of the American College of Surgeons: Chicago.
18. Grimm, E., *Resolution by Mr. Schupler. Attachment to letter from Eleanor K. Grimmm to Henry W. Cave, MD.*, in *Colored Surgeons, 1946-1980.* 1946, Archives of the American College of Surgeons: Chicago.
19. (1945) *Surgeons' Color Line.* Time Magazine.
20. Wright, L.W., *Letter from Lydia W. Wright to Henry W. Cave, January 29, 1951*, in *Colored Surgeons 1946-1980.* 1951, Archives of the American College of Surgeons: Chicago.
21. (December 8, 2001) *Helen Dickens, 92, Pioneering black physician.* Los Angeles TImes.
22. *Minutes of the meeting of the Board of Regents of June 10-12, 1983.* 1983, Archives of the American College of Surgeons: Chicago.
23. *Minutes of the meeting of the Board of Regents of June 23, 1945.* 1945, Archives of the American College of Surgeons: Chicago.
24. *Minutes of the meeting of the Board of Regents of February 2,3, 1990.* 1990, Archives of the American College of Surgeons: Chicago.
25. *Minutes of the meeting of the Board of Regents of June 7,8, 2002.* 2002, Archives of the American College of Surgeons: Chicago.

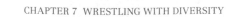

CHAPTER 8
Creating the Infrastructure for Graduate Training in Surgery

Threaten effectiveness of the American Board of Surgery (ABS) to meet the country's needs for competent surgeons was in question because an insufficient number of newly minted surgeons met the eligibility requirements for the board's examinations. The problem was a dearth of high-quality residency programs. The certification process would not bring about major improvements in surgical care without revision and expansion of the graduate education system. The board had neither the resources nor the expertise to address this problem. The American Medical Association (AMA) had published standards for residencies in surgery and had opted out of the proposed Joint Council with the College, contending that it was not needed. The AMA had set standards for internships and residencies in the late 1920s and had an approval program that it was attempting to upgrade. As new certifying boards were established, the AMA worked with them to approve hospital residencies in their specialties. The problem was that their standards for residencies were very general, leaving the hospitals with wide latitude, and resulting in significant variations in the quality of the programs. The AMA program was not rigorous enough to meet the standards of the ABS or the College.

≈✴≈

The Problem

The College had not planned to take on the approval of residencies. There was no obvious source for funding, and the Great Depression already made it difficult to fund ongoing projects. It would be a major departure for the organization, which had focused only on postgraduate education by holding the Clinical Congress and sectional meetings annually. These were major commitments for the staff and the leadership, which spent weeks just roughing out the program for the Clinical Congress, a growing enterprise that included technical exhibits, symposia, panel discussions, lectures, and courses. Dozens of speakers had to be lined up and cared for. Convention centers needed to be scheduled years in advance as did hotels to house thousands of attendees, their spouses, and other guests. An academic convocation with the initiation ceremony for new Fellows had to be planned and executed.

Other College staff was busy producing publications, maintaining a library of 40,000 volumes, and servicing Fellows from all over the world who requested medical information to assist them in caring for patients. Each applicant for fellowship had to be vetted in the central office and information had to be exchanged with the state and regional credentials committees. Communication with the Governors and the growing number of chapters was ongoing. The hospital standardization program alone was a major undertaking, requiring visits to hundreds of hospitals each year, compiling the results, and granting or denying approval. But it was the hospital standardization program that would make it possible for the College to take on the standardization of graduate medical education in surgery.

Malcolm MacEachern, the architect and leader of the hospital standardization program, had visited thousands of institutions over the years, including those with training programs in all specialties of medicine and surgery. He probably had a better understanding than anyone in the country of what makes a good residency. He organized a session on graduate medical education at the 1937 Clinical Congress to promulgate his thinking that the College should use its expertise in hospital standardization to accredit hospitals for graduate education. (Figure 8.1)

At the same Clinical Congress, MacEachern asked the Regents to establish a department of graduate training for surgery and the specialties in the College, headed by an officer of the College and supported by a strong advisory committee of five or six surgeons. Board Chairman George Crile, picking up on this suggestion, favored a strong committee, asserting that the College should act independently in graduate medical education. Regent John Jennings, of Brooklyn, believed the College should assume responsibility for the training of surgeons. Another Regent, Dr. Irvin Abell, said that it would take several years for the AMA to develop its residency standardization program. He believed the College was in a position to do what no other organization could do for graduate training in surgery. Dr. Dallas Phemister agreed that the College was the logical organization to set up a system to train young surgeons in hospitals. He and Jennings pointed

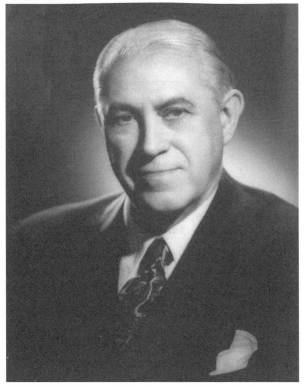

FIGURE 8.1 Dr. Malcolm T MacEachern, ACS Associate Director and architect of its hospital standardization program.

out that internists, whose board was established in 1936, also needed a program to standardize and expand residencies and that a combined committee of the American College of Surgeons and the American College of Physicians (ACP) was desirable. (Figure 8.2) Subsequent efforts to enlist the ACP were unsuccessful.[1,2,3]

The Regents voted to create a new committee on graduate training for surgery with Phemister, who had always been interested in graduate medical education, as chairman. Crile said that for a long time some specialties had complained that the College was run by general surgeons who paid little attention to other specialties. He recommended that specialists should be included, so they named it the committee on graduate training for surgery and the surgical specialties.[4] In addition to Chairman Dallas Phemister, the members were Drs. Donald Balfour of Rochester, Minnesota; John Fraser, of Montréal, Canada (obstetrics and gynecology); Evarts Graham of St. Louis (thoracic surgery); Allen O Whipple of New York (general surgery); Albert Rustenburg of Ann Arbor (otorhinolaryngology); Harry Gradle of Chicago (ophthalmology); Howard Naffziger of San Francisco (neurologic surgery); Alexander Randolph of Philadelphia (urology); and Philip Wilson of New York (orthopaedic surgery).[5]

MacEachern Proposes the Solution

MacEachern then gave the Regents a document he had prepared, entitled Criteria for Graduate Training for Surgery.[6] He specified that the hospital had to have a well-organized medical staff with department chiefs responsible for the graduate training program. The hospital also had to have an adequate patient census, complete laboratory and x-ray facilities, and other diagnostic and therapeutic facilities. Weekly departmental conferences in surgery and the surgical specialties, in which the resident was encouraged to take an active part, were required, as was a weekly clinical pathology conference. The hospital was required to have an outpatient department with a follow-up clinic in which the resident could work, a medical library, and an affiliation, if possible, with a medical school to provide the resident with opportunities for basic science study and study using cadavers or animals.

The hospital must have assigned personnel responsible for active and personal supervision and direction of the residents. The hospital should be approved by the College and appear on a list of approved hospitals for surgical residencies, which included general surgery and the surgical specialties. MacEachern's wisdom and foresight in setting forth the basic requirements for surgical residencies in the 1930s is confirmed by their current use as the basic pillars of the modern surgical residency.

MacEachern listed the qualifications of residents as honesty and evidence of high character. College training, preferably culminating in a degree, was desirable. Graduation from a medical school approved by the AMA and the American Association of Medical Colleges (AAMC) was required, and it was preferable that the medical school be rated in the higher brackets on the approved list. Another prerequisite was an internship of 18 months in a hospital approved by the ACS and approved for intern training by the AMA. The duration of residency training was to be three years, with six months spent in another institution. For those entering a surgical specialty at least one year in general surgery and two years in the selected specialty were required. The resident should devote time to the study of gross and microscopic surgical pathology, roentgenology, and the auxiliary basic sciences. The surgical service should provide sufficient patients for study and experience and the resident should be the responsible surgeon for at least 100 major operations with satisfactory results.

The resident was to have the opportunity to observe autopsies and study the findings. He should devote as much time as possible to reading scientific literature under the direction of his preceptor. It was advisable to have a journal club to stimulate this. The resident should carry out anatomical dissections on cadavers and animals, should be encouraged to participate in research, and should keep records of all his work and educational activities. He was to actively participate in medical staff and clinical pathological conferences and in department meetings. He should engage in some teaching activities for nurses and students. A record of progress should be kept by the resident and reviewed monthly by his preceptor.

At the termination of residency the resident should be examined by the Advisory Committee on Graduate Training for Surgery, which examination should consist of a thesis jointly selected by the resident and his subcommittee, or a written or oral scientific and clinical examination, or both, if deemed advisable. MacEachern's wisdom and expertise was remarkable. Even today, surgical residents who had these qualities and carried out the specified duties would emerge as ethical, competent practitioners of surgery.

Using MacEachern's proposed minimum standards for rating hospitals for graduate training, Dr. Melville Manson, of the College's hospital standardization program, had surveyed a sample of hospitals with and without residencies to obtain information about the quality of their programs or their suitability for residency programs. The bottom line was that the facilities, personnel, and diagnostic resources were mostly adequate in the hospitals that had residents. Organization of the surgical staff was lacking, however. The medical staff did not have a systematic method to supervise residents or to direct their activities and there was no consistent program or curriculum for residents.

Without revision and expansion of the graduate education system, Manson estimated that 50 percent of those surveyed could be put on an approved list. Nearly 36 percent of the remainder had everything necessary

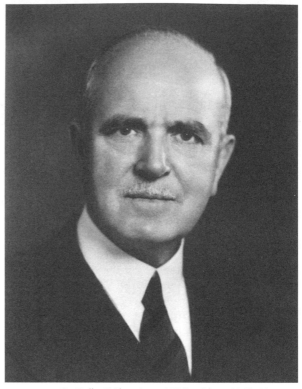

FIGURE 8.2 Dr. Dallas B Phemister, ACS President, 1948–49.

to conduct adequate graduate surgical training except for sufficient organization of the medical staff. They had well-equipped diagnostic departments with competent technical and professional personnel and surgeons who could effectively conduct a training program. Among the deficiencies were the libraries, books, journal clubs, organized provision for reading and study, and cadaver dissection. Residents were required to attend conferences of the medical staff, but many of these conferences were unsuitable for learning.[7] Nevertheless, these deficiencies could be easily rectified in most of the institutions. The outlook for standardizing graduate training in surgery and its specialties was good.

The committee on graduate training had its first meeting in November 1937. They revised the criteria and the manual for graduate training in surgery for publication in the *Bulletin of the American College of Surgeons* in January 1938, a resource that stimulated many hospitals to develop residency programs. Dr. Harold Earnhardt, who was put in charge of surveying hospitals for residency programs, and his associates Dr. MN Newquist and Dr. EW Williamson, surveyed a large number of hospitals in late 1937 and early 1938 to increase the number of approved hospitals and address the critical need for more residency positions. By February, the committee on graduate training had 70 of the surveyors' reports to review for approval or denial.[8]

Nevertheless, the Committee on Graduate Training remained concerned that the number of hospitals qualified to have training programs was still too small for the number of individuals seeking training in surgery. To ameliorate this, the Regents changed the College's policy to read that applicants for fellowship who received the medical degree after January 1, 1938, must have completed three years of hospital service in one or more acceptable hospitals (rather than hospitals approved by the American College of Surgeons) of which two years shall have been spent in training in surgery in hospitals approved by the American College of Surgeons for graduate training in surgery.[9] This reflected the fact that in the 1937–38 academic year, only 31 percent of all residencies were for three years or longer, meaning that the opportunities to train in a three-year approved program were very limited.[10]

The College Takes the Lead

Malcolm MacEachern, with the approval of the Committee on Graduate Training for Surgery and the Surgical Specialties, began the task of recruiting more hospitals into the graduate medical education of surgeons by creating a "Graduate Training Number" in the January 1938 *Bulletin of the American College of Surgeons*. This issue contained most of the papers presented at the October 1937 symposium on graduate training as well as MacEachern's "Criteria for Graduate Training in Surgery and a Manual of Graduate Training for Surgery," which set forth explicitly the requirements for surgical residency programs,[8,11] MacEachern's long-time assistant, Dr. Harold Earnhardt, and his colleagues Dr. MN Newquist and Dr. EW Williamson, went on the road to survey as many hospitals as possible for graduate training in 1938.

On May 14, 1938 the staff gave the Executive Committee an article by Phemister, entitled "Graduate Training for Surgery, General Surgery, and the Surgical Specialties," which was to be published in the *Bulletin* and in *SGO*. In discussing it, committee members ruminated about the slow progress in graduate medical education. They noted that Allen B Kanavel, who was present and probably embarrassed by his mention, had presented a paper on the use of hospitals for graduate training purposes ten years previously.[12]

Kanavel's foresight and wisdom would be missed, for less than two weeks later this loyal confidant of Martin, Crile, and Graham was killed in an automobile accident near Pasadena, California where he spent most of his time. A founder, Regent, and President of the College, Kanavel also was for many years the associate editor and, at the time of his death at age 59, editor of its journal, *Surgery, Gynecology, and Obstetrics*. He was skilled and meticulous in neurologic surgery, and developed a novel approach to the pituitary through the nose, but he is best remembered for his expertise in hand surgery and his classic text, *Infections of the Hand*. He preceded his student and mentee, Loyal Davis, as professor and chairman of the department of surgery at Northwestern University.

For a while it appeared that Alfred Blalock's prediction that establishment of the ABS would create dire consequences for the College was being realized, because young surgeons blamed the College for the establishment of all the surgical boards. They believed that if the College's standards had been higher, the boards would not have been formed. The rumor was that young surgeons would not be eligible for staff positions in local hospitals and medical schools unless they were certified by the specialty boards and many were worried that their training would not be accepted by the boards.

Fellows of the College resented having to take the board examinations. They thought their status was diminished because young surgeons who were not Fellows seemed convinced that certification by a board led to a higher standing than fellowship in the College. Adding to the concern was that the Maryland Crippled Children's Commission, administered by federal funds provided through Social Security legislation, required certification by the American Board of Orthopaedic Surgery for all surgeons doing this work in Maryland. Young surgeons resented this ruling and blamed the College for it.

Many older surgeons who performed the gamut of surgical procedures believed they needed no recognition beyond fellowship in the College, and they resented the ABS and all specialty boards. Despite the rancor of young surgeons and the fellowship, there were no wholesale resignations from the College, nor did the number of applicants for fellowship decline. Soon doctors would worry more about the possibility of war in Europe than the College and the boards.

The College had other concerns about extending the training requirements. Besley, the College's long-time Treasurer, believed that in time fewer surgeons would seek fellowship in the College and the corresponding decrease in revenue from initiation fees would be distressing.

Furthermore, the College was spending an estimated $30,000–$35,000 per year to inspect hospitals for graduate training and had no revenue from this activity.

Dallas Phemister, chair of surgery at the University of Chicago and chairman of the Committee on Graduate Training, insisted on adding four months of laboratory work in pathology to the requirements, which not all hospitals could provide; a majority of hospitals did not have facilities and expertise for the required training in basic sciences. Specialty boards such as urology and neurosurgery required two years of general surgery before specialization and these residents occupied slots that were needed for general surgery residents. Phemister believed that residents would need a small salary to sustain them for the lengthened period of training. He saw this as a major problem because hospitals would have to find this money, and many were still reeling from the Depression.[9] All these factors restricted the output of competent surgeons.

～※～

More Programs Are Needed

By October 1938, 374 hospitals had been surveyed in 1937–38, of which 89 were fully approved for graduate training. There were two types of programs, one providing two years of training for residents who would obtain additional training in the surgical specialties, and the other for three years or more of training in general surgery, with increasing surgical responsibility and greater emphasis on training in the basic sciences. Nevertheless, the consensus of the Committee on Graduate Education was that at least twice the number of available resident positions was needed to meet the demand.

MacEachern reported that surveying the hospitals for graduate medical education was a much bigger job than anticipated. Hospitals were begging for accreditation. Crile worried that the program was taxing the personnel in the College as well as its phone system.[13]

The *Bulletin of the American College of Surgeons* published another "Graduate Training Number" in January, 1939.[14] The featured article was "Criteria for Graduate Training for Surgery and a Manual of Graduate Training for Surgery." This spelled out the flexible guidelines for establishing residencies in general surgery and the surgical specialties. Also included were the proposed minimum standards. But aspiring residents and hospitals focused on that part of the issue listing the 123 institutions approved for training and their 335 programs in general surgery and the surgical specialties. Medical students and practicing physicians had, for the first time, comprehensive information on where they could apply for training, and hospitals that were not on the list were stimulated to develop programs. How to do so was in the same publication. Also included were outlines of seven types of training programs culled from the approved hospitals.

Institutions interested in developing residencies could use these templates to establish their programs.

The publication of this timely information signaled the College's new and significant leadership in graduate medical education. The *Bulletin* had been sent to hospital executives for many years, and they were accustomed to reading it for news about the hospital standardization program. As regular readers, their interest in establishing residency programs was piqued by the information in the *Bulletin*. The new role of the College as the accrediting agency for residency programs was confirmed and solidified when the ABS notified the College that, with few exceptions, it would accept training only in those institutions on the College's list as acceptable for admission to their examination process.[15, 16]

The rapid expansion in the number of residency programs, stimulated by the requirements of the certifying boards, would enable the training of outstanding physicians and surgeons for the last half of the 20th century and beyond. But this professional endeavor was not without difficulty and compromise in its early years. For example, in Chicago some prospective residents, as a condition of their appointment, had to agree that they would not locate in Chicago when their training was finished.[12] Many hospitals were unable to meet the basic science criteria of the standards. They were asking medical schools for help, but their requests often fell on deaf ears.[15] Medical schools, especially state schools, were not interested in taking the lead in graduate medical education. For this reason, residencies became an undertaking of hospitals and remained so for many decades.

≈ ✳ ≈

Hospitals Respond

Hospitals responded to the need for more residencies. There was little downside, and their better graduates could be enticed to stay on the medical staff, elevating their status and reputation in the community. The process of accrediting hospitals for graduate training was not highly organized and it was not very thorough. There was too much work to do in a very short period of time. Many of the standards and criteria were arbitrary. At the College's Centennial, residency programs approved by the Accreditation Council on Graduate Medical Education would almost certainly produce competent physicians and surgeons, but in mid-century this was not the case for all programs.

By October 1939, 185 hospitals of approximately 400 surveyed were on the approved list for training in general surgery and the surgical specialties, an increase of 96 in one year. In all the surgical specialties, 1,606 residents were in training, and approved hospitals were turning out 580 surgeons annually. There were 81 medical school affiliations.[17,18] The College's best guess was that an annual output of 500 to 600 trained surgeons was needed to maintain the surgical workforce, so the 1939 production appeared to be sufficient.

Despite the rapid increase in the number of surgeons produced, some of the Regents and staff believed that the many of the new surgeons were not competent. Regent Arthur Shipley pointed out that the public was attacking the profession because there were not enough well-trained doctors.[19]

According to statistics compiled by the medical historian Rosemary Stevens,[20] in 1940 42.3 percent of full time specialists were board certified. Only 20.9 percent of full time specialists in general surgery, colorectal surgery, neurosurgery and plastic surgery were certified. Most surgery was performed by physicians who were not full time surgeons; rather, they were general practitioners who performed surgery.

The status of surgical practice prior to World War II was summarized by Dr. Mont R Reid, professor and chairman of the department of surgery at the University of Cincinnati, in his invited address to the AAMC in 1939. He agreed that the improvement in surgical education was essential to improve the care of patients, but he sounded an alarm about the existing state of surgical practice:[21]

> It is no secret that many of our hospitals countenance unethical and unsatisfactory surgical work because they are faced with the necessity of filling beds in order to bring in revenue. Some will frankly admit that they can see no reasons for denying themselves this revenue when the barred doctors will take this revenue to other hospitals.

He then recounted the story of a "brilliant young man who had just completed his training..." and went to a community where he wished to practice, where he was told that he could not make a living unless he was willing to split fees.

Reid called on all medical organizations to help regulate the practice of medicine, and concluded by stating, "This business of unregulated and uncensored surgical practice is a matter for serious consideration ...; the public is paying an enormous toll in the unnecessary loss of lives."[21]

Use of the new infrastructure for surgical training, put into place by the board and the College in less than five years, was brought to an abrupt halt by World War II. By December 1942, residencies longer than one year after internship no longer existed because the government had taken control of medical education. Sooner or later, the Regents opined, the country would be without an adequate number of surgeons. The problem was even more serious in Canada, which geared up for war earlier than the United States.[22] The need for medical manpower to care for the sick and wounded among the 12 million Americans who served in the war and the care of the civilian population at home became the predominate issues. The academic leaders and the leadership of the College either were deployed in the armed services, many overseas, or were too busy taking care of patients to worry much about education and training. The federal government boldly took over and controlled medical education, and medical educators yielded to the country's immediate needs.

REFERENCES

1. *Minutes of the meeting of the Executive Committe of January 9, 1938. Letter from ER Loveland to George Crile, December 30, 1937. In.* 1938, Archives of the American College of Surgeons: Chicago.

2. *Minutes of the meeting of the Executive Committee of January 9, 1938. Letter from JH Means to George Crile.* 1938, Archives of the American College of Surgeons: Chicago. p. 1-43.

3. *Minutes of the meeting of the Executive Committee of October 9, 1937.* 1937, Archives of the American College of Surgeons: Chicago.

4. *Minutes of the meeting of the Board of Regents of October 24, 1937.* 1937, Archives of the American College of Surgeons: Chicago.

5. *Minutes of the meeting of the Board of Regents of October 29, 1937.* 1937, Archives of the American College of Surgeons: Chicago.

6. *Minutes of the meeting of the Board of Regents of October 29, 1937. Exhibit D.* 1937, Archives of the American College of Surgeons: Chicago. p. 1-22.

7. *Minutes of the meeting of the Board of Regents of October 29, 1937. Exhibit C.* 1937, Archives of the American College of Surgeons: Chicago.

8. *Minutes of the meeting of the executive committee of January 9, 1938.* 1938, Archives of the American College of Surgeons: Chicago. p. 1-43.

9. *Minutes of the meeting of the Board of Regents of May 1, 1938.* 1938, Archives of the American College of Surgeons: Chicago.

10. *Graduate Medical Education. Report of the Commission on Graduate Medical Education.* 1940, Chicago: University of Chicago Press.

11. MacEachern, M., *Criteria for graduate training for surgery and a manual of graduate training in surgery.* Bulletin of the American College of Surgeons, 1938.

12. *Minutes of the executive committee meeting of May 14, 1938.* 1938, Archives of the American College of Surgeons: Chicago.

13. *Minutes of the meeting of the Board of Regents of October 16, 1938.* 1938, Archives of the American College of Surgeons: Chicago.

14. MacEachern, M., *Criteria for graduate training for surgery and a manual of graduate training in surgery.* Bulletin of the American College of Surgeons, 1939(January).

15. *Minutes of the meeting of the Executive Committee of July 29, 1939.* 1939, Archives of the American College of Surgeons: Chicago.

16. Stephenson, G., *The American College of Surgeons and graduate education in surgery: A chronicle of surgical advancement.* Bulletin of the American College of Surgeons, 1971. **56**: p. 1-83.

17. *Minutes of the meeting of the Board of Regents of October 29, 1939.* 1939, Archives of the American College of Surgeons: Chicago.

18. *Minutes of the meeting of the Board of Regents of October 20, 1939.* 1939, Archives of the American College of Surgeons: Chicago.

19. *Minutes of the meeting of the Board of Regents of February 11, 1940. Exhibit B. Graduate training for general surgery and the surgical specialties.* 1940, Archives of the American College of Surgeons: Chicago.

20. Stevens, R., *American Medicine and the Public Interest. A History of Specialization.* Updated Edition ed. 1998, Los Angeles and Berkley: University of California Press.

21. Reid, M., *The training of surgeons: Method in use at the Cincinnati General Hospital.* Academic Medicine, 1940. **15**: p. 163-168.

22. *Minutes of the meeting of the Board of Regents of December 13, 1942.* 1942, Archives of the American College of Surgeons: Chicago.

CHAPTER 9
The War Years

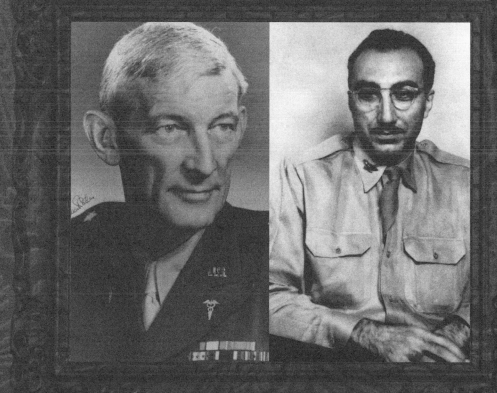

Finding Doctors for World War II

By 1939, the military was planning for war. The Surgeon General of the United States Army, Dr. James C Magee, attended the October meeting of the Board of Regents. Dr. George Crile told him that the American College of Surgeons (ACS) would be happy to put its resources at the disposal of the U.S. Army or Navy. Magee explained that there were currently 100,000 men in the armed forces, and the plan called for several million men. The 32 base hospitals that were currently authorized would not be sufficient; 70 would be needed. Magee said that the same plan used for World War I would be in effect. That meant that academic units would sponsor the hospitals and organize them. The authorities of the academic institution would then designate the personnel by name and position. Every staff member of a general hospital would be a member of the staff of the institution sponsoring the hospital. The authorized 32 hospitals at that time would be formed from the same institutions that formed the original 50 base hospitals in World War I. Magee already had many requests from medical schools, asking for the privilege of organizing hospitals.

He said he wanted to work through the organized medical societies to obtain information. He was especially interested in physicians who held reserve commissions because they were trained and could be put on active duty quickly.[1]

Indeed, the faculties of medical schools were assigned to hospital units under the command of leaders of their medical schools and hospitals. In this manner the army had experienced teams of experts in place to provide the best possible care of injured and sick soldiers throughout the war. Some of the young men entering the military after their abbreviated internships and residencies were also assigned to these hospitals, where faculty could supervise them and round out their training. During World War II almost all of the 52 general hospitals and 20 evacuation hospitals were staffed by medical school faculty.[2]

In the spring of 1940, Magee and Admiral McIntire of the U.S. Navy asked the American Medical Association (AMA) to draw up and distribute questionnaires to all physicians and to record the findings as a database for the enlistment and recruitment of health professionals for the war. Surveys were made in every county to determine the personnel needed for civilian health care. Every man under age 45 was subject to the draft under the Selective Service Act, including physicians. The plan was for the civilian population to be cared for by physicians age 45 and older and women physicians of all ages.

President Roosevelt created the Procurement and Assignment Service in October 1941 to maintain a list of all physicians, dentists, and veterinarians and their ages, physical condition, professional qualifications, and availability for service in the various military, civil, and industrial agencies of the country. The basis for the database of doctors was the information previously collected by the AMA. The Procurement and Assignment Service was the vehicle through which physicians under the age of 45 enlisted in the armed forces. They made their availability known to their state chair of the Procurement and Assignment Service, often through their local medical society, and they were commissioned in the army or navy by their local recruiting boards as they were needed. [3]

The Procurement and Assignment Service also made known the needs to meet its quotas, and this stimulated enlistments. Through the altruistic call to national service for doctors, the physician personnel needs of the army, navy, and the army air force were met without a physician draft. The depth of their altruism and the fullness of their devotion to their country will forever reflect glowingly on that generation of physicians and serve as an example for future generations.

The National Research Council, established by President Woodrow Wilson in 1916, was also instrumental in assisting the government in the early preparation for war and in promoting scientific research related to the war effort, such as research on shock, blood substitutes, and war neuroses. Approximately 220 leading scientists representing about 85 scientific organizations composed this Council; its Division of Medical Sciences was dominated by prominent Fellows of the ACS with Alfred Blalock as its vice chairman.

Wartime Education and Training

In December 1942, the army established the Army Specialized Training Program (ASTP), in which high school graduates who had achieved specified academic standards and scored well on an achievement test were selected for an accelerated college program that included military officer training followed by active duty. Most received additional specialty training prior to assignment to a unit.

Included in the ASTP was premedical education for two years, following which students competed for entry into medical school. The United States Navy's V12 program was similar. Students who met the requirements were allowed to apply for a commission as a second lieutenant in the army or ensign in the navy, and thereby came under the jurisdiction of those services, which deferred them from active duty through medical school and their internships. The army wanted authority over who would be admitted, but the medical schools refused. A series of meetings was held between government officials and the Association of American Medical Colleges (AAMC), representing the schools, which resulted in restoration of medical school autonomy in the admissions process.

Students drawn from the ASTP were paid $132 per month to cover both living expenses and the cost of military uniforms while in medical school. The schools were under contract to produce them as army physicians. The wartime needs created a remarkably altered medical education system. To accelerate the production of physicians, at the urging of the AAMC, medical schools compressed each year of their standard curriculum to nine months, thereby graduating each class in three instead of the conventional four years. Thus, a class graduated every nine months. Internships were also slashed to nine months. Half of those who finished internships were conscripted for army duty and the other half either entered civilian practice or residency training in a specialty. Half of those who completed residency were conscripted for army service and the other half entered practice. Residencies were limited to two years, even if they were customarily longer.

These changes in undergraduate and graduate medical education provided both the military and the civilian sector with the necessary number of physicians. This training model, which accelerated the production of physicians for military and civilian service, was known as the 9-9-9 program because throughout internship, the assistant residency, and residency, each year of training was shortened to nine months.

Some faculty of medical schools had been exempted from service because of the critical need for educators in the many institutions where faculty had been deployed as part of a medical school hospital unit. The government allowed deans to decide who would be deferred. Those left behind had to take care of large numbers of patients and teach the same number of medical students, but in an accelerated curriculum. They worked day and night with few, if any, days off for the duration of the war. Much of the curriculum was delivered by the most efficient medium, the lecture. This method of teaching persisted for years after the war until it was recognized that other methods, such as problem-based learning, were more effective.

Students had little vacation time and practically no time for outside activities. The schools compressed the curriculum but did not eliminate much material, so they had to learn almost the usual amount of material in less time. There was little time for discussion or for digestion of lectures. Students no longer had three months of vacation each year, during which they could work to pay tuition and expenses. It was for this reason that the monthly stipend was provided. The army and navy required military training alongside the academic activities, and students resented having to drill and, sometimes, to march to class.

Students were assigned to internships, and because few were available at those hospitals affiliated with medical schools, a majority was sent to private hospitals, where the number of medical staff members had been reduced because of enlistments and the draft. Consequently, interns were used to provide much needed clinical services at the expense of their educations. The situation was lamented by Regent Frederick Coller in his presidential address to the American Surgical Association (ASA), when he said, "Graduate training worthy of the name has ceased. After the war there will be 20,000 to 30,000 men educated inferiorly to those before the war."[4]

≫ ✳ ≪

The College and the War

The nation was still reeling from the attack on Pearl Harbor and alarmed by its proximity to the mainland when the Board of Regents met on January 18, 1942. Originally scheduled for San Francisco, the meeting was moved to College headquarters in Chicago out of fear of another attack. The Clinical Congress had been planned for Cleveland in October. Several other College meetings that had been planned for San Francisco were moved to Chicago. They thought the Midwest was safer.

Malcolm MacEachern, who was attuned to what the fellowship was thinking from talking to surgeons during his travels, recommended cancellation of the sectional meetings for the coming year. He wanted to replace them with "War Sessions," a series of 20–30 meetings between February and April in different communities that would focus on war wounds, wound care, burns, fractures, and other injuries. Most of the physicians and surgeons who were about to enter the army did not know how to care for military wounds, yet they would be expected to know how to do so. MacEachern wanted the College to assume responsibility for preparing them for military duty.

Participants were not charged a fee for the War Sessions. The resulting deficit was ameliorated by the generosity of several donor corporations. The Becton-Dickinson Foundation for the Advancement of Scientific Knowledge provided personnel, equipment, and projection services without cost to the College. They requested in advance that they receive no publicity for this. Deknatel, which made silk sutures, sent the College the same amount of money it would have spent for a booth for its technical exhibit, even though the College was not holding a Clinical Congress. This was representative of the generosity of the many organizations that supported the College, in part because of their gratitude for the high standards set by the Board on Industrial Medicine and Trauma Surgery, designed to improve the care of their workers, and the effort of the entire country to win the war.

Evarts Graham recommended that the College invite AMA president Dr. Fred Rankin, a surgeon from Lexington, to attend some of these War Sessions to explain his new job. Commissioned as a Colonel, Rankin had been asked to work in the surgeon general's office to take charge of allocating men with special training to military jobs where their training would be used to best advantage. Rankin's AMA presidential address in 1942 reflected the country's commitment to the war, which was shared by the ACS and the entire medical profession, when he exclaimed, "War is now our principal business; all national efforts are ancillary to its successful termination in a permanent peace by decisive victory. In this struggle the entire nation is mobilized and, as an integral part of its citizenry, the medical profession cheerfully and enthusiastically offers its all."[5]

Many surgeons were worried whether they would be able to perform surgery in the army, and others simply wanted information about what was going to happen to them. Another suggestion was to invite British physicians to talk about their experience with war wounds, which had been the subject of many articles in the British surgical journals. The Regents agreed to have a few of these meetings as early as February and "see how it goes."

The War Sessions program put together by MacEachern and his staff began with motion pictures from the U.S. Army and Navy with footage of the actual medical, surgical, and hospital activities in the various theaters of operation. Then medical officers gave talks on the scheme for triage and evacuation, and their experiences at field and evacuation hospitals. They included statistics on the number of casualties they treated, the locations of wounds, how they were managed, and their results. This was followed by a talk on communicable diseases as wartime problems. At lunch a representative from the Procurement and Assignment Service, responsible for medical personnel, talked on "Medical Education and Manpower Problems in Medical and Nursing Service for the Armed Forces, Hospitals, and Civilian Population." After lunch there were 30-minute scientific presentations, followed by a talk on the current and projected postwar programs of the United States Veterans Administration.

The afternoon program was concluded by discussions on emergency medical services in wartime disasters (civilian defense) and the role of industry in supporting medical services in wartime. A forum was held at dinner, during which participants and the audience interacted with questions and discussions ranging from wartime medical education to the treatment of specific wounds. War Sessions covered the latest methods of treating wounds, burns, and fractures. Speakers gave the latest information on chemotherapy (sulfa drugs and penicillin), aviation medicine and surgery, transportation of the wounded, and rehabilitation of injured soldiers. A parallel program was provided for hospital administrators, stressing the organization, facilities, equipment, and administration of the various types of military medical facilities, such as field, evacuation, and general hospitals.

Between 21 and 24 War Sessions were held each year from 1942 through 1944. Attendees were enlisted medical officers, civilian practitioners, and administrators of hospitals, the latter selected from institutions that had problems identified through the hospital standardization program. The College advertised the sessions by listing the locations and programs in the *Bulletin*. All the sessions were held between February and April. The program was similar for every meeting. For the staff, this was a traveling show for which they went from one meeting to the next. Attendance at each of the very popular sessions ranged from 750–1,500. Practicing physicians appreciated that they were not pulled away from their practices for more than one day because the depletion of physicians from communities due to military service had left them overworked. The War Sessions for 1945 were cancelled because of the extreme restrictions on travel as the entire country focused on the final push for victory.[6, 7]

Another educational effort was a series of Wartime Graduate Medical Meetings, made available by a joint committee of the AMA, the American College of Physicians (ACP), and the ACS. Committees representing each of 24 regions of the country developed an impressive six-hour curriculum for a one-day meeting consisting of clinics, demonstrations, and lectures targeted to doctors in the armed forces stationed in the United States. Most of the material presented was on war problems but some civilian disorders were included. The curriculum included sessions on burns and reconstructive surgery, head, spine and nerve injuries, malaria, digitalis, sulfa drugs, penicillin, and short wave diathermy and ultraviolet treatments. The meetings were held in areas in which there was a concentration of military personnel, but they were open to all physicians in the region.[8]

The College was not the only surgical organization committed to the war effort. In 1940, the ASA established a Committee on National Preparedness that made its services available to the Surgeon General of the Army for any purpose he desired. The Association devoted 15 papers at its 1941 annual meeting to a symposium on war surgery, entitled "Surgical Preparedness,"[9] even though the United States had not yet entered the war. A year later, the program featured a symposium on burns, inspired by the devastating burns suffered in the attack on Pearl Harbor. Subsequent programs were dominated by reports on treatment of war injuries and papers describing research on wartime issues such as infection, shock, and surgical nutrition.

A seminal contribution of the College staff to the war effort was the publication of an annual War Issue of the *Bulletin*, organized by Mrs. Marion Farrow, originally hired by Franklin Martin as a secretary, which provided all physicians with indispensable information about College activities and changes that impacted the profession, such as the 9-9-9 program for medical education. The *Bulletin* listed times and locations of the War Sessions and the Wartime Graduate Medical Meetings. The lectures and proceedings of the War Sessions were published verbatim throughout the war years.

Miss Marguerite Prime and her staff in the library and the Department of Literary Research compiled and published in the War Issue an annual, up-to-date bibliography of all published articles and books on medical problems in wartime.[10] (Figure 9.1) Miss Prime's staff took requests from physicians for information on specified topics, searched the literature, and sent the requester the relevant material. This was an invaluable resource to civilian and military physicians and surgeons; however, the staff was disappointed that they received many requests from physicians in the service overseas but were unable to get the material to some of them because of mail service problems created by the war. Three translators on the staff responded to requests for information from international Fellows.[6]

Another important contribution was a detailed curriculum and syllabus for interns and residents on the care of trauma patients, which was put together and published in the *Bulletin* by the New York and Brooklyn Regional Fracture Committee.[11] Each year the *Bulletin* also published the list of medical motion

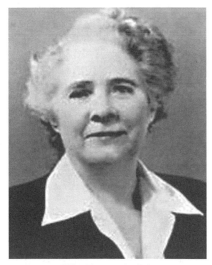

FIGURE 9.1 Miss Marguerite Prime, Director, Department of Library and Literary Research. Courtesy of the Medical Library Association.

pictures approved by the College, many of which covered war problems. They were available for loan to physicians and institutions.

The Fracture Committee, which met in January 1942, recommended the use of sulfonamides in open wounds even though no scientific study had proved that they were useful. The National Research Council was studying the question, and eventually numerous reports suggested that there was no advantage to this practice. Primary debridement of wounds, with secondary closure three to five days later was adopted as the standard treatment. Penicillin had been used only for research in the early days of the war, but its effectiveness prompted the development of techniques to manufacture it in large quantities, and it was used extensively.[12]

The 1942 Clinical Congress

Planning for the October Clinical Congress in Cleveland was around the war effort. The highlight would be a general assembly for all attendees on Monday morning, featuring presentations by the Surgeons General of the United States Army, Navy, and Public Health Service as well as by Colonel Rankin, representing the Office of Civilian Defense. Panel sessions dealing with subjects that are important under war conditions were scheduled. Because there were so few surgeons available in communities and so much time was needed for sessions on war surgery, no operative clinics were planned. Capt. Frederick R Hook, a member of the United States Navy who later was the U.S. Navy Force Medical Officer, South Pacific Area, was scheduled to give the Annual Oration on "Wounds in Combat."

Associate Director Crowell, increasingly aggressive in promoting his areas of responsibility, told the Regents that it would be a mistake not to put cancer on the program. He said, "Cancer will continue whether we have a war or not." (Figure 9.2) The Regents were unmoved; they saw that the need to educate surgeons in war surgery was acute and directly related to our winning or losing the war. There would be nothing to stop the College in doing what it could to secure victory. Losing would bring disaster to our country and to the world.

Planning for the Clinical Congress continued into October when Board Chairman Irvin Abell called a special meeting of the Board to discuss whether the Clinical Congress should be held. Already, 42,000 of the nation's 170,000 physicians and

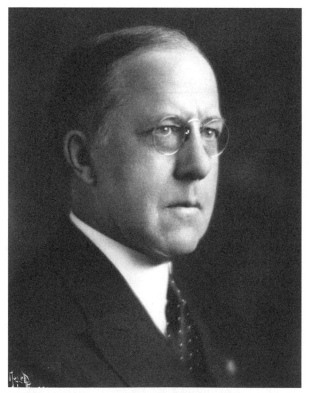

FIGURE 9.2 Dr. Bowman C Crowell, ACS Associate Director and Director of Clinical Research, 1926–49.

surgeons were in the armed forces, and another 18,000 were needed to reach maximum strength. He told the Regents that transportation was so difficult that he had been put off airplanes twice within the past month and had to wire Washington for priority to stay on the planes, an attestation to the importance attached to the ACS and its President.[13]

George Crile had wired Miss Grimm that he could not host the Clinical Congress in Cleveland, one of six areas in which large army training centers were about to be established, because the army had taken over the main auditorium in the city and the two largest hotels. The hospitals and doctors were overtaxed taking care of sick military personnel. He noted that the Southern Surgical Association (SSA) and the Society of Clinical Surgery (SCS) had cancelled their meetings.

Regent Henry Gradle said the American Academy of Ophthalmology held their meeting in Chicago. Of the 207 new men taken into the Academy, only 12 were present. The College would have the same problem at its convocation.

The Regents were unanimous in voting for cancellation—even those not present, who sent telegrams. Graham's telegram summarized the sentiment: "Strongly urge cancellation of meeting this year because of difficulty of travel and because nearly everybody is too busy to attend meeting not essential to war effort. I consider cancellation more patriotic then holding meetings."[14]

Because the College officers were elected and took office during the Clinical Congress, and recognizing the need for stability in the College leadership during the war, the officers agreed that the President, Vice Presidents, Secretary, and Treasurer would continue to serve until their successors were appointed and accepted. All standing committees would remain in place without changes in membership or chairs, although some substitutions were made for members serving overseas.

President W Edward Gallie said he was uncomfortable with this ruling because he was a Canadian, and did not feel it was appropriate for a Canadian to lead an American College during wartime. Irvin Abell said, "I think we would all take exception to your reference to us as Americans, for you also are an American. The bylaws specify that the officers-elect shall assume their offices at the annual session. Following their election they cannot take office, because the meeting has been canceled." Thus did a Canadian preside over the American College of Surgeons for five years, until 1946, when he was succeeded by the President-Elect, Irvin Abell.[13] (Figure 9.3) The Regents agreed to confer fellowship in the College on the initiates in absentia, but not on the proposed honorary Fellows.

Help for Surgeons in the Armed Forces

Throughout the war, men in the service who were applying for fellowship, especially those overseas, were having difficulty putting together their case histories, which the credentials committees scrutinized. In 1942, the Regents agreed that they should do the best they could under the circumstances and they allowed the local credentials committees to determine the adequacy of the list.[15] Later, they waived the requirement of a list for men in service because many had no access to their records.[16] These actions were very significant. The case histories were used by credentials committees to examine the candidates on their knowledge and surgical judgment, and were important indicators of their patient outcomes. In addition, the credentials committees collected information on the candidates' education and training, hospital appointments, and, most importantly, ethical standing among the Fellows of the College in his community. The College viewed this process as a comprehensive examination of the candidate.

This concept of examination was so ingrained in the College leadership that they later had difficulty understanding why the military services, the Veterans Administration, and even hospitals would regard board certification superior to College fellowship. It seemed to the Regents and College staff that the process for admission into the College was far more rigorous than that used by the boards to convey certification. It measured the full gamut of the candidate's qualifications, whereas the board dealt only with training and knowledge. Once a surgeon was

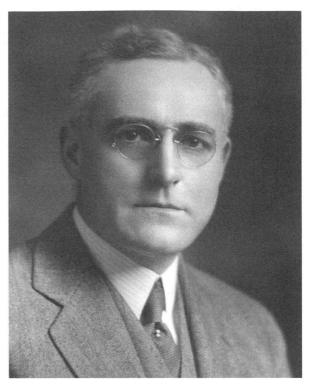

FIGURE 9.3 Dr. W Edward Gallie, ACS President, 1941–46.

admitted to fellowship in the College, he would have a lifetime relationship with the College; after an individual was certified he would have no further contact with the board. Although the Regents valued certification, they thought this lifetime relationship was more valuable than a one-time certification.

During WWII, the American Board of Surgery (ABS) did not compromise its standards except to give applicants full credit for the nine-month internship if they were serving in the military and to give one year of credit toward the required five years of postgraduate training to military surgeons who performed operations. Toward the end of the war, however, when military and veterans groups requested that the board adjust its training requirements for surgeons who had served, the board did not capitulate. Instead, it reestablished its prewar standards.[17] In addition, surgeons who had nine months of internship during the war, but did not serve in the military, were required to make up the three months, which was virtually impossible and eliminated them from certification.[18]

The College, being a membership organization dependent on the good will and happiness of the Fellows for its well-being, was more generous than the ABS, whose mission was only to determine the suitability of candidates to practice the art and science of surgery. The Regents waived dues for the year in which Fellows entered the military and during their subsequent service. They also waived the $5.00 registration fee for the Clinical Congress, a long standing irritant, for Fellows who were not in arrears on their dues. No analysis of the impact on the College's finances was requested or provided, a typical lack of concern about finances on the part of the Board and staff.

Back at the Office

Encouraged and supported by the Regents, the staff of the College was heavily involved in wartime activities. Malcolm MacEachern was at the pinnacle of his career. He was regarded as one of the foremost experts on hospital administration in the country, a reputation that led Northwestern University to convince him to start and head its degree program in hospital administration in 1943 as a part time undertaking. The annual MacEachern Symposium at Northwestern, established by his students and fellow faculty, has attracted outstanding speakers and a large audience even through to this day. To ensure the quality of the facilities for their workers, the Standard Oil Company asked MacEachern to inspect privately two of its hospitals in eastern Venezuela and in Aruba, and paid all of his expenses. Ever prudent, MacEachern sought and received approval from the Board to do this.[7]

The College had functioned for almost 10 years without a Director, and Board Chairman George Crile, who had functioned as a part time Director, was dead. The staff leadership had gradually fallen on Malcolm MacEachern, the workaholic, who willingly accepted it. Associate Director Bowman Crowell, of equal rank, devotedly and competently supervised the cancer programs and everything else that MacEachern did not. A humble man, he was content to remain as second fiddle despite his occasional crankiness. Fortunately, the personalities of MacEachern and Crowell allowed them to not only coexist, but to excel in their indispensable roles within the College, while working in a leadership structure inadvertently designed to create animosity and trouble. MacEachern was chairman of the Committee on Hospitals of the Procurement and Assignment Service and a member of the Subcommittee on Hospitals for the Office of Defense. He was also an *ex officio* member of the Allocation Committee of the Procurement and Assignment Service, a consultant to the United States Office of Civil Defense, secretary of the Medical Council of the United States Veterans Administration, and a member of the Special Committee on Nursing. Dr. Charles Waltman, who ran the cancer clinics program, had left for military service and Crowell assumed his duties.[19]

Under MacEachern's leadership, the hospital standardization program was expanded to include 94 military hospitals throughout the country, a major accomplishment in a very short time. In addition, the Veterans Bureau asked the College to bring 15 veterans hospitals, to be selected by the College, up to the standards for approval.[19]

By 1943, the number of hospitals under survey was 4,045, which was an increase of 258 hospitals over 1942. Of this number, 2,875 were fully approved and 378 were provisionally approved. Approval was denied to 792 hospitals. The four surveyors, all physicians, including one woman, were led by Earl Williamson, who had been MacEachern's first assistant in the program. They were on the road constantly.[16]

Care of crippled children using state or federal funds required participation in the hospital standardization program, as did maternal care for enlisted men's spouses; both types of care were instituted by several states. This added to the cachet of the program.[20]

Citizens were increasingly discriminating in the selection of their hospital. The standardization program was so popular that the impetus to be on the list of approved hospitals was frequently pressure from community leaders, responding to citizens' desire to improve their community hospitals. The College received many probing inquiries from hospitals and community leaders by letter, telephone, and telegraph about the ratings it assigned to hospitals. The public now knew more about approved hospitals than ever before; its interest in maternal care was especially intense.

The College was now a presence in the lives of ordinary Americans. In 1942 alone, hundreds of newspapers published announcements by or editorials about the College. Articles about the approved list of hospitals were published in 132 newspapers, and 1,810 newspapers published one or more articles on the 1941 Clinical Congress in Boston. Announcements or reports on the War Sessions appeared in 655 newspapers. *Time, Newsweek, Science Newsletter, Harper's Magazine*, and many other magazines published material related to the College.[21]

Miss Marguerite Prime, College Librarian, received a gift of more than 1,000 volumes from Dr. WW Pierson of Des Moines. By late 1944 she was two years behind in recording acquisitions in her catalog because of so many requests for articles and information from surgeons in the armed forces.[20] Everyone on the College staff was working at full capacity, six days a week.

Hospitals in Wartime

The war made it difficult for hospitals, in large part because of the shortage of physicians, nurses, and other professional personnel lost to the armed forces. The absence of young, well-trained surgeons put the burden of surgery on older men, many of whom had poor training or were general practitioners. Supplies and equipment were scarce because of wartime regulations for conservation, allocations, and priorities. Hospitals in some communities survived by sharing—for example, using a common facility for preparation of intravenous fluids, which were not supplied by manufacturers in the 1940s. Government regulations required recycling of all rubber products, especially gloves, because of a shortage of natural rubber and the need for tires on military vehicles.

Despite their administrative headaches, hospital administrators, like almost everyone in charge of something during the War, remained resolute and optimistic, as expressed in a speech by Arthur H Perkins, superintendent of a Newport News, Virginia hospital:

> Let me assure you that standards of hospital service can be maintained during the war if we remember to put first things first, to build high morale, to reward our loyal workers with pay sufficient for the increasing cost of living, and to serve the needs of our patients under a wartime economy which of necessity must cause us to trim our sails so that our ship, The Hospital, will weather the storm and be ready to go on with its service to mankind when peace again shall urge men to build and not to destroy.[22]

By 1943, a severe nursing shortage was compromising medical care at both military and civilian institutions. An estimated 65,000 women were needed in 1943 alone. Responding, Congress created the Cadet Nurse Corps program, which subsidized nursing schools and provided scholarships. The schools were required to be within hospitals approved by the ACS. Nurses graduated in 30 months and were expected to provide essential nursing services in the United States or overseas for the duration of the war. During the five years of its existence almost 125,000 nurses, including 3,000 African Americans, were added to the workforce, most of whom replaced experienced nurses who had gone overseas with the military. The 1943 goal of 65,000 was exceeded. Like many other organizations, the College responded by sponsoring and preparing a film, "RN--Serving all Mankind," designed to recruit young women into nursing, which during six months had 2,500 showings throughout the country and 150 copies constantly in circulation. The Cadet Nurse Corps, administered by the Public Health Service, was the most successful nursing recruitment and education project in history.[23]

At their meeting in June 1945, the Regents cancelled sectional meetings and regional meetings for 1945 and 1946.[24] Two months later on August 15, the Japanese surrendered after the devastation of Hiroshima and Nagasaki by the atomic bomb. Spontaneous celebrations broke out in every village, town, and city. The country was euphoric. The boys would be coming home, and the young doctors who had been snatched from their training and mustered into military service could make plans for civilian practice or additional training. Those who left practice or academia would return to begin again, many to face competition from their colleagues who annexed their patients during the war.

At war's end the major issues for the College were dealing with problems created by the returning physicians who wanted to resume their careers or advance them, and the threat of government control of medicine, which detractors snidely called socialized medicine. Nevertheless, the outlook for young men (and a few young women) in medicine was never better. Doctors were needed everywhere, and specialization would flourish. A culture of research, its beginnings stimulated before the war by the availability of federal funds, had grown during the war, and was to become permanently imbedded within the academic community. Investigators in all fields of science would have access to unprecedented funds, which would lead to discoveries that advanced their fields beyond imagination and gave them satisfaction and recognition. Physicians and surgeons in private practice would use the products of this research to diagnose and treat patients, who would look on their doctors as miracle workers. The outlook for surgery and surgical patients had never been better.

REFERENCES

1. *Minutes of the meeting of the Board of Regents of October 17, 1939.* 1939, Archives of the American College of Surgeons: Chicago.

2. Richards, A., *The impact of war on medicine.* Science, 1946. **103**: p. 575-576.

3. Seely, S., *Procurement and assignment service.* Bulletin of the American College of Surgeons, 1942. **27**: p. 159-165.

4. Coller, F.A., *The state of the association. Address of the President.* Annals of Surgery, 1944. **120**: p. 257-267.

5. Rankin, F.W., *The responsibilities of medicine in wartime.* Science 1942. **95**: p. 611-614.

6. *Minutes of the meeting of the Board of Regents of November 19, 1944.* 1944, Arcives of the American College of Surgeons: Chicago.

7. *Minutes of the meeting of the Board of Regents of June 17, 1944.* 1944, Archives of the American College of Surgeons: Chicago.

8. *Minutes of the meeting of the Board of Regents of June 27, 1943.* 1943, Archives of the American College of Surgeons: Chicago.

9. Ravitch, M.M., *A century of surgery. 1880-1980.* 1981, Philadelphia: J.B. Lippincott Co.

10. *War issue.* Bulletin of the American Colllege of Surgeons, 1944. **29**: p. 40-56.

11. Bulletin of the American College of Surgeons, 1944. **29**: p. 28-43.

12. *Minutes of the meeting of the Board of Regents of January 18, 1942.* 1942, Archives of the American College of Surgeons: Chicago.

13. *Minutes of the meeting of the Board of Regents of October 14, 1942.* 1942, Archives of the American College of Surgeons: Chicago.

14. *Minutes of the meeting of the Board of Regents of October 14, 1942.* 1942, Archives of the American College of Surgeons: Chicago.

15. *Minutes of the meeting of the Board of Regents of June 17, 1942.* 1942, Archives of the American College of Surgeons: Chicago.

16. *Minutes of the meeting of the Board of Regents of December 12, 1943.* 1943, Archives of the American College of Surgeons: Chicago.

17. Griffen, W.O., Jr., *The American Board of Surgery---Then and Now.* 2004, Philadelphia: American Board of Surgery.

18. Rodman, J.S., *History of the American Board of Surgery. 1937-1952.* 1956, Philadelphia: J.B. Lippincott Co.

19. *Minutes of the meeting of the Board of Regents of December 13, 1943.* 1943, Archives of the American College of Surgeons: Chicago.

20. *Minutes of the meeting of the Board of Regents of November 10, 1944.* 1944, Archives of the American College of Surgeons: Chicago.

21. *Minutes of the meeting of the Board of Regents of June 7, 1942.* 1942, Archives of the American College of Surgeons: Chicago.

22. *Twenty-fifth annual hospital standardization report.* Bulletin of the American College of Surgeons, 1942. **27**: p. 262.

23. *The cadet nurse corps 1943-1948.* www.lhncbc.nlm.nih.gov/apdb/phshistory/resources/cadetnurse/nurse.html.

24. *Minutes of the meeting of the Board of Regents of June 23, 1945.* 1945, Archives of the American College of Surgeons: Chicago.

CHAPTER 10
Who's in Charge, the Board or the College?

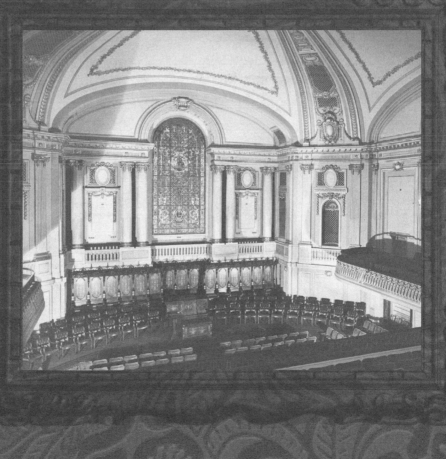

John B Murphy Auditorium

Their war was over, but not all the returning doctors found it easy to reenter civilian practice. Physicians who had stayed at home were correctly concerned that the "invasion" of their communities by discharged medical officers would heighten competition and reduce their incomes. An acute shortage of hospital beds already made it difficult for doctors to serve their patients. Returning physicians exacerbated the shortage, and in some communities the existing medical staffs dealt with it by denying hospital privileges to the newcomers, effectively barring them from practice. This added to the resentment the returning veterans had toward those who had not served and who they perceived had profited during the war while not having to endure the stress of battle and separation from their families.

Many men who had served overseas had not seen their families for several years, and some of them had never seen children who were born after they were deployed. They felt that those who stayed home enjoyed the financial fruits of their labor and had a satisfying family life without the stress or grief of separation and the poor military pay. To be denied hospital privileges was the last straw, and they turned to the American Medical Association (AMA) and the College for relief. Both organizations passed resolutions decrying this practice and asserting that well-trained, competent, and ethical individuals should be given similar opportunities as offered to established medical practitioners in the community.[1,2] Neither organization had any direct authority over local medical staff matters, but the practice gradually disappeared as more beds were added.

Board Certification, the New Gold Standard

Most of the returnees were not board certified. Either they were denied admission to the certification process before the war because the boards held that their training was inadequate, or their abbreviated training during the war made them ineligible to sit for the exams. Some who were eligible for certification were unable to take the exams because of their military assignment, and others simply had not yet submitted their applications to the board. Allen Whipple, as chairman of the American Board of Surgery (ABS) in 1941, had encouraged the board to lobby the U.S. Surgeon General to give board certified surgeons special consideration for rank and assignment. The board did not approve an overt lobbying effort, but several board members influenced the armed services to give ABS diplomates a higher rank and to assign them to surgical duties exclusively.[3] Many non-certified surgeons who enlisted were assigned duties other than surgery.

In addition to the Founders Group of 1,152, only 770 surgeons had been board certified by April 1942.[4] Many of the founders were ineligible for military service because of age, so those who enjoyed higher rank and better assignments were an elite minority whose status was resented by the rank and file. Their displeasure was an unwelcome, but obvious sign of the importance of board certification, and they resolved to obtain the requisite surgical training and become certified after the war. They became convinced that during their professional lifetime, the full benefits of practicing surgery might not be available to them without board certification.

President Truman signed a bill in 1946 that added insult to injury. The legislation gave board certified Veterans Administration (VA) physicians an additional allowance equal to 25 percent of their base pay. This created some bizarre situations. A newly certified physician made more money in the VA system than his chief of surgery who was trained before the board existed and had many years of surgical experience.[5] The differential pay by the government helped to solidify board certification as the gold standard for preparation for practice.

≈≈ ✳ ≈≈

The Regents React

During the Board of Regents meeting in April 1946, Alfred Blalock pointed out that the attractiveness of membership in the American College of Surgeons (ACS) was lessened by the legislation emphasizing certification by the boards. The Regents were beginning to understand that surgeons were focused on board certification, not College fellowship, as the marker of surgical qualification.[6] MacEachern, fanning the flames, told the Regents that the bill also qualified osteopaths to take care of veterans, and designated them as specialists. "This can hamstring the College if it isn't handled strongly soon," said W Edward Gallie.[6]

Regent Alfred Blalock said, "This is perfectly natural. Everyone is in favor of more training and the board requirements for training are stricter than those of the American College of Surgeons, and a more vigorous examination is required."[6] He thought it was understandable that the Veterans Administration would choose the organization that had more rigorous standards. He said, "I think it is going to ruin the College; that is, the certifying aspects of it. It has already been severely damaged. There has to be some getting together on that aspect (examination) if the College is to be preserved."[6] (Figure 10.1) Dallas Phemister agreed: "There should be a renewed effort to bring the two groups together and get a consolidation of them. As Gallie has said, it is ridiculous to have men go through two sets of examinations to be certified as surgeons."[6]

The Regents believed the process of admission to fellowship was a rigorous examination of the candidate. The surgeon's application was vetted by a local credentials committee, which verified his training and experience. The state or regional committee on applicants requested information from senior local and regional surgeons about the nature of the candidate's practice and his competence. Special emphasis was placed on his ethical standing as a surgeon and as a member

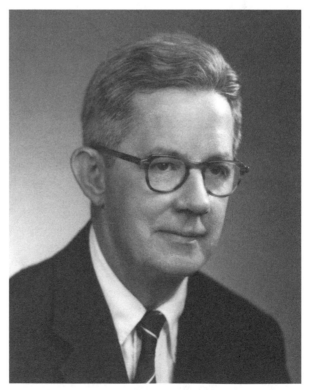

FIGURE 10.1 Dr. Alfred Blalock, ACS President, 1954–55.

of the community. Usually, some members of the committee were familiar with the candidate and if questions arose, they made personal inquiries to obtain an accurate, comprehensive portrayal of the candidate. Candidates were required to submit abstracts of 50 cases they managed, and at an interview the cases were used to quiz the candidate on his knowledge and judgment. Finally, the candidate's dossier was reviewed by the central credentials committee at College headquarters prior to submission of his name to the Board of Regents for final approval. Understandably, the Regents thought this "examination" by the College was competitive with that of the boards and even wider in scope, especially with regard to ethical standing, which the boards did not investigate. This contributed to their frustration over the growing appeal of board certification.

The Regents tended to overlook the less rigorous training requirements of the College, the local medical politics that sometimes influenced decisions of the committees, the variability of standards between committees, and the subjective nature of the "examination." These factors, thought by some to be flaws in the process, allowed some fee splitters and surgeons of borderline competence to slip through the process and motivated those who founded the board.

Seeking a Solution

Having brought the problem into the open, the Regents now began to seek a solution. Vice Chairman Arthur Allen said, "We are unprepared and have been shortsighted in that we should have made our qualifications for fellowship a little harder over a shorter period of time and by now have been in a position not to accept anyone who was not certified by a board. As soon as that comes about, the probability is that the power of these examinations will be given over to the College—certainly on the fundamentals, and probably more than that."[6] He erroneously believed that if the College would accept board certification as the primary criterion for admission to the College, the board would be willing to yield its authority to the College.

Evarts Graham declared that the College should set up its own examination if the board was unwilling to amalgamate with it, but Allen cautioned that the College should not compete with the boards. Blalock posed questions. "Why there should be two bodies? Why can't there be a fusion of them so that the boards take over most of the examination and perhaps we could put a greater degree of energy into the meetings?"[6] Vernon David, both a Regent and a member of the board, asked rhetorically whether the ABS would be interested in getting together with the College.

Malcolm MacEachern replied that the two organizations already worked together on hospitals. The board continued to use the College's list of approved hospitals as accreditation of sites for surgical training. "I would like to see us examine the men in the local credentials committees first and then let them be eligible for taking the board examination," he said, reflecting his belief that the College's process for vetting candidates was superior to that of the ABS.

The Regents now understood that the power of the College was gradually slipping away and the ABS was picking it up. They still viewed the College as an examining body. Their view that the committees of practicing surgeons should examine candidates conflicted with the view of the academics, who favored rigorous training requirements and objective, structured examinations by the academic elite. The ABS was uncompromising in its training requirements and its insistence that diplomates restrict their practices to surgery.

To swell its membership, the training requirements of the College were less rigorous and Fellows were permitted to do some general practice. The College understood that surgeons in small communities could not survive economically without doing some general practice, and in some areas the surgeon was the only physician available. It was better to compromise so that competent surgeons would practice in small towns and rural communities. The focus of the ABS was on surgical excellence, which promoted exclusivity, whereas the College acceded to the practical realities of community practice throughout the country, tilting it toward inclusivity.

For a half-century, fellowship in the College was the gold standard for surgeons. But now, the country was hungry for specialists, so young surgeons had opportunities to limit their practices to surgery in many communities. They were mindful that in the future hospitals would probably require board certification for medical staff membership. Board certification would secure their futures as surgeons. Membership in the College was a luxury, but not an essential. After a half-century of steady growth and increasing influence, the future of the College was uncertain. To the Regents, the situation was frightening.

They continued to wrestle with the problem. Graham, the foremost advocate for creating the ABS and its first chairman, said, "It isn't necessary for the American Board of Surgery to retain that name, nor is it necessary that they remain under the wing of the Advisory Board of Medical Specialties. It was put there originally simply because nobody else would have us."[6] He was not convincing. Several Regents commented that the board would never divorce itself from its umbrella organization for fear of losing its identity.

Blalock sounded the alarm:

> In another six or twelve months, from the viewpoint of credentials with candidates, I think the American College of Surgeons is through. I think something has got to be done and be done now or we will simply have an annual meeting and survey hospitals; and that is a most useful function, but the young men coming up are not going to be seeking membership in the American College of Surgeons, they are going to seek certification by the Boards.[6]

Regent Allen added that there were 4,000 returning veterans hoping to be certified by the American Board of Surgery. "That means that practically all the men who will do surgery in this country in the future are going to be certified by a specialty Board or the ABS. Any hope for the College has got to come from men who are certified in the future."[6]

Blalock then laid out a strategy, one that other Regents were reluctant to accept.

> Something should be done, such as making certification by the American Board of Surgery a prerequisite for membership in the American College of Surgeons. In addition to that there could be an examination by the College for ethics, etcetera. The College could also continue its educational activities and its hospital (standardization) activities and the examining part could be taken over by the American Board of Surgery. I think it would help both organizations.[6]

Most of the Regents were unaware that Graham had brushed protocol aside and invited several members of the ABS to meet with them. They were waiting outside the room. He had felt the need to bring the two organizations together before the war and had advocated this in 1941, when he completed his term as director and chairman of the ABS.[3] Graham sensed that now was the time to strike. He introduced the invitees from the board: Drs. Vernon David, Robert Dinsmore, Arthur Elting, Warfield Firor, J Stewart Rodman, and Nathan Womack.

Graham began by explaining that when the board was organized many men felt that the College had "muffed the ball." It was too easy to get in, and men who were not qualified were admitted. Those who controlled the College were not taking it in a direction that would appeal to the young generation. The board was organized as a "protest organization," he said. Nevertheless, there was hope that the two organizations would get together at some later time in an "intimate relationship." Graham reviewed the preferential hiring of certified physicians and the proposal in the Wagner-Murray-Dingell bill that gave military physicians a bonus for board certification, and the presumption that the same would hold true in the socialized medicine system that the bill, then under consideration by Congress, would create.

Many young men were writing the headquarters office to ask what the College was going to do about this. The Regents believed, he continued, that they will seek certification rather than fellowship. A serious decline in the membership will hamper and perhaps eliminate the activities of the College, especially the hospital standardization program. Graham said that it would be admirable for the group to agree to a plan that would stop the antagonism and competition between the two organizations.

Graham then proposed that the ABS separate itself from the Advisory Board for Medical Specialties and become the admitting board to the ACS. All candidates for admission to the College would be required to meet the College's prerequisites and present the certificate issued by the ABS. He conceded that the board delegation might object because some current members of the College could not pass the board's exam, but after a certain date the new rules would be applied. Graham believed that the American Board of Orthopaedic Surgery and the other specialty boards would follow suit.[6]

In the ensuing discussion, all agreed that both organizations were committed to elevating the standards of surgery. Frederick Coller, who had been elected to a six-year term on the board in 1941, pointed out that his committee on relations between the College and the board had agreed on several occasions that certification by the board should be accepted as the professional qualification for membership in the College.[3] He had been promoting this to members of the board for three years, but progress was slow. He had hoped that passing the first examination of the board would qualify the young surgeon as a junior member of the College, and passing the subsequent exam would qualify him as a Fellow of the College.[4] (Figure 10.2)

The respected Arthur Elting, a charter member and the immediate past chairman of the board, was called upon to speak. He began by saying, "I suppose my particular excuse for being here is one of antiquity (he was 74)."[6] He agreed that the ABS was formed because the standards for admission to the College were too low, and that it was hoped that certification by the ABS would be used as the standard. "In the early years there was so much antagonism between the two organizations that we hardly dared to mention this, but now is the time to consider it. The other boards have been unwilling to have a common, single basic examination before a second exam in their specialties so they are unlikely to amalgamate with the College."[6] He then proposed a committee of six, three from each organization, to work out the details of a plan to amalgamate.[6]

Regents Gallie, Naffziger, Ochsner, and Blalock agreed with Elting, but ABS member Warfield "Monty" Firor, a member of Blalock's faculty at Johns Hopkins, noting that this would be good for the College, asked what was in it for the board. Graham, struggling, pointed out that the board did not have the capacity to check on the qualifications of candidates that the College had; the ABS used only their academic qualifications. He said MacEachern had information that the College did not admit two surgeons who the board had certified.

Firor responded, "Out of a total of about 1,400, that is not bad,"[6] MacEachern pointed out that in the previous year ten percent of College initiates were not certified. Gallie noted that the board turned down some applicants because their training was inadequate, but did not counsel them on where to obtain satisfactory training. He suggested that the College could raise the standards for training programs to bring them in line with the requirements of the boards.

Dinsmore and Rodman, sensing an opportunity for the ABS to gain advantage, asked if the Regents were

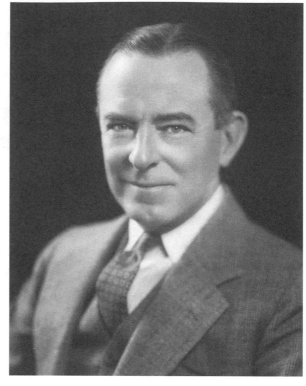

FIGURE 10.2 Dr. Frederick A Coller, ACS President, 1949–50.

willing to say that the only portal of entrance to the College would be through the boards. Abell and Allen, the chair and vice chair, respectively, affirmed it. Warming to the prospect of a better relationship, the group then decided to have Elting's proposed committee of six work on a proposal. As the College contingent, Graham appointed himself, Allen, and as chair, Coller. The Board appointed its chief executive, Secretary-Treasurer J Stewart Rodman; Samuel Harvey, and as chair, Fordyce St. John.

Committee Work

The committee of six never met, but the three board representatives met at the annual meeting of the ABS in May 1946 and developed a proposal for the full board to consider. Later, Frederick Coller, chair of the College's contingent and a member of the board, provided the proposal to the College's committee.[3,7]

The board unanimously agreed that the proposal represented the views of the American Board of Surgery. It read:

1. In the first place, it is felt that the American Board of Surgery has a real responsibility to the constituent societies which elected members to the Board and that therefore in a matter of such importance, no final action should be taken by the Board without referring that action back to the respective organizations for their

consideration and approval.

There are three members of the Board elected by the American Surgical Association, three members from the American College of Surgeons, three from the Surgical Section of the American Medical Association, and one each from the respective regional groups, viz.: the New England Surgical, the Southern Surgical, the Western Surgical and the Pacific Coast Surgical societies.

2. The difference in the fundamental concepts of the American Board of Surgery and the American College of Surgeons must be considered. The object of the American Board of Surgery is to determine what surgeons are competent both by virtue of their training and by actual examination to practice surgery.

Our understanding of the purpose of the American College of Surgeons is to induct into the College those men active in the practice of surgery, but not confining their work to that specialty necessarily, with the purpose of continuing a further education program in the field by sectional and annual meetings and other like procedures. (An example of this is the education program carried on in the treatment of fractures.) Furthermore, the College has been highly effective in improving the standards of hospitals, an essential step toward proper practice in itself.

On the basis of the policy of the College, some 14,000 men had been inducted into its membership. Only 1,497 of those men, who have been accepted into the College but who have applied to the Board, have been able to meet the requirements of the American Board of Surgery. It is but fair to assume that of the 14,000 odd men who have been admitted to the College, a very considerable number could not have satisfied the American Board of Surgery requirements either by training or by examination, or both.

3. It would be unfair, obviously, to the diplomates of the American Board of Surgery to depreciate the importance of the training and the qualifications, which have been required of them by any action of the Board which is directed in an attempt a fusion of different standards.

4. Notwithstanding the fact that the American Board of Surgery has made no attempt to bring pressure to bear toward recognition of its diplomates, at the present time an increasing number of the better hospitals, and recently, those of the Veterans Administration, are requiring qualification by the Board for appointments to their staffs.

5. Your committee feels that the great opportunity of the College of Surgeons is in the development of a continuing educational program. The obligation of the American Board of Surgery, on the other hand, is that of determining the adequate qualifications of one's fitness to practice general surgery. In principle, there is no

basic conflict in these two objectives and, indeed, to the minds of your committee they should complement each other.[3]

The committee's proposal represented the board as the source of standards higher than those of the College. It goes on to say that a huge majority of members of the College could not meet the board's training requirements or pass its examination, ignoring the fact that most of the College members were admitted to fellowship before the ABS existed, when there were no training requirements, and when there were few institutions that provided adequate training. Furthermore, most of the 1,497 diplomates of the board did not meet its training requirements or even take the examination, for they were admitted as the Founding Group on the recommendations of 60 medical schools and the seven societies that sponsored the board. The Founding Group was the elite of American surgery. The average community surgeon who was not a member of an elite society or on a medical school faculty had little chance to be included. The statement that it would be unfair to the diplomates of the board to attempt "a fusion of different standards" closed the door on any negotiation with the College about the "amalgamation" that board founder Graham envisioned. The committee then bullied the College by stating that the better hospitals and the Veterans Administration required board certification (but not College fellowship). Finally, the committee recommended that the College develop a continuing education program, ignoring the extensive continuing education provided by the College for more than 30 years.

The College's committee, Drs. Graham, Coller, and Allen, to which was added Dr. Gilbert Thomas, who was a member of the American Board of Urology, drew up a response that was sent to the ABS. The committee pointed out the different procedures used by the two organizations in evaluating candidates and concluded that the College's system was superior because the scope and specialty of the candidate's practice was determined and his ethical standing was elucidated.[8]

After the Regents heard the statement of the ABS committee, they discussed a written proposal by MacEachern[7] that would consolidate the two organizations' activities: Candidates would apply either for fellowship or for board certification. The application would go through the local and central credentials committees of the College. If approved, the board examination would be given by the board. If the candidate passed, he would be admitted to fellowship in the College. The College would survey hospitals for graduate training in surgery, including general surgery and the surgical specialties and underwrite the expenses of that program. Obviously, this would put the College in charge of determining who could sit for the board's exam.

Graham saw that this proposal would go nowhere: "The time is not yet ripe to try to amalgamate with the boards. There is a certain amount of antagonism based on old prejudices and lack of information."[7] He recommended that the College ask each of the six surgical boards to appoint a representative, preferably the board chairman, to be a Regent of the College. This would educate the boards about the College. He said, "This current situation cannot be allowed to exist for very much longer."[7]

Blalock did not think Graham's proposal would work because there was too much antagonism between the boards and the College. Arthur Allen then formally proposed that by January 1948, all applicants should be certified by one of the specialty boards before being accepted for fellowship in the College. He said, "This is a big step and it will cost us some money, but we will have to face it sooner or later. If we had been on this problem as we should have been for the past 10 years, we would be in that place already."[7] The solution that might save the College was now on the table.

Phemister spoke against it because given the slow rate at which the board certified surgeons, the rate of membership in the College would decline. Fewer Fellows paying dues would create a financial problem and reduce the prestige of the College.

Blalock continued to support the idea of certification before fellowship. The Regents were now actually wrestling with a solution and not just talking about the problem. MacEachern, representing the view of the staff, wanted the College to manage the entire process of certification and fellowship.

Lurking in the background was the understanding that the College had no leverage. The ABS was in the driver's seat and had no reason to negotiate anything. This was the College's problem, not theirs.

Finally, his proposal to elect board chairs as Regents rejected, Graham moved that representatives of the various specialty boards be invited to the next meeting of the Board of Regents as guests. They would be present when the Regents discussed Allen's proposal that made board certification the gateway to fellowship. Graham thought this would help to bring the boards and the College together in the "amalgamation" he had envisioned soon after the board was formed.[7]

An Attempt to Amalgamate

The Regents met again in March 1947 in the presence of their invited guests, the representatives of the ABS and the surgical specialty boards. They were Drs. Nathan A Womack, surgery; John J Shea, otolaryngology; Robert E Ivy, plastic surgery; Guy A Caldwell, orthopaedic surgery; and George F Cahill, urology. Regent Howard Naffziger represented the American Board of Neurological Surgery.

Regent Frederick Coller, chairman of the committee appointed to improve relations with the ABS, began by reviewing the history of the College and stated that the first specialty board (the American Board of Ophthalmology) was organized in 1916 and the most recent (the American Board of Neurological Surgery) in 1940. Meanwhile, the College's main activities were continuing education, hospital standardization, and advising on graduate training. He stated that the College was very strong and did its work through the Clinical Congress, the sectional meetings, fracture committees, and medical motion pictures.

"At the present time," he said, "we need make no apology for the College as an educational institution."[9] He pointed out that some years prior the Regents recognized that the standardization of surgery had developed along a number of different lines and believed that those activities should be coordinated, so a meeting was held in Chicago with the various boards. The meeting was interesting but not fruitful because of the multiple difficulties of getting action. The need for coordination persisted.

Coller reminded the guests that a year ago, at the American Surgical Association (ASA) meeting, some representatives from the ABS met with the Regents. Committees were appointed from each organization, but the two committees had not met. Coller, not wanting to affront the guests or create more animosity, did not mention the acerbic proposal of the board's committee or the equally caustic response of the College's committee.

The College has been criticized for bringing in certain members, Coller said. He felt this criticism was not as valid as it was years ago. The boards realized that their screening procedure was not perfect either. Not a few men who pass the boards are in other types of practice (in violation of their 100 percent surgical practice rule). Some people have applied to the College and passed the boards but are not eligible for admission to the College. In short, he said, the College has a better means of finding out what a surgeon is doing in the community and many of the boards do not have the capacity to follow through on this.

Coller related that the boards had been critical of the College's evaluation of hospitals, but the boards did not have the resources to initiate their own surveys, and the College would welcome suggestions. He said, "We now recognize the professional standard provided by the passing of a board (examination) as professional qualification for entrance to the College. However, the College reserves the right to scrutinize the record of these men and they might be kept out of the College."[9]

Although Coller's statement was true, the College had no policy for using board certification as a gateway to membership. The only benefit for the certified applicant was exemption from submitting case histories or a reduction in the required number of histories from 50 to 25. Furthermore, the published policy was that this special treatment of certified applicants "does not imply that the College declines to admit to fellowship candidates...who are not certified by one of the special [sic] boards."[10]

While their guests were still present, the Regents went on to approve a policy advancing junior members to senior membership on successful completion of the basic examination (Part I, now the Qualifying Exam) of the surgical boards. But Coller's advocacy for admission to the College on successful completion of Part II (now the Certifying Exam) was not discussed.[9]

The chairman asked for discussion. There was none, not even an acknowledgement of the Regent's action. The ABS representatives were not interested in giving any of their authority to the College, nor was there anything to negotiate. There would be no amalgamation.

≈≫✳≪≈

Learning to Live with One Another

The College leadership had been embarrassed and humiliated by the academic elite who formed the ABS. Franklin Martin and his colleagues on the Board of Regents had been out of touch with the new surgical academia, where scientific methodology was being applied to the surgical treatment of patients. Young surgical scientists were studying how operations disrupted normal physiology and how operations could modify the pathophysiology of disease to restore health. The classic example was that division of the vagus nerves to the stomach reduced the amount of acid secreted by the stomach, facilitating the healing of an ulcer in the first part of the small intestine, then believed to be caused exclusively by exposure to excessive acid.

The academics learned that the health of patients, including such aspects as their nutritional status, was important in preoperative and postoperative care, and they were studying methods to improve it. They were exploring the best means to prevent surgical infection, ranging from mounting ultraviolet lights in operating rooms to dusting wounds with sulfa powder. In many of these endeavors the pharmaceutical and medical device industries were collegial partners. Surgical scientists were developing new operations and making older operations safer.

The academic elite understood that poorly trained surgeons had poor outcomes. They could not understand why the leadership permitted less than capable surgeons to become fellows of the College, which purported to exist to elevate the standards of surgery. They could not countenance fee splitting or understand how fee splitters slipped through a vetting process the College leaders touted. Contemporaneous with the rise of the young academics was the aging of the Board of Regents and their contemporaries, and the general impatience and cheekiness of youth exacerbated the schism between the ABS and the College.

Although the College was officially supportive of the formation of the ABS, its leaders had reason to dislike the board. The board's founders did not seek rapprochement with the College, whose leaders perceived that they were the elite of American surgery. Instead, they simply formed the board.

The College believed the process leading to fellowship was a complete "examination" of the individual. State and local credentials committees collected education and training data on candidates, reviewed the opinions and recommendations of local surgical leaders about them, and interviewed them, quizzing them about cases, a process through which they thought they were able to determine their competence and ethical footing. College leaders believed that the "examination" of the board tested only their fund of knowledge and some aspects of surgical judgment, whereas the College examined the entire constellation of an individual's characteristics, including the quality and ethics of their practice.

It boiled down to a contest over who decides whether an individual is or is not worthy of the appellation "surgeon." The two organizations had different methods and processes for determining who should be a surgeon; each believed its was best.

Despite the best efforts of the College's leadership, the two organizations would remain permanently separate. Eventually, the Board became most effective in determining and measuring the qualifications of surgeons for practice. The College continued and expanded its fundamental mission of advancing the ethical and competent practice of surgery through education and advocacy. Neither the Regents nor the members of the Boards could have predicted that their failure to amalgamate, permanently separating the roles of the two organizations, bequeathed to subsequent generations a workable, some would say ideal, arrangement for surgeons, surgery, and the public. Although the roles of the Board and the College are combined in the Royal Colleges that had been established in the days of the British Empire, that model is probably precluded by antitrust law in the United States. The natural tension between the boards and the College stimulates these organizations to be creative, to move into uncharted waters, and to use one another's expertise to advance the profession for the benefit of patients.

The College's failure to gain complete control of standard setting for surgeons and surgery was a bellwether event, for it signaled to the College that working with other organizations would always be essential to accomplish its mission of promoting the ethical and competent practice of surgery. But before the turmoil between the ABS and the College abated, the question of who controlled the education and training of surgeons became another critical issue.

REFERENCES

1. *Minutes of the meeting of the Board of Regents of March 24, 1947.* 1947, Archives of the American College of Surgeons: Chicago.
2. *Board of Regents of American College of Surgeons considers delays in appointments to hospital staffs.* Bulletin of the American College of Surgeons, 1947. **32**: p. 149.
3. Griffen, W.O., Jr., *The American Board of Surgery---Then and Now.* 2004, Philadelphia: American Board of Surgery.
4. Rodman, J.S., *History of the American Board of Surgery. 1937-1952.* 1956, Philadelphia: J.B. Lippincott Co.
5. *Minutes of the meeting of the Board of Regents of September 7, 1947.* 1947, Archives of the American College of Surgeons: Chicago.
6. *Minutes of the meeting of the Board of Regents of April 1, 1946.* 1946, Archives of the American College of Surgeons: Chicago.
7. *Minutes of the meeting of the Board of Regents of December 17, 1946.* 1946, Archives of the American College of Surgeons: Chicago.
8. *Report of committee on relations of the American College of Surgeons with the American Boards.*, in *Executive Department correspondence, American Board of Surgery, 1941-1969*, Archives of the American College of Surgeons: Chicago.
9. 1947, *Minutes of the meeting of the Board of Regents of March 23, 1947.*, Archives of the American College of Surgeons: Chicago.
10. *Requirements for fellowship. American College of Surgeons, January 1, 1949.*, in *Member services. standards and requirements for fellowship, 1913-1980.*, Archives of the American College of Surgeons: Chicago.

CHAPTER 11
The Postwar Years

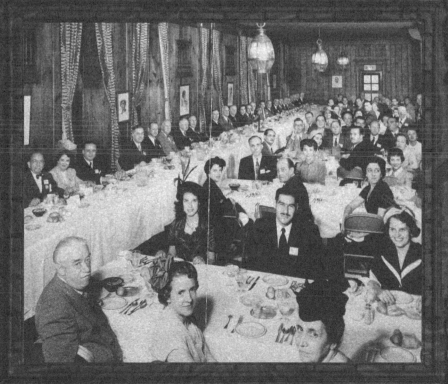

Inter-American Congress Luncheon, Chicago, Lake Shore Club, October 21, 1949

The end of the war and the return of the men and women who served elevated the mood of the country. The country had been mired in the Great Depression and World War II for 15 years, and the citizenry, especially the young veterans, were eager to create better lives for themselves and their children, which meant securing a good job, owning their own home, and having adequate and pleasing leisure time. They were willing and able to work hard to achieve these goals, and the country's industry and businesses were eager to meet their needs. Factories that had been geared for the production of military equipment and supplies retooled to make appliances, automobiles, clothing, and other items that had been scarce, unavailable, or unaffordable during the Depression and the war. Low interest loans for veterans stimulated unprecedented growth in housing and the development of entire communities that included schools, fire departments, and other necessary infrastructure. The migration of young people to Western states led to a youthful lifestyle and experimentation in science, education, social policy, and technology development, especially in California. Later this experimentation extended to the health maintenance organization (HMO), a new model for the delivery of health care, led by the Kaiser Foundation.

The Staff Struggles to Keep Pace

The return of surgeons to civilian life shook the College out of its wartime state of near-hibernation. Suddenly, the College staff was overworked because several key employees who had been called to military service did not return to their old jobs and personnel budgets were too tight to hire others. The hospital standardization program and requests for graduate medical education surveys by hospitals were growing, requiring more on-site surveys, coordination with the American Medical Association (AMA), and administrative work. The process of admitting new Fellows became more complex because so many applicants had been postponed by local credentials committees from one year to the next because of the war. The Central Credentials Committee, composed of staff, appraised the cases that had been repeatedly postponed and eliminated those who could never obtain fellowship, so as to reduce the workloads of the local credentials committees.[1]

Although Associate Directors MacEachern and Crowell were the highest ranking staff, they did not share the role of chief executive officer. The Regents, by not appointing a Director after Martin died, left them to manage the College, but without portfolio. Their duties within their respective departments took almost all of their time. MacEachern managed the hospital standardization program and Crowell all the activities related to cancer and trauma. Of the two, MacEachern was the better manager and much more aggressive.

But it was Miss Eleanor Grimm who saw to it that the publications were edited, correspondence answered, the officers and Regents tended to, and problems solved. Her long history with Franklin Martin spawned a deep devotion to the College that continued to grow after he died. Because of her close association with him as the College grew, she understood the need to maintain pleasant, professional relationships with the officers and Regents, to communicate with the Fellows respectfully, and to create a culture of hard work and devotion within the College for the benefit of the surgical patient. She knew what had to be done and did much of it herself, but she too was without portfolio to manage the College and its staff.

The dedication of its individual employees and the devotion of supervisors, such as Miss Marguerite Prime in the library and the Department of Literary Research and Mrs. Marion Farrow, the bookkeeper, kept the College functioning during the difficult war years. When the war was over, they had to work harder to meet the needs of the organization but they had little guidance. Crile's plan that the staff would report to the Board of Regents worked while he was Chairman of the Board because he made frequent, regular visits to the College, but his successor did not, so the staff had little direction.

The aftermath of the war created some unanticipated problems for them. They realized early in 1946 that the first convocation in five years, scheduled for December in Cleveland, would be attended by about 2,000 of the 2,600 initiates who had been approved for fellowship during the war years, in contrast to the usual 500 to 600. Although these surgeons had been admitted to the College in absentia, they had not had the honor of being formally recognized and congratulated by the College at the stirring convocation ceremony held during the Clinical Congresses, which were not held during the war. Staff worked through the difficulties of obtaining the use of a large auditorium and securing housing for the initiates. Then another problem surfaced. The Moore Company could not supply 2,000 graduation gowns because of a shortage of the velvet material used in their manufacture. Undaunted, the staff sent out a letter asking Fellows who had gowns to lend them to the initiates. The situation was so acute that the staff also asked Fellows to send in the gowns of any dead Fellows they might have known.[2] In the end, none of the initiates knew whose gown they were wearing, and all went well.

Postwar Hospital Problems

Hospitals had difficulties adjusting to the returning physicians. In 1947, MacEachern reported on the hospital standardization program and noted several ongoing problems. Graduates of non-approved medical schools were working in approved hospitals, and there seemed to be no immediate solution to this. General practitioners were being marginalized in hospitals and were complaining. Many of them performed surgery, but trained surgeons were gaining control and imposing restrictions of privileges on those without formal training, reducing their incomes. Some hospitals required that surgical procedures be performed by board-certified surgeons. The question of who decides who can perform surgery was a very contentious issue in many hospitals.[3]

Responding to MacEachern's report, the Regents passed a resolution that membership on the active medical staff of a hospital was for physicians and surgeons who are ethical and competent in their fields, though not necessarily exclusive specialists and diplomates of American boards. The resolution also stated that membership in the College and American Board of Surgery (ABS) certification were valuable criteria in selecting medical staff members and clinical department heads, but such appointments were not to be restricted to those individuals.[3] Again, the College was reluctant to lend its full support to the boards, recognizing that many members of the College were not board certified, and that the number of board certified surgeons was insufficient to meet the needs of the country. It was clear that it would be some time before more rigid rules for medical staff privileges could be applied. In 1945, only 251 of the College's 581 initiates (43 percent) were board certified.[1,3]

Recruiting Strategies for Fellowship

Nevertheless, the College acknowledged board certification as an indicator of professional achievement. Part of the power of the board was to set standards for training; this was enforced by requiring applicants for certification to meet the training requirements in order to sit for the examination. In this manner the Board controlled the standards for training as well as those for the knowledge required to practice the specialty. Shortly after the war, the College clarified its training requirements for fellowship. Applicants whose medical degrees were obtained after January 1, 1944 had to complete not less than one year of internship in a hospital approved for the training of interns and not less than three additional years in hospital service, which must include graduate study of the basic medical sciences as they pertain to surgery and graduate training in general surgery or the surgical specialties in hospitals approved for such training by the College. This brought the College's requirements in line with the minimum requirements of the ABS, and gave young surgeons a common training pathway that would lead to board certification and fellowship in the College.[4,5]

Many physicians who performed surgery applied to the College but were rejected by the local and state credentials committees. For example, in 1947, 489 of the 1,279 applicants (38 percent) were not approved by the College's credentials committees.[3] Only about 50 percent of the initiates had been Junior Candidates, an early affiliation with the College designed to make them familiar with training requirements and, through mentors, to provide advice on training and their progress toward fellowship. Junior Candidates were more likely to achieve fellowship than their counterparts who had not joined the Candidate program, but the program had languished during the war.

Newly appointed Assistant Director Dr. H Prather Sanders, a Fellow of the College who had been president of the Chicago Medical Society, revised the junior program, and included the requirement that Junior Candidates prepare an annual report on their progress in training for the Central Credentials Committee, which then provided advice and counsel.[2] This eliminated the sporadic and sometimes unwise counseling by mentors and centered the mentoring within the central administration. This greatly improved the value of the Junior Candidate program, and eventually led to other programs and strategies designed to engage residents and medical students for eventual recruitment purposes.[6]

The reasons that so many applicants for fellowship were turned down by the local credentials committees were related to the transitions surgical training and credentialing were undergoing. Before the establishment of the ABS in 1937, there were no absolute requirements for surgical training. General practitioners, who had only an internship, often made both surgery and obstetrics part of their practices, especially in communities that were underserved by specialists. Difficult surgical patient problems were sent to specialists in larger cities or medical school hospitals, but the economic incentive to perform simple operations such as herniorrhaphy, appendectomy, or cholecystectomy were too compelling to resist.

In addition, the ethic of the doctor was to care for the patient without fail, and many communities were served by a single general practitioner, who felt responsible for all the medical needs of his community. Some of these practitioners eventually limited their practices to surgery. Many had become good surgeons, but some were not, and the local credentials committees acted accordingly. The training requirements of the board excluded many practicing surgeons, who then applied for College fellowship.

Some of those who did not meet training requirements were acceptable for fellowship, but others were not.

Board certification or College fellowship was used as criterion for surgical privileges at large hospitals in large cities, but many community hospitals struggled to have enough competent surgeons to serve their needs. The granting of surgical privileges was a function of the medical staff of the hospital, obligated to follow the bylaws of the medical staff in the process. Often, these rules were not very specific and the medical staff was left to make final judgments about the quality of applicants. In some hospitals, the need for additional surgical help was so acute that marginal applicants were accepted; in others, more surgeons meant more competition, and only the most highly qualified survived the process. This process, akin to natural selection, widened the disparity between good and bad hospitals.

Although the College had streamlined its admission process, not all the problems had been anticipated. In 1947, Dr. Sanders brought the matter of Dr. Lloyd Irving Ross, a Fellow of the College, to the attention of the Regents. A Harvard graduate in his forties, Ross was admitted to fellowship in 1938 and paid his annual dues regularly, including those for 1947. After learning that his investment banker, Willard York, with whom he had entrusted $150,000, had declared bankruptcy, Ross ambushed and gunned down York, and his wife, son, and mother while they were on their way to church. He turned himself in, was tried, found guilty, and given the death penalty. Subsequently, he was declared insane and sent to a mental institution.[7,8] Dr. Sanders said that as far as he knew his only option was to report this to the Regents because, according to Section 7, Article III of the bylaws, before any action was taken by the Regents toward expelling a Fellow, 30 days written notice must be sent to that Fellow, informing him of the intention, so that he might have the opportunity to appear before the Board if he wished. James Monroe Mason, the southern Regent, said, "I think it would be best to ignore something like this." Gilbert Thomas said, "I think the only thing which should concern us is whether or not any mention is made in the press of his being a Fellow of the College." Phemister settled it: "I move that Dr. Ross be suspended from fellowship in the College immediately; this action to be effective until such time as further action may be taken by this Board." The motion carried, no further action was taken, and the matter was settled forever.[9]

Television at the Clinical Congress

In 1947 the newly appointed Regent Alfred Blalock, who held the prestigious chairmanship of surgery at Johns Hopkins, told MacEachern about transmitting closed circuit television from the operating room to 20 television sets at the recent Hopkins alumni meeting. He recommended that the College use this technology at the next Clinical Congress in New York.[10] The local arrangements committee there engaged RCA to try it on an experimental basis. They successfully televised operations to television monitors in the Waldorf-Astoria Hotel.[9] At the 1948 Clinical Congress, operations were carried by black-and-white closed circuit television to an eight-foot by ten-foot screen in a large meeting room at the Biltmore Hotel. The cost was covered by the *Los Angeles Times*, General Electric, RCA, and the Pacific Telephone and Telegraph Company. The College was learning to use sponsors for special projects. This was the largest and most expensive Clinical Congress ever, with 101 commercial exhibits, but no profit resulted because the registration fee had been eliminated to encourage attendance.[11] The College soon dropped the operative clinics in favor of televising operations with a voice linkage between the surgeon and the auditorium so panelists, and even members of the audience, could ask questions. Often, distinguished panelists bantered with the equally distinguished surgeon, to the delight of the audiences.

In 1949 and thereafter, the pharmaceutical firm Smith, Kline, and French sponsored the television program, which was in color for the first time and led to its regular use until 1975, when closed circuit television was dropped because of cost and the potential liability to the surgeon and the College if the cause of a bad result was documented by televising a poorly performed operation publicly.[12,13]

The Surgical Forum

The Surgical Forum, one of the great contributions of the College to surgical science and to young surgical investigators, was the idea of Dr. Owen H Wangensteen, chairman of the department of surgery at the University of Minnesota. An outstanding investigator whose residency program was very research oriented, Wangensteen contacted Dr. Irvin Abell, Chairman of the Board of Regents in 1940, about establishing a forum where young men could present their research work. He believed it unfair that the American Surgical Association (ASA), the Southern Surgical Association (SSA), and other surgical organizations did not accept papers from young surgeons unless the work

was done in association with an older colleague, who usually was required by the organization to present the paper. He pointed out that young faculty members in the basic medical sciences could present their research work at meetings of the Federation of American Societies for Experimental Biology, which included the American Physiological Society, the American Society of Biological Chemists, and others, but there was no organization that allowed young surgeons to present their work.[14] (Figure 11.1)

Evarts Graham, whose surgical training program also was research oriented, told the Regents he had proposed this to the ASA, which "turned down the idea bluntly and coldly." He said, "Surgery locks its doors against the younger man," and cited the German Surgical Congress, which had hundreds of papers on its program with a membership of only 1,500. He felt that a forum would attract younger men and make

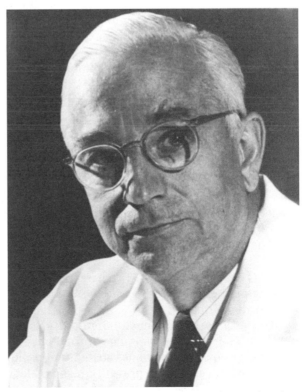

FIGURE 11.1 Dr. Owen H Wangensteen, Surgical Forum founder; ACS President, 1959–60.

them enthusiastic supporters of the College, a prediction that was fulfilled. During the discussion, Rudolph Matas, the eighty-year-old, beloved surgical leader from New Orleans, said,

> The greatest reverence should be paid to the child. The older man should have the respect of youth. It is flattering for a man of my years to be able to participate in your meetings here. I am flattered to be here and to share your plans and enthusiasm.

With this blessing, the Regents approved the idea, noting that the 2,000 Junior Candidates of the College could participate.[14]

Wangensteen and MacEachern met in 1941 and decided that three mornings would be reserved for Surgical Forum sessions at the Clinical Congress in Boston. They would notify the Junior Candidates and deans of the medical schools of the request for papers.[15]

Associate Director Bowman Crowell suggested that the Forum be called the "Forum on Fundamental Surgical Problems," and so it was until 1993, when the name was changed to the Owen H Wangensteen Surgical Forum in honor of the visionary man who had founded it 50 years previously.[16]

Wangensteen formed a Surgical Forum Committee of Graham, Alexander Brunschwig, who did basic research on the functions of the stomach and later pioneered radical cancer surgery, Coller, Mason, and himself.[17] They solicited papers from young surgeons through a letter to the professors of surgery at medical schools and received a surprising 150 submissions, from which the committee chose those that were presented at the Clinical Congress in October 1941. Presenters were limited to 10 minutes and there was no discussion.[17]

The Forum resumed in 1946, after the cancellation of the Clinical Congresses during the War. In 1948, comments and questions from the audience were permitted after each paper, and this tradition has continued as one of the most important interactions the College has facilitated.[18] Young investigators, aware of the famous senior investigators who would be in the audience, honed and practiced their presentations to perfection. Public commendation of their work and the quality of their presentations by senior surgeons exhilarated young presenters, stimulating them to continue their research. Less than stellar work was justifiably criticized, but usually in a constructive manner.

By 1949, the Forum had become one of the most popular features of the Clinical Congress. Sessions for the surgical specialties were phased in, beginning with neurological surgery.[13] Wangensteen and Loyal Davis pushed to have abstracts of the presentations published in a separate volume,[13,19] and, in 1951, Wangensteen proudly showed the Board of Regents the first volume containing the abstracts from the 1950 presentations, published by the reputable WB Saunders Company.[20-24] Mindful of his hard work and the popularity of the Forum, they formally expressed their gratitude to him.[25]

The Forum filled an academic void in the College and brought respect to it from scientists in other medical disciplines. Since its founding, the heads of surgery in medical schools have read the Surgical Forum program to see which institutions are represented, measuring their own in the process, and have resolved to improve the research activities of their departments.

Discussing the Forum stimulated the Regents to think of other ways to bring basic medical science to the meetings of the College. Graham pushed for having lectures on recently discovered hormones such as cortisone and estrogen, and vitamins, including vitamin K, necessary to prevent massive bleeding during surgery, pointing out that "sex hormones (research) is going along so fast we have difficulty keeping up with the progress." Crile commented, "We don't appreciate how outmoded we are by repeating ourselves year after year, and wearing out our welcome." In other words, the programs of the College did not reflect the recent innovations in science, and attendees were beginning to notice.[15]

The growing importance of surgical science led to the appointment of a committee on Nutrition of the Surgical Patient in Relation to Pre- and Postoperative care. Isidore Ravdin, Chairman of the Department of Surgery at the University of Pennsylvania, agreed to serve as its chair, and the membership included the young, notable surgical physiologists, a growing breed of scientists who sought to understand the biochemical and physiologic effects of surgery on the human body in order to ameliorate those that were deleterious.[12]

≈✴≈

International Relationships

Regent Howard Naffziger, the prominent neurosurgeon from San Francisco, was invited to the Philippines to give a series of lectures. Their surgical leaders had formed the Philippine College of Surgeons, patterned after the ACS, and asked him to facilitate a close relationship between the two Colleges, noting the close relationship between the College and the Royal College of Physicians and Surgeons of England. The Regents, undoubtedly influenced by the bravery of Filipinos during the wartime occupation of their country and the close relationship between the United States and the Philippines, decided to invite the leadership of the Philippine College of Surgeons to the next Clinical Congress as special guests, beginning an enduring special relationship between the two Colleges.

Naffziger said that after teaching in the Philippines he took a trip around the world and visited medical schools in Siam, India, Egypt, and Greece, among other countries. He said that most of those he met spoke English moderately well and read it quite well. They were looking toward America for leadership in surgery, and he proposed that the journal *Surgery, Gynecology, and Obstetrics* be sent to selected medical societies and medical schools around the world. Miss Grimm said that the *Bulletin* should be sent as well, and the Regents agreed to this after a discussion of the cost, which was minimal. These were the first efforts of the College to reach out beyond South America and England. Soon, these international relationships flourished, and positioned the College as the world's leading surgical organization, eventually with 33 chapters outside North America.[12]

Unfortunately, the College's longstanding relationship with Latin American surgeons was becoming rocky. The Sixth Inter-American Congress of Surgery, a gathering of surgeons from Latin American countries, was to be held for the first time in conjunction with the College's Clinical Congress, scheduled for Chicago in October 1949. The Inter-American Congress officials had requested that the College pay the expenses of delegates to the Congress. The College had reluctantly set aside $5,000 for this purpose despite grumbling from most of the Regents. They talked about how wealthy the Latin American surgeons were and that they were able to travel all over the United States and Europe with their families, whereas U. S. surgeons could not. Evarts Graham commented that the College was Santa Claus, and everybody was asking for gifts.[26]

Responding to the displeasure of the Regents, Miss Grimm and other staff members sought funds from the government to cover the costs of the Congress. They met in Washington, DC with the surgeon general, the State Department, the physician to the president, and others, but were unsuccessful. By this time, $25,000 had been committed to the Latin Americans. At their April 1949 meeting, Miss Grimm suggested to the Regents that the College have a banquet for the Latin Americans, with the cost paid by the attendees, except for the Latin American guests. Phemister, who was easily provoked, asked, "Why should we have a different banquet for them than we have for ourselves? Let them learn something by coming up here, and that is that they can get along without their Latin frills." Alton Ochsner explained, "They have been brought up on it."

Phemister retorted, "When you go to England, you don't ask them to put on an American dinner, do you? You take what they have." They voted not to authorize any more money for the Congress.[12] There was no banquet, but the staff hired interpreters to translate from English into Spanish and Portuguese, and a young woman was hired to interpret for the ladies on their tours.[27]

Problems with the Hospital Standardization Program

Despite the College's success in improving hospitals and the care provided in them, several ethical issues continued to confront the profession and the public. Unnecessary surgery, ghost surgery, and fee splitting were still commonplace. Evarts Graham, whose early small town Iowa experiences as an ethical surgeon in an unethical practice environment had sensitized him, asked MacEachern whether the College would know if unnecessary surgery was done in the hospitals it approved. He replied that the standardization program required that every piece of tissue, normal or abnormal, including a circumcision, must be examined by a pathologist, who was required to produce a written report that described its characteristics. For example, a removed uterus would be examined to determine if it was normal or abnormal. Hospitals established "tissue committees," consisting of internists, surgeons, and pathologists who reviewed these reports, and some of them used the results to determine who could perform surgery. He pointed out that based on the results some physicians were limited to surgery outside the abdomen.[18]

MacEachern reported that during inspections in some hospitals the field staff would pull about 100 medical records and examine them to determine, for example, if the hospital's high rate of normal appendices resulted from appropriate incidental appendectomies performed during other operations or from the misdiagnosis of appendicitis. He complained that this was not routine because the College could not afford an adequate field staff.

The performance of surgical procedures by general practitioners was a major issue, and the College received many complaints from its Fellows about it. Some hospitals were using fellowship in the College or board certification as a criterion for medical staff membership or surgical privileges but the hospital community was concerned that this could bring charges of monopoly from the Federal Government.

Coller and Graham urged MacEachern to require tissue committees for approval in the standardization program. Sensing that it might be supported, MacEachern made a motion that every hospital must have a tissue committee and mandatory consultation on every case performed by physicians who were not board certified or Fellows of the College, but nobody seconded the motion. This was becoming a frequent outcome of

Regents' meetings; the tendency was to complain about problems, but to take no action to rectify them. In this case they probably did not want to offend the AMA, whose membership included most of the general practitioners in the country.

Both the AMA and the American Hospital Association (AHA) were interested in accrediting hospitals. The AMA was already inspecting them for their internships and some residency programs, and taking on the College's program would give the AMA control over hospitals and presumably stop them from employing anesthesiologists, radiologists, and pathologists, which the AMA decried.

The AHA also wanted to take over hospital accreditation. Obviously, it would take control away from a physician-oriented organization, opening the door to reducing the influence of the medical staff in hospital policies and procedures. The College did not emphasize inspection of non-professional services, such as housekeeping and the dietary department, which hospital administrators knew were integral to the quality of care delivered. Furthermore, many of the postwar administrators had been trained in new degree-granting hospital administration programs, such as the one started by MacEachern at Northwestern University in 1943, and they were critical of the College's standardization program for its important omissions.[19]

The Threat of Socialized Medicine

Harry Truman, who as Vice President assumed the presidency on the death of Franklin Roosevelt in April 1945, espoused a national health care system during his campaign for the presidency in 1948. President Roosevelt had included national health insurance in the Social Security Act in 1935, but he soon removed it, fearing it would jeopardize passage of the entire Social Security bill. Thereafter, although he favored the concept of national health insurance, he never fully supported its implementation. Senator Robert Wagner (D-NY), a liberal Democrat, introduced an amendment to the Social Security Act in 1939 that would have provided federal funds, administered through the states, for a variety of medical services, but it died in committee. In 1943, Wagner, Senator James Murray (D-MT), and Representative John Dingell (D-MI) introduced a bill for national compulsory health insurance, but it also died in committee. Wagner, Murray, and Dingell tried again in 1945, but Republicans branded it as "Socialism" and support faded. Republicans gained control of Congress in the November 1946 elections, and while both parties put forth health care initiatives, none gained traction.

Harry Truman made mandatory national health insurance, to be funded by a payroll tax, a key feature of his campaign for election in 1948. During the campaign, Oscar Ewing, head of the Federal Security Administration, released a report documenting the poor health of the nation and the large number of preventable deaths. The report recommended mandatory national health insurance as a solution. The Ewing Report was widely circulated by the media and became the central focus of a national debate.[28] Truman's surprising victory over the Republican candidate, Thomas Dewey, and the election of a Democratic Congress alarmed the country's physicians. Most of them were members of the AMA, on which they depended to defend their interests.

The AMA made a special assessment for a war chest to fight what they branded as "Socialized medicine" and hired a California public relations firm, which indoctrinated the public at many levels, including doctor's offices, where pamphlets were handed to patients and the doctor discussed the "evils" of socialized medicine. The administration's bill, sponsored by Senators Murray and Dingell, was fiercely debated, but did not move out of committee despite efforts by Ewing to make it more palatable. Eventually the debate turned to a proposal to convert the Federal Security Administration to a cabinet level Department of Welfare, to be headed by Oscar Ewing, whose agenda would be to implement compulsory national health insurance. The AMA and its public relations firm went into action again, and the proposal was defeated in 1950.

Ewing then scaled down the administration's proposal to include compulsory health insurance only for those ages 65 and older and their dependents. This, too, was blocked by the AMA campaign, and Truman's efforts waned as he was forced to deal with the Korean Conflict, which began in June 1950.[29] To keep the ball in the air, Truman appointed a President's Commission on the Health Needs of the Nation, which was headed by Dr. Paul Magnuson, a Regent of the College and Chief Medical Officer of the Veterans Administration, where he conceived and implemented the affiliation of veterans' hospitals with academic medical centers. Later, he founded the Rehabilitation Institute of Chicago. Magnuson's Commission recommended a joint federal and state program in which the federal government would provide matching funds for those in need, such as the elderly and the indigent. The plan remained dormant until it served as the basis for the Medicare Act signed into law in 1965.[30]

The leadership of the College spoke disparagingly of the Ewing Report. Board Chairman Arthur Allen believed the profession should develop an alternative proposal, rather than simply oppose the administration's plan. General Paul Hawley, who headed the effort to unite the many individual Blue Cross and Blue Shield health insurance plans, had urged the AMA to support a national private health insurance plan as an alternative to the administration's plan, but the AMA declined, believing that the government would take it over.[27]

As part of its strategy, the AMA planned to send a resolution opposing compulsory health insurance to the president and all senators and representatives. They asked many medical organizations, including the College, to endorse it. Mr. Beverly Vedder, the College's attorney, recommended against endorsing the resolution because it was committing Fellows, who had not even seen it, to support it. Vedder was afraid that the Fellows of the College would not have a unanimous opinion about the resolution, and he believed this could jeopardize the College's tax-exempt status. He recommended that the Regents not support the AMA resolution. The Regents voted twelve to four to support the resolution. That they would be willing to jeopardize the College's tax status was a measure of their determination to fight what they believed was socialized medicine. Vedder pleaded with the Regents not to risk their tax-exempt status, adding that the AMA resolution was not well done. They capitulated and asked him to work with Dr. Warren Cole to come up with a better resolution.[27]

After a great deal of discussion with Mr. Vedder, two days later the Regents approved the following resolution:

> Whereas, the great advances which have been made in surgery under the stimulus of private enterprise may be impeded by federal control of the practice of medicine. Now, therefore, be it resolved, that the American College of Surgeons does hereby go on record as being opposed to the principle of the federal control of the practice of medicine.[19]

The Regents had been constrained from speaking out for surgeons by their agreement in 1935 that the College leadership would speak through the AMA on economic issues, and that the College would limit itself to addressing the advancement of surgery. Fourteen years later that principle was ignored over the issue of government control of health care, and since then the College has spoken for surgeons on many issues, advocating for their interests and those of surgical patients.

The College and Health Insurance

In the midst of the national debate over a national health plan, private insurance plans were gaining popularity. In October 1949, Mr. Frank Smith, director of the Associated Medical Plans, the members of which were the country's 67 Blue Shield plans, was invited to speak to the Regents. Each Blue Shield plan, which covered physician services, was sponsored by a state medical society, a county society, or a group of county societies. They functioned in 40 of the 48 states, Hawaii, Puerto Rico, the District of Columbia, and four Canadian provinces. There were 13 million subscribers and their dependents, and the plans were adding one million new subscribers every three months. Most of the plans were affiliated in some manner with the Blue Cross plan, which covered hospitalization, operating in the same area. The 67 Blue Shield plans generated $125 million annually, approximately 80 percent of which was paid out to surgeons.

The AMA, through its constituent state, county, and local medical societies, was behind the growing Blue Shield enterprise and nominated members of the Associated Medical Plans' governing board. But the interlocking directorate was disbanded in 1949 because the AMA was afraid of losing its tax-exempt status, leaving the Associated Plans as an independently incorporated agency. The Blue Cross Commission was a parallel organization under the auspices of the AHA. General Hawley was employed by the Associated Plans of Blue Shield and by Blue Cross to bring the two commissions together and to the extent possible, standardize the offerings of the various plans across the country.

Mr. Smith asked the Regents to appoint a committee with whom Dr. Hawley could work to keep surgeons informed about the Associated Plans and to offer advice. They wanted the College to speak for surgeons, which would make their communication efforts easier, and deflect some criticism of the plans to the College.[19] Regent Warren Cole said that it was insurance plans that would "lick" socialized medicine. Phemister emphasized that it must be "voluntary insurance."

Allen commented, "The College represents approximately 15,000 surgeons in the United States and 10,000 to 12,000 are really interested in this. They are now receiving some fee for the semi-private patient that they used to get no fee for, and they like it." He pointed out that they were using private patients for training in Massachusetts (he practiced at the Massachusetts General Hospital) and that the department of surgery was collecting insurance fees for professional services that could be used for experimental work or anything they chose, provided it was agreed on by the staff. The Board approved the formation of a liaison committee, and Allen appointed William Estes Jr, Chairman of the Board of Governors, and Regents Warren Cole and Alton Ochsner as the committee, with Cole as chairman.[19]

The Regents in their dual roles as doctors and leaders of the College hoped that private insurance plans would stem the tide of socialized medicine. The tension between advocates of private insurance on one hand and publically funded health plans on the other has been a constant since the enactment of Social Security, and grew to a head in 2010 with the debate over the "public option," a plan to provide compulsory health insurance funded by the government.

As the political battles over health care heated up, Regent Howard Naffziger advocated for hiring a person to be based in Washington, DC, who would serve as a "listening post" for the College. Several retired admirals were discussed as candidates, but eventually the Regents were concerned that the person would be identified as a lobbyist and jeopardize the College's tax-exempt status. Despite the increasing influence of politicians in the health care system, the College was not yet able to get beyond its role as a professional organization dedicated to surgeons and quality surgical practice. The tension between behaving like a professional organization and a trade organization has pervaded the College ever since.[31-33]

The Looming Financial Crisis

Mr. Edward G Sandrok, described at age 32 as "a man who had wide experience in business and accounting," was hired as the College's controller in 1945.[34] He had been an auditor and senior investment analyst for the Continental Illinois National Bank and Trust Company in Chicago. Many Fellows were excused from dues during the Depression, and those who served overseas during World War II were also excused. Sandrok immediately went to work to collect dues, and by 1947 almost all of the 8,000 dues-paying Fellows were current. Nevertheless, he recognized and reported to the Regents that the income of the College, which was essentially fixed, was no longer adequate to meet the expenses.[3] (Figure 11.2)

The expenditures were escalating, yet most of them seemed absolutely necessary. Pension plans were established for the eight senior College staff in 1945. Because of the Great Depression, the salaries of Miss Grimm and Dr. Bowman Crowell had been reduced in 1932, and were not restored until 1945. Obviously, this was not a frivolous expenditure. Their willingness to work at reduced salaries for 14 years was a testimony to the extraordinary devotion of Grimm and Crowell to the College and their work. No other example is needed to demonstrate the change in relationships between employer and employee during the past half-century.

Naffziger, then in his thirteenth year as a Regent, complained that more than 97 percent of College funds were in bonds, noting that most

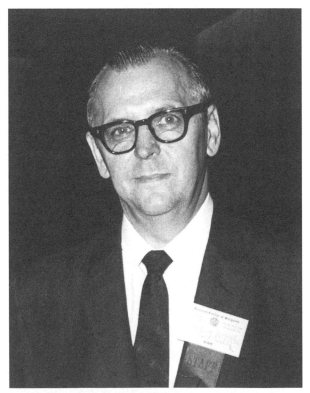

FIGURE 11.2 Mr. Edward G Sandrok, Assistant Director and Controller, 1951–67.

universities had begun to invest in equities.[35] His concern drew no attention. Prior to Sandrok's arrival, there was no analysis of the financial impact of actions by the Board of Regents. Furthermore, the Regents did not respond to Sandrok's warnings; instead, they gave themselves reimbursement for travel, and a ten dollar per diem for attendance at College meetings, later raised to $20.[36] The Regents approved a new lunchroom for the College staff and a plan to rewire the facilities. They also approved a recommendation from the finance committee for a Christmas bonus, not to exceed $25, for each member of the staff.

MacEachern told the Regents that he was short on field staff and office staff. He suggested a $5 million fundraising campaign to meet the needs of the College.[11] This was considered by an external consultant, who concluded a year later that raising that amount of money was not feasible.[33]

The fundamental problem was that the College's revenue consisted almost exclusively of dues, which were static, while the College was constantly taking on costly programs that generated no revenue. The brash Wangensteen, present only because he was chair of the Surgical Forum Committee, told the Regents that the inspection and approval of hospitals should be paid for by the hospitals. He said, "We are putting too much money in that and nothing is coming back."

MacEachern pointed out that charging hospitals has been discussed before. He believed strongly that not charging enabled the College to be independent in its judgments. MacEachern believed that the board should try to get the money from a foundation.

Wangensteen's comments represented the opinion of young surgeons: the College was spending too much money on hospital standardization and not doing much of anything for the fellowship. Even before he was brought on as a Regent in 1950, Wangensteen asserted that the College should improve and expand its programs, and "encourage the interest and have the interest of every man in surgery in this country." Board Chairman Allen, the elder statesman, responded that it was primarily a question of money and facilities. Alton Ochsner reinforced the fact that there was not enough money to do everything the College wanted to do.[19]

From the beginning, the Regents and the staff had been wedded to the increasingly expensive hospital standardization program. Because of it, they had seen spectacular improvement in the quality of surgery and of medicine in general. Jettisoning it was unthinkable, but it was clear that the College could not sustain it.

≈✳≈

Hitting Bottom

To the College leadership, everything seemed to be changing in the late 1940s. Illustrious leaders and staff who were guiding lights for many years passed away, including Dr. John Jennings, who had been a Regent for fourteen years, and Dr. Frederic Besley, a former President and the long-time Secretary of the College. From nearby Waukegan, Illinois, Besley attended all the meetings of the Administrative Group after his close friend Franklin Martin died. As a practicing surgeon, his advice and counsel to the staff was invaluable. Dr. EW Williamson, who had worked at the College for 28 years, and was the senior hospital inspector in the hospital standardizations program, died suddenly on a train after attending a credentials committee meeting in Kansas.[31] Dr. Fraser Gurd, a Canadian Regent, died on the train in Chicago after adjournment of a meeting of the Board of Regents at the College in 1948. Mr. Albert D Ballou, general manager of the Surgical Publishing Company, from 1907 to his retirement in 1945, died in 1949.[34] The company published the College's journal, *Surgery, Gynecology, and Obstetrics*. Dr. Charles R Reynolds, a valuable staff member who had been surgeon general of the United States during the 1930s, retired in 1948,[37] and Mrs. Marion T Farrow, executive secretary, who was with the College since its organizational meeting, retired in 1945.

Dr. Bowman Crowell, who with Dr. Malcolm MacEachern was associate director of the College, took a leave of absence because of illness from January through April 1949 and retired in November of the same year.[19,38] He was hired by Martin in 1926 and served the College for 23 years. He died in 1951 at age 72.

The College, like most institutions, did not make much forward progress during World War II. Other than those related to the war effort, no new programs were initiated. The Regents were not fully engaged, and the most visible and exciting College event, the Clinical Congress, was not held. After the war, the surgical environment became more complex and difficult. Board certification was seemingly more important to young surgeons than College fellowship. The surgical specialties and subspecialties were establishing their own societies and educational forums. The AMA was attempting to monopolize the inspection of hospitals for residency training programs. The American Boards of Surgery and Orthopaedic Surgery complained that the College's surveys of hospitals for residency programs were not done well, giving rise to the fear that the College's program was in jeopardy. Socialized medicine was on the federal government's agenda, and the popularity of health insurance was putting insurance companies between doctors and their patients. The College was gradually losing its preeminent position as the arbiter of all things surgical as the external environment changed, and there seemed to be nothing the College could do to change the course of events.

Internally, the leaders of the staff had grown old, retired, or died.[32] From 1946 onward, meetings of the Regents were increasingly unfocused, with more and more irrelevant discussion and fewer decisions. The Board Chairman, Irvin Abell, in his early seventies, had difficulty keeping the discussion on track and moving the agenda along. Several Regents complained that there was insufficient time at their meetings to get the business of the College done. The appendix to the agenda had grown to almost two inches in thickness, and was not sent out in advance.[26]

The Regents spent too much time discussing matters that staff should have handled. Often, Miss Grimm had to step in to correct inaccuracies or to review the history of an issue so that the discussion would be relevant.[37] MacEachern clearly was not functioning as a leader, nor was he getting direction from the Board Chair. He seemed to be overwhelmed.

As external events chipped away at the prestige of the College, its internal problems prevented it from responding and charting a new course. Suddenly, the decision of the Regents in 1935 not to hire a Director after Martin's death was having serious consequences. As associate Directors, neither MacEachern nor Crowell had the authority to chart the course of the College, nor were either of them capable of doing so. They were consummate staff members, but not visionaries or charismatic leaders. And now Crowell was retired, leaving MacEachern as the leader without portfolio. The younger Regents had little confidence in him, and those who were older no longer had high expectations of him.

Irvin Abell, Chairman of the Board of Regents, died suddenly on August 28, 1949, at age 72. He had served as Chair for ten years, having succeeded George Crile, as the second Board Chair in the 36-year history of the College. This was the lowest point in the history of the College.

Two months later the Regents met to elect a new Board Chairman. Arthur "Jimmy" Allen, who had been Vice Chairman of the Board of Regents for 10 years and a member of the Board for 12 years, seemed to be the logical choice. A Kentuckian, he received his medical degree from Johns Hopkins and his surgical training under George Brewster at the Massachusetts General Hospital, where he practiced and taught for his entire career. In 1936 he was named Chief of the East Surgical Service there and because of his uncanny judgment and superior technical skills, was called on to operate on large numbers of patients, including many physicians. His friend Gordon Gordon-Taylor said he "radiated happiness and kindness."[39] Alton Ochsner, who served with him as a Regent, said about him: "He was an extremely kind person, had a rare sense of humor, and had a faculty of expressing himself in the most lucid and pleasing manner.[40]

The Regents also thought that Jimmy Allen would be able to devote the necessary time to the College, given that he had retired from surgery a year earlier.[41] But when nominated on Monday, October 18, he demurred, stating that Boston was a long way from Chicago and the College would be better off with a Chicago person. Graham asked to postpone the election until Friday, but Miss Grimm reminded him that the bylaws required action then and there. They agreed to suspend the bylaws until Allen could discuss his issues with the nominating committee, and then made him temporary chairman.[27]

But Arthur Allen and some of his colleagues on the Board had another agenda. Allen recognized that the College had no leader. He had been a Regent when Crile was Chairman of the Board, and saw how Crile met with the staff in Chicago on a regular basis. Although the Director General, Franklin Martin, was dead, Crile functioned as the director of the College. Crile was never given this title, nor did he seek it, but he listed himself as the "Director, American College of Surgeons" in his biography.[42] Abell did not function as the director or even spend much time in Chicago. Given the problems facing the College and its fellowship, Allen knew that a full-time director, as well as a strong Board chair would be needed to get the organization back on track. After accepting the temporary chairmanship, he announced that he wanted the meeting to end in time for him to have dinner with Dr. and Mrs. Loyal Davis and General Paul Hawley at the Casino Club, a few blocks away. Although there are no records of the dinner conversation, Davis and Allen clearly were recruiting Hawley to be the director.[43]

But what about MacEachern, who had given his entire professional life to the College? Bowman Crowell had announced his retirement, so MacEachern expected to be named the director. Although there is no record of how it transpired, MacEachern was named Director of the ACS on October 22, 1949, even as Allen was recruiting Paul Hawley for the position.[44]

At the Board meeting six weeks later Arthur Allen, now the permanent Chairman, announced,

> We have obtained the services of Dr. Paul R Hawley to come to the College when he can terminate his commitments with the Blue Shield commission. It was not possible, for reasons beyond our control or which we felt were beyond our control, to give Dr. MacEachern the sort of position we think he should have had, namely director of the American College of Surgeons. I think everyone understands, and Dr. MacEachern understands it. Time has gone on too long, and we have been very remiss in our duty as Regents not to have found a way out of that situation, even though it did not seem possible. Dr. Abell did not think it possible to do it. We have gone along with a dual control [MacEachern and Crowell], and that the organization could run and could have accomplished anything, shows that the people involved with the peacemakers and

the administrative board have done a very outstanding job, and they think this is the time to mention it. The Regents are widely scattered and they have about four meetings a year. The only time they are informed concerning the central office is through the literature that comes as a result of the administrative board meetings, occasional letters, telephone calls, etc. This means a loosely tied together organization, which I am sure cannot go on indefinitely. It seemed to the Regents that the very best way we could handle the situation was to get a fresh start by bringing in a complete outsider with nationally known executive ability, and who would with the help of the people now in the College see if we could not perhaps attain a more firm footing. The Regents know the whole story, and Dr. MacEachern knows the whole story, and Miss Grimm knows the whole story. Dr. MacEachern has been fine about the whole subject. The only satisfaction we could get was to make him director of the College during the intervening months, so that he could retire from the College with a dignified title. .... Dr. Hawley said he fully appreciates how important Dr. MacEachern is to the organization. I am sure they will get on well together ... we hope this change is going to make for happiness and proper coordination in the administrative group and turn out to be the sort of change that we believe is essential at this time. I know the Regents have talked this over and mulled over the possible effect on Dr. MacEachern, and that has worried us no end. I am sure it is for the best interest of the College. It is never possible to make radical changes without having it hurt someone. It is a dreadful thing that we have been so derelict in not correcting Dr. MacEachern's situation before. But it did not seem to some to be possible. It is wonderful the way Dr. MacEachern has taken this. I know he will do all he can for the College as long as he can, and I know that goes for Miss Grimm, too.[13]

In his sorrowful, but hopeful discourse, Allen demonstrated the qualities he would use to lead the College out of its predicament: honesty, clarity of thought, compassion, resolve, optimism, and vision. His first move was to hire Paul Hawley.

REFERENCES

1. *Complete Minutes of the meeting of the Board of Regents of November 30, 1945.* 1945, Archives of the American College of Surgeons: Chicago.
2. *Minutes of the meeting of the Board of Regents of April 1, 1946.* 1946, Archives of the American College of Surgeons: Chicago.
3. *Minutes of the meeting of the Board of Regents of September 7, 1947.* 1947, Archives of the American College of Surgeons: Chicago.
4. *Complete minutes of the meeting of the Board of Regents of December 17, 1946.* 1946, Archives of the American College of Surgeons: Chicago.
5. *Complete minutes of the meeting of the Board of Regents of September 6, 1947.* 1947, Archives of the American College of Surgeons: Chicago.
6. *Minutes of the meeting of the Board of Regents of December 15, 1946.* 1946, Archives of the American College of Surgeons: Chicago.
7. *Crime: Entranced,* in *Time* 1947.
8. James, L., *Letter box,* in *Clews. Your home for historic true crime.* August 17, 2006.
9. *Complete minutes of the meeting of the Board of Regents of December 15, 1947.* 1947, Archives of the American College of Surgeons: Chicago.
10. *Complete minutes of the meeting of the Board of Regents of March 24, 1947.* 1947, Archives of the American College of Surgeons: Chicago.
11. *Minutes of the meeting of the Board of Regents of October 16, 1948.* 1948, Archives of the American College of Surgeons: Chicago.
12. *Complete minutes of the meeting of the Board of Regents of April 23, 1949.* 1949, Archives of the American College of Surgeons: Chicago.
13. *Complete minitues of the meeting of the Board of Regents of December 5, 1949.* 1949, Archives of the American College of Surgeons: Chicago.
14. *Minutes of the meeting of the Board of Regents of October 25, 1940.* 1940, Archives of the American College of Surgeons: Chicago.
15. *Minutes of the meeting of the Board of Regents of February 16, 1941.* 1941, Archives of the American College of Surgeons: Chicago.
16. *Minutes of the Executive Committee of the Board of Regents of April 30, 1941.* 1941, Archives of the American College of Surgeons: Chicago.
17. *Minutes of the meeting of the Board of Regents of November 4, 1941.* 1941, Archives of the American College of Surgeons: Chicago.
18. *Complete minutes of the meeting of the Board of Regents of December 5, 1948.* 1948, Archives of the American College of Surgeons: Chicago.
19. *Complete minutes of the meeting of the Board of Regents of October 18, 1949.* 1949, Archive of the American College of Surgeons: Chicago.
20. *Complete minutes of the meeting of the Board of Regents of April 21, 1950.* 1950, Archives of the American College of Surgeons: Chicago.
21. *Complete minutes of the meeting of the Board of Regents of September 10, 1950.* 1950, Archives of the American Colege of Surgeons: Chicago.
22. *Complete minutes of the meeting of the Board of Regents of October 27, 1950.* 1950, Archives of the American College of Surgeons: Chicago.
23. *Complete minutes of the meeting of the Board of Regents of November 20, 1950.* 1950, Archives of the American College of Surgeons: Chicago.
24. *Minutes of the meeting of the Board of Regents of April 13, 1951.* 1951, Archives of the American College of Surgeons: Chicago.
25. *Complete minutes of the meeting of the Board of Regents of November 4, 1941.* 1941, Archives of the American College of Surgeons: Chicago.

26. *Complete minutes of the meeting of the Board of Regents of December 6, 1948.* 1948, Archives of the American College of Surgeons: Chicago.

27. *Complete minutes of the meeting of the Board of Regents of October 16, 1949.* 1949, Archives of the American College of Surgeons: Chicago.

28. Fuchs, J.R., *Oral history interview with Oscar Ewing.* 1969, Harry S. Truman Library and Museum: Independence, MO.

29. Doherty, K., Jenkins, J.A., *Examining a failed moment: National health care, the AMA, and the U.S. Congress, 1948-50.* 2009, University of Virginia: Charlottesville, VA.

30. (1952) *Medicine: For the nation's health.* Time Magazine.

31. *Complete minutes of the meeting of the Board of Regents of May 27, 1948.* 1948, Archives of the American College of Surgeons: Chicago.

32. *Complete minutes of the meeting of the Board of Regents of October 19, 1948.* 1948, Archives of the American College of Surgeons: Chicago.

33. *Complete minutes of the meeting of the Board of Regents of July 24, 1949.* 1949, Archives of the American College of Surgeons: Chicago.

34. *Minutes of the meeting of the Board of Regents of November 30, 1945.* 1945, Archives of the American College of Surgeons: Chicago.

35. *Minutes of the meeting of the Board of Regents of June 23, 1945.* 1943, Archives of the American College of Surgeons: Chicago.

36. *Minutes of the meeting of the Board of Regents of December 1, 1945.* 1945, Archives of the American College of Surgeons: Chicago.

37. *Complete minutes of the meeting of the Board of Regents of February 2, 1947.* 1947, Archives of the American College of Surgeons: Chicago.

38. *Complete minutes of the meeting of the Board of Regents of October 22, 1949.* 1949, Archives of the American College of Surgeons: Chicago.

39. Gordon-Taylor, G., *In memoriam, Arthur W. Allen, FRCS (Hon) (1887-1958).* Annals of the Royal College of Surgeons of England, 1958. **22**: p. 357-60.

40. Ochsner, A., *In memoriam: Arthur Wilburn Allen, 1887-1958.* Surgery, 1958. **44**: p. 1116-17.

41. Ottinger, L., *From Warren to Warshaw.* The Massachusetts General Hospital Surgical Society Newsletter, 1999. **1**(No. 1).

42. Crile, G.W., *An Autobiography. Edited, with Sidelights by Grace Crile.* Vol. 2. 1947, Philadelphia: J.B. Lippincott.

43. Davis, L., *Fellowship of Surgeons. A History of the American College of Surgeons.* 1960, Chicago: American College of Surgeons.

44. Grimm, E., in *Notebooks.* 1950, Archives of the American College of Surgeons: Chicago.

CHAPTER 12
Formation of the Joint Commission

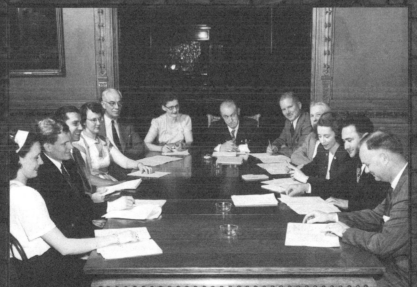

General Paul Hawley

Hawley was born in 1891 in West College Corner, Indiana, on the Ohio border, the son and grandson of small-town physicians. He received his MD in 1914 from the University of Cincinnati, interned at Cincinnati General Hospital, and returned to his hometown to practice medicine.

After less than a year, too energetic and restless for general practice, he joined the United States Army. By June 1918, he had advanced to the rank of major and was sent to France as a surgeon with an infantry regiment.

After World War I, he obtained a PhD in public health from Johns Hopkins University. Then he was assigned to several duty stations in the United States and the Philippines. Destined to become one the few general officers in the Medical Corps, he was selected for the Command and General Staff School and the Army War College, where he excelled.

When World War II began, he was sent to England to organize medical support for the invasion of France. After D-Day, by then a major general, Hawley directed the entire medical department in the European theater, which eventually reached the strength of 254,000 officers and enlisted men, including 16,000 physicians, 4,500 dentists and 18,000 nurses. He built a system of hospitals that ranged from 200 to 3,000 beds each for the care of the sick and wounded.[1] (Figure 12.1)

Modeled after the Civil War example of the medical chief of the Army of the Potomac, Dr. Jonathan Letterman, Hawley's philosophy was to quickly move the most severely wounded to the largest available hospital behind the lines, where the professional

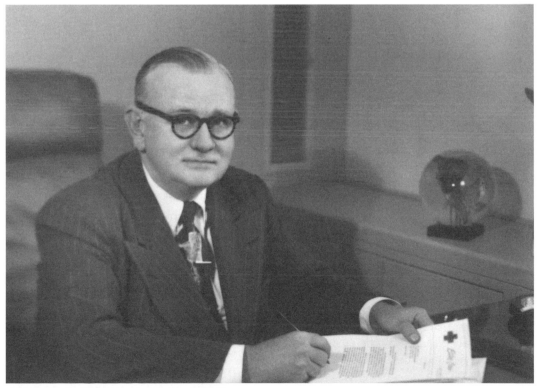

FIGURE 12.1 Dr. Paul R Hawley, Director, 1950–61.

expertise and equipment was at the highest level. Hawley's implementation of a modernized version of Letterman's system led to the low mortality and morbidity rates for U.S. Army personnel in Europe during World War II. The use of the helicopter as an air ambulance in the Korean, Vietnam, and Middle East conflicts extended this concept and, combined with the advances in surgery and medical equipment, reduced wartime mortality even further. Later, Hawley noted in a speech that Letterman died in obscurity, but his contributions made those of Florence Nightingale seem small.[2]

After the war, the newly appointed administrator of the Veteran's Administration, General Omar N Bradley, who had worked with Hawley in Europe, hired him as medical director of the Veterans Administration (VA) system, which was languishing because of its antiquated health care, inadequate facilities, and its bureaucratic, politicized administration. President Truman was worried that the VA would be overwhelmed by the large number of veterans returning from the war and jeopardize his chance to be elected president in 1948.[3] Hawley recruited an expert in rehabilitation, Dr. Paul Magnuson, chair of orthopaedic surgery at Northwestern University, and Dr. Elliot Cutler, who had experience with the VA in Massachusetts. The VA had only 500 career doctors, but needed 3,500. The number of hospitals was insufficient to accommodate the returning veterans. Many of them were in inconvenient, rural areas, distant from other medical facilities because congressmen had located them in small towns in their districts to provide employment and economic growth.

Hawley and Magnuson devised a brilliant solution to these problems. They created formal affiliations between the VA and academic health centers, building new hospitals on their campuses and involving the medical school faculties in the care of veterans by supervising interns and residents, who rotated through the VA hospitals. This provided injured veterans with many of the best doctors in the country. Within months, veterans began to receive the high-level, scientifically based care delivered at academic health centers. The involvement of faculty and trainees solved the physician deficit. Academic centers were eager to have additional facilities for education and training on their campuses, built and financed by the federal government.

VA funds were also allocated for faculty and resident salaries. By early 1946, the VA had 97 hospitals.[4] Twenty-nine more were opened in the next two years, a remarkable feat of planning, bidding, constructing, and organizing that probably could not be duplicated today. Continuing construction brought the total to 151 by 1950, 70 of which were affiliated with academic medical centers. At the College's centennial, an estimated 30,000 medical students and 20,000 residents rotate through VA hospitals annually as part of their education and training, including many future surgeons.[5] Tens of thousands of practicing surgeons are grateful for the opportunities they had to learn their craft as students and residents at a VA facility.[6]

Their missions completed, Bradley and Hawley left the VA in 1948. Bradley was appointed Army Chief of Staff and, later, the first Chairman of the Joint Chiefs of Staff. Hawley was named chief executive officer of the Blue Cross and Blue Shield Commissions. His task was to unify the two commissions, sponsored by the American Hospital Association (AHA) and the American Medical Association (AMA), respectively. Many physicians and their organizations had concerns about the interposition of insurance carriers between doctors and patients, potential intruders in the doctor-patient relationship, often described as "sacred." Hawley's two-year experience with private health insurance, which was experiencing phenomenal growth, would prove invaluable in ameliorating the ethical concerns of surgeons and the College leadership about this method of payment for physician services.

⤙✦⤚

"The Director" Takes Over

Hawley, the first Director of the American College of Surgeons (ACS) since 1935, began his duties in March 1950. He made his presence known immediately by bustling about and signing letters and memos as "The Director." Behind his desk at the College's offices in the elegant, but somewhat impractical Nickerson Mansion on the corner of Erie and Wabash Streets in Chicago, was a beautiful fireplace with a mantel on which sat his general's helmet. One of a succession of plants was in the helmet; the lack of water drainage and sunshine killed them after a few months. Miss Marion Rapp was delegated to carry the helmet to a florist on State Street for replanting on a regular basis. Finally, she suggested that she drill a hole in the helmet for water drainage. Hawley said, "Marion, that helmet has been used for many purposes for which it wasn't intended. It went through several wars and I was lucky enough that nobody put a bullet hole through it. And I'd hate, by God, I'd hate you to be the first one to do it."[7]

⤙✦⤚

Problems with the Hospital Standardization Program

Hawley quickly learned from Controller Sandrok that the College's revenues could not sustain the expenses of its programs. Chief among these was the hospital standardization program, which had cost the College more than $2 million. Hospitals were not charged for accreditation, so the financial burden of the program fell on the Fellows through their dues to the tune of approximately $75,000 annually. Hawley believed their dues should be used for accreditation of graduate training programs and the continuing education and professional development of surgeons, not for the improvement of hospitals. He decided to find a way to get the College out from under the hospital standardization program.

During World War II, the program languished because the College was short of staff, and hospitals were focused on dealing with shortages of supplies, equipment, and doctors. After the war, the frequency of inspections was reduced to save money, and the added burden of inspecting hospitals for their graduate medical education programs stressed the capabilities of the staff. During the same period, the expansion of hospital services and the rapid development of graduate programs in hospital administration led to better management and organization of the non-professional services of the hospital. Hospital administrators adopted the modern view that departments such as dietary, medical records, laundry, and housekeeping were integral to the care of patients, and began to criticize the College's standardization program because of its emphasis on the professional activities of the hospital's staff, and its less intense attention to the supporting services. Members of the AHA lobbied the Association leadership to develop its own standardization program that would include rigorous scrutiny of nonprofessional services, but the AHA Council did not assent because it would be too costly.[8]

Late in the spring of 1950, the AHA learned that the College might discontinue its hospital standardization program and concentrate its efforts on graduate training in surgery. The AHA Committee on Structure then imposed a dues increase that would provide $100,000 in additional revenue for a hospital standardization program.

The committee met with Hawley to discuss the possibility of transferring the hospital standardization program to the AHA, and a tentative outline of the terms of the transfer was developed. Hawley polled the Regents by phone and found the majority sympathetic to the transfer.[8]

On June 5, 1950, Hawley formally summarized the situation in a letter to Arthur Allen, Chairman of the Board of Regents, stating that the budget problems created by the recent agreement with the American Board of Surgery (ABS) and the Council on Medical Education and Hospitals was giving the staff and the Regents great concern. He said, "The plain fact is that we must either curtail our expenses or raise dues, and the latter course would seem to be impracticable, and probably unproductive because of expected resignations."[9] Hawley said he had been engaged in "tentative" discussions with the AHA and that their trustees may approach the Regents with a proposal to take over the hospital standardization program. The agreement would be structured "somewhat as follows:" A commission would be appointed to set the hospital standards, determine the policies, and supervise the program. One half of the commission would be nonmedical people, one fourth physicians and surgeons, and one fourth people active in the hospital field. The program would be financed by the AHA at $100,000 per year. Malcolm MacEachern would be employed by the AHA, at least during the period of transition. The entire College staff engaged in hospital standardization would be employed by the AHA, and the AHA would rent from the College its space at 660 North Rush Street. Hawley continued,

> We are faced today with this inescapable fact: The College cannot continue to spend $75,000 a year on this program and meet other essential needs of surgeons and surgery. We must now decide whether the American College of Surgeons should be devoted primarily to the interests of surgeons or that of hospitals. We cannot meet both requirements.[9]

He requested permission to continue negotiations, stressing that there would be no agreement without approval by the Regents. Subsequently, Hawley detailed the proposed agreement to the Board of Regents.[10]

The AHA Plan

The AHA Board of Trustees discussed the proposal on June 10. They favored a commission of 25 members, to include a standards commission of 13 members, including the chairman. Six of the 13 would be hospital administrators and six would be outstanding physicians and surgeons, three appointed by the ACS and three by the American College of Physicians (ACP). The other 12 members would be hospital trustees and hospital administrators. The commission would have final authority to establish hospital standards and inspection procedures, and it would recommend hospitals for approval by the AHA. Final approval would be by the Association's Board of Trustees. MacEachern and his staff would be invited to join the staff of the AHA.

Temporarily, the Association would rent the Chicago office building that housed the College's standardization program. Records would be transferred to the AHA. Clearly, the AHA planned to take over the College's program and make it their own. With only six physicians among the 25 members of the commission and authority for final approval by the AHA trustees, the AHA control of hospital standardization would be absolute. This plan was approved by the AHA board.[8]

A joint committee of the board of trustees of the AHA and representatives of the College, who were Hawley and Regents Warren Cole and Henry Cave, reviewed the plan on July 21. The committee agreed that the medical component of the commission should have power to act in the setting of standards covering medical practice in the hospital, but that the full commission should approve the definition of those items that constituted medical and surgical practice in the hospital.[10] The College representatives were more interested in standard setting than in controlling the entire process. The plans were moving smoothly and swiftly, and the AHA was in the driver's seat.

≈✳≈

The AMA Reacts

The Board of Regents of the College was to meet on August 4 to approve the plan, but no one had anticipated the virulent reaction of the AMA when its leadership learned that the College was giving the standardization program over to the AHA. They saw this as another attempt by the AHA to deliver a major blow to the autonomy of physicians that would compromise the doctor-patient relationship. This added fuel to the fire because they believed hospitals were already destroying physician autonomy by hiring pathologists, radiologists, and anesthesiologists.

The AMA believed this violated the doctor-patient relationship, as did many physicians in these specialties. They argued that all physicians should be in a fee-for-service relationship with patients, without an intervening third party. Any other financial relationship was unethical. The ongoing battle around this ethical issue intensified the alarm and anger exhibited by the AMA on learning that the College was giving control of the standardization program to the AHA. Allowing the AHA and its hospitals to have complete control of the hospital environment through standard setting and accreditation could reduce or even eliminate the role of the medical profession in hospital affairs.

In a meeting with College officials, the leadership of the AMA expressed its disapproval of the proposed arrangement with the AHA in no uncertain terms. Believing they were morally obligated to preserve physician control of the standardization program, the AMA delegation proposed that they take it over and carry it on their own budget. They pointed out that they and the ACS had already agreed on a combined effort to survey graduate training programs and that hospital standardization could be dovetailed with this.[11] It was clear that the AMA would go to any length to prevent the AHA from gaining control of the program.

The College Backs Off

ACS Board Chairman Allen briefed the Regents on the AMA reaction. (Figure 12.2) He did not want to transfer the program to the AMA, nor did he want to jeopardize the friendly relationship between the AMA, the College, and the ABS that flowed from their recent collaboration on the graduate training program in surgery. Knowing that the College would lose face by giving the program to the AHA, and having his own concerns about the wisdom of it, he raised the possibility that the four most powerful organizations, the ACS, ACP, AMA, and AHA, could together take over the program. In an equal partnership, this would give three-fourths of the representation to doctors. His suggestion was satisfactory to everyone, but Vice Chairman Frederick Coller and Hawley doubted that the AMA would accept the proposal or that the AHA would put money into the commission with only one-fourth representation.[11]

The Regents tabled Hawley's proposal that the AHA take over the program. They formally agreed that unification was desirable and financially wise, and that a cooperative effort and financial stability should be sought. Allen appointed a committee to give further study to the problem and directed that the trustees of the AMA be informed of the action of the Board of Regents.[12]

The Board of Trustees of the AHA met in special session on August 4 and 5 and was told that the Regents had tabled Hawley's proposal that the AHA take over the program. Determined to control hospital standardization, the AHA board passed a resolution that the AHA would establish a hospital standardization program and invite interested organizations of the medical profession to cooperate in the development of standards relating to the practice of medicine in hospitals. Thus, the AHA Board of Trustees resolved to establish their own hospital standardization program without regard to the College and the AMA.[8]

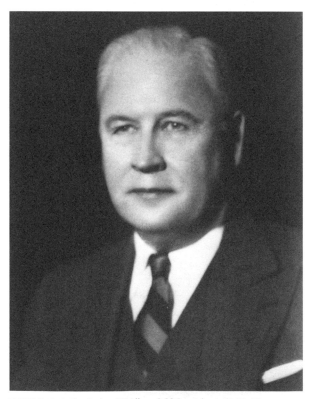

FIGURE 12.2 Dr. Arthur W Allen, ACS President, 1947–48.

ACS and AMA Representatives Meet

On September 9, 1950, Allen reported to the leadership of the AMA that the College's Board of Regents did not want to give the program to the AHA; rather, the Regents believed the four organizations should form a commission. When this idea was taken to the AHA, Allen said, "They blew their top." He continued, "These birds are going to start it (a standardization program)."[13] They all agreed that the Hospital Association was just as dangerous as the federal government. They believed that the goal of the AHA was to take over the medical profession. Allen said that if the AHA was unwilling to compromise there was no choice but to combine with the AMA and run a separate hospital standardization program, which would be a dreadful choice. Hawley believed that the AHA would influence professional standards in the hospital and weaken the authority of the profession. In Hawley's original proposal, the six physicians on the commission would have absolute authority for professional standards, but others pointed out that the entire commission of 25 members could vote out anything these six physicians wanted.

After lengthy discussion, Hawley said, "I agree with everything that has been said, but we are broke."[13] They discussed the possibility of the AMA and the College starting their own program, but no one really wanted to do that. The AMA representatives reiterated that they would be happy to take over the entire program and combine it with the graduate medical education standardization program, but this was not acceptable to the College leadership.

A Contentious Meeting

The stalemate continued until, at the invitation of Arthur Allen, five representatives of the AHA leadership met with leaders of the College, the AMA, and the ACP on September 30, 1950. Allen, who chaired the meeting, recounted that the College's original plan was to turn the program over to the AHA, but at their meeting in August the Regents were not ready to make a final decision.[14]

AMA president Dr. Elmer Henderson asked AHA president Dr. Charles Wilensky if the AHA was willing to enter into a joint program administered by the representatives of the ACS, the ACP, the AHA, and the AMA. Wilensky replied that the AHA trustees wanted the total administration of the program to rest with the AHA. Henderson said this practically precluded any discussion. He said, "What I mean is that if you folks are going to take that attitude, then I don't see why we should waste our time."[14] Wilensky assured the group that the AHA did not want to set standards for the professional aspects of patient care; this would be done by the six physician members of the commission. Dr. Donald Anderson, an AMA representative, countered that any board of 25, with six doctors and 19 hospital administrators reporting to the AHA board cannot protect the medical profession.

The meeting continued in a very contentious manner until Dr. Evarts Graham, who had been uncharacteristically quiet, proposed the formation of an independent commission, with representatives from the AHA, AMA, ACP, and the ACS. The organizations would contribute money to support this independent board. It could have its headquarters anywhere it wanted, not necessarily in Chicago. Certificates of approval would be given to hospitals by the joint board. Graham said an alternative was that the College continue to administer the program, but with financial support from the other organizations. If there was equal representation of the four organizations in Graham's proposal, the governing body would have at least three physicians to every hospital administrator.[14]

After much discussion, all the participants agreed that the current standardization program needed improvement in the nonprofessional areas. Henderson expressed his support for Graham's proposals, but said the AMA was totally opposed to giving the program and its control to the AHA.

Wilensky stated firmly that the AHA would create a standardization program in keeping with its board's concepts of what is good hospital care. They all understood that Wilensky's position meant there would be two programs, one for the hospital side run by the AHA, and the other for the professional side, run by the College and perhaps with the other physician organizations.

With no solution in sight, the participants agreed to meet again in about two weeks.[14] Despite the impasse, they all wanted to continue to work on a solution. Each organization had a stake in the outcome: the College desperately needed to eliminate or reduce its financial commitment to hospital standardization. The AHA wanted to control hospital standardization to win the battle over employment of physicians and to improve the nonprofessional aspects of standardization. The AMA wanted to ensure physician control of the entire process. The ACP wanted to be a player in standardization.

❦

Another Meeting of Representatives of the ACS, AMA, ACP, and AHA

The next meeting was on October 8, 1950 at the Statler Hotel in Washington, DC. Again, Arthur Allen presided. Pushing for an agreement, Allen said that the ACS Regents want to make a decision about the program at their meeting on October 21 in Boston. He said they would not accept the proposal that the AHA manage the hospital aspects and another organization the professional aspects. He reminded the group that Evarts Graham had proposed a separate commission with equal representation from the four groups, but that the AHA was concerned that three representatives from each group could frequently come to a vote of nine physicians to three non-physicians.[15]

❦

A New Proposal from the AHA

Wilensky, who had obviously been in contact with the AHA board, now proposed a commission of 12 members of the medical profession, six members of hospital boards of trustees representing the public, and six hospital administrators, for a total of 24. All of the 12 physicians would be AMA members, although they would be representing the ACP, the ACS, and the AMA. Chairman Allen raised the question of finances and suggested that the AHA pay half the amount and the medical groups pay the other half. During this meeting, Mr. George Bugbee, executive director of the AHA, introduced the phrase "joint commission."[15]

≈⨳≈

The Regents Are Updated

At the October 21 meeting of the Board of Regents of the College, Chairman Allen reported that after three "discouraging" meetings, a fourth meeting of four representatives from each of the four organizations was "very rewarding." He said that there was a lot of give and take between the AHA and the AMA, which were previously at "swords' points," and he briefed the Regents on the progress to date of the meetings of the representatives of the four organizations.[16]

The next day, Drs. Henderson and Gunderson of the AMA appeared before the Regents and said that the standardization of hospitals was for the medical profession and that the program should not be shared with hospital people on an equal basis as the AHA had proposed. Henderson said he had received hundreds of letters opposing going in on an equal basis with the AHA, and several state medical societies had gone on record opposing this. He did not believe that he could sell the House of Delegates on any kind of a program giving the AHA equal partnership.[15]

On the last day of the Regents' meeting, Dr. Wilensky, president of the AHA, told them the AHA did not want to intrude on the practice of medicine. He said that the job of performing surgery and practicing medicine was the responsibility of physicians and surgeons, whereas the job of administrating the hospitals was the responsibility of the administration. He said,

> Any plan for transfer of the program, a joint effort, or any plans for the creation of a commission ...will meet with the approval of the AHA. Any plans you might want to consider for a joint effort of the College and the American Hospital Association meets with our hearty desires. We are ready to finance the program and we are ready to develop a commission including representatives of those organizations you may want to select with us. It is only by a joint effort, only by working together, that we can make better hospitals and better workshops. We should not quibble over the numbers (of representatives on the commission), whether it is 3, 6, 9, or 12. We spoke at one point of six physicians against a total of 25. If anybody's mind would be eased by a more equal division it is all right with the AHA.[17]

His generous remarks were in contrast to his testiness at the initial meetings of the representatives, and with those of the AMA officials a few days earlier. Wilensky clearly had the green light from the AHA Board of Trustees to negotiate a more conciliatory agreement.

Coming Together at Last

Representatives of the four organizations plus an observer from the American Psychiatric Association met on November 19, 1950.[18] Allen told the group that the Regents decided at their last meeting that the College would continue the standardization program until the matter could be settled amicably and in the best interests of the public. But, he said, the Regents preferred that a commission, a separate organization with adequate representatives from all interested groups, take over hospital standardization.

Dr. AJ O'Rourke, an AHA representative, asked if the College was planning to do it on as large a scale as it had previously, and Hawley answered, "Even larger." Allen chimed in, "We are really going to go to town on it."[18] They were putting pressure on the AHA to compromise, giving the impression that if there was no compromise, the AHA would be out of it completely. O'Rourke challenged Allen about where the money was going to come from, and he responded that they would add ten dollars to the dues to handle it.

Allen then said, in skillful compromise, "I don't believe it is right for one group such as the American College of Surgeons to continue to have the sole responsibility for this great program in which every doctor ought to be interested, and in which every hospital administrator ought to be interested. We really ought to be able to get together on it in some way or other."[18]

Bugbee, being very polite and respectful of Allen, then asked how he felt the commission should be financed. Allen replied that he did not think it should be based on who had the most power, rather that the hospitals which are accredited should pay for the service.

Dr. Warren Cole, a College Regent, said that the medical profession knew about the proposed fifty-fifty arrangement and did not like it. They were more interested in each of the four organizations having one-fourth of the representatives. Allen asked whether the House of Delegates of the AMA would accept, as a compromise, a one-third representation by the AHA instead of one-half. Both Gunderson and Henderson said that would be possible.

College Regent Fred Rankin, chairman of surgery at the University of Michigan, picked up on this and said the administrators of the organizations should be sent off to a private room to work on something concrete. He proposed that they consider a plan in which the AHA and the AMA each have a third of the representatives to the commission and furnish a third of the funds, and that the College of Surgeons and College of Physicians together have the other third of the representatives and furnish a third of the funds. Rankin said,

> A lot of us don't know about the details, but we certainly could get a small body of men together to offer us something to chew on instead of fighting all the way around. I know all these speeches. You can call me Bugbee or Father (Msgr. Healy, an AHA trustee) or anybody else, and I can get up and give you his speech. I've heard them six or eight times.[18]

There was uproarious laughter, and Rankin's comments broke the ice. Henderson said he heartily agreed. Allen asked if Rankin had made the one-third/one-third/one-third proposal in the form of a motion and Rankin responded that he had. Henderson seconded the motion and Allen asked the executives of the organizations, Hawley (ACS),

Dr. George Lull (AMA), Mr. George Bugbee (AHA), and Dr. LeRoy Sloane (ACP), to get together and draw up a plan based on Rankin's proposal.

There was discussion about accreditation of psychiatric hospitals and representation for American Psychiatric Association (APA), accreditation of Canadian hospitals (because all the physician organizations had Canadian members), pediatric hospitals, and general practitioners, whose organization was not represented. Under Allen's skillful maneuvering, the group finally decided that the four organizations involved would work together to appoint psychiatrists, pediatricians, general practitioners, and Canadians on their groups of representatives to the putative commission. Eventually, they approved Rankin's motion unanimously, a historic decision that led to the continuous improvement in the care of patients in the United States, and later, throughout the world.[18]

The Board of Regents of the College was briefed on the following day, November 20, 1950. To stem the College's financial hemorrhage resulting from the standardization program, they agreed that non-dues-paying Fellows, of which there were about 8,000, would receive a letter requesting a pledge for five years of an amount ranging from $25–$100 per annum for the standardization program. Letters would be sent in each of the five years to members whose dues were paid up in perpetuity during that year.[19]

The Joint Commission Is Formed

For the next three months, the committee of four organization executives met frequently to develop a final proposal for the organizations' representatives, who met again on March 4, 1951, at the offices of the ACS.[20] Arthur Allen presided. They were presented with articles of incorporation and bylaws for a joint commission on hospital standardization. After long discussion, they agreed that the organization should be named the Joint Commission on Accreditation of Hospitals, and that this would be the only body that would give accreditation to hospitals meeting the established standards, eliminating the possibility that the AHA would develop their own accrediting organization, as originally planned.

The four organizations would be the corporate members, and the Canadian Medical Association would be invited to be a member. If the Canadians participated, there would be three commissioners from the ACP, three from the ACS, seven from the AHA, six from the AMA, and one from the Canadian Medical Association. A director, who must be a physician, and a small staff would be hired. Inspections would be made by field staff employed by the participating organizations. All inspections were to be made in the same manner and reported on a form prescribed by the commission. Accreditation was to be granted by the Joint Commission, not by individual members of the corporation. The budget was to be shared in proportion to the number of representatives. The acrimony evident in previous meetings had dissipated, and the participants moved through the document with very few changes and additions. At the end of the meeting, they made a special effort to thank Dr. Arthur Allen for his determined and fair leadership, giving him a round of applause. They left as friends, in good spirits.

They met again on July 15, 1951, to report on the decisions of their respective parent organizations. The Regents of the ACP and the ACS approved the program as outlined, and the House of Delegates of the AMA agreed to leave approval authority with the AMA delegation. The Canadian Medical Association joined the commission, only to resign in 1958 when the Canadian Council on Hospital Accreditation began to survey hospitals in Canada. In November 1951, the AHA House of Delegates approved the document and authorized incorporation. The Joint Commission on Accreditation of Hospitals was immediately incorporated in the state of Illinois and its first organizational meeting, as much a celebration as a business meeting, was held on December 15, 1951.[21]

An operating budget of $70,000 was approved, funded by assessment of the corporate members at $3,500 per seat. Malcolm MacEachern's contributions to hospital standardization were celebrated, and the Board agreed to rotate its chairmanship between the corporate members, a practice that continues as the College celebrates its Centennial.

The Joint Commission's first president was Dr. Edwin L Crosby, president elect of the AHA. He was widely respected for his public health background and as executive director of the Johns Hopkins Hospital. The offices were rented from the College at 660 North Rush Street. In 1953, the Joint Commission grandfathered all the approved hospitals in the Colleges' standardization program, and began its own inspection program.[21]

Throughout the Joint Commission's history, its board, leadership, and employees of have remained passionate about their mission to improve the health care delivered in hospitals and other venues. The organization has remained true to the principle that guided the hospital standardization program of the College when the program was initiated in 1917: knowledgeable professionals should assess hospital conditions and achieve consensus among themselves on standards that would have the greatest effect on improving patient care.

The founding of the Joint Commission is a story that began as warfare between leaders of medical organizations. The warfare gradually morphed to compromise and consensus, then friendship, and, finally, decisions made solely in the best interests of the public. In the fast-moving health care field, disagreements between leaders of health care organizations surface frequently. The story of the founding of the Joint Commission serves as a reminder for leaders to work with one another, and together do what is best for the public.

REFERENCES

1. *Medical News, Maj Gen Paul R. Hawley, MC, USA Dies.* JAMA, 1966. **195**.
2. *Medicine: All - American Surgeon,* in *Time Magazine.* 1947.
3. Bradley, O., Blair, C., *A General's Life.* 1983, New York: Simon and Schuster.
4. *History of the Department of Veterans Affairs. Part 5,* United States Department of Veterans Affairs.
5. Blank, A., *Sixty years later, academic - VA health care affiliation still strong.* AAMC Reporter, 2006(July, 2006).
6. Rege, R., *Why should the VA continue academic affiliations?* Am J Surg, 2004. **188**: p. 453-458.
7. Hanlon, C., *Interview of Marion E. Rapp.* 2001, Archives of the American College of Surgeons: Chicago.
8. *Proceedings of the House of Delegates of the American Hospital Association. 52nd annual convention.* in *52nd annual convention.* September 17, 20, 1950: American Hospital Association.
9. *Letter from Paul R. Hawley to Arthur W. Allen, dated June 5, 1950.,* in *Joint Commission on Accreditation of Hospitals, Minutes of origination.,* Archives of the American College of Surgeons: Chicago.
10. Hawley, P., *Memorandum from Paul R. Hawley to the ACS Board of Regents of August 1, 1950. In minutes of the Board of Regents of August 4, 1950.,* Archives of the American College of Surgeons: Chicago.
11. *Abstract of the minutes of the Board of Regents meeting of August 4, 1950.,* in *71-90 collaboration. Joint Commission on Accreditation of Hospitals.* 1950, Archives of the American College of Surgeons: Chicago.
12. *Minutes of the meeting of the Board of Regents of August 4, 1950.* 1950, Archives of the American College of Surgeons: Chicago.
13. 1950, *Minutes of the meeting of the Board of Regents of September 9, 1950,* Archives of the American College of Surgeons: Chicago.
14. *Minutes of the joint meeting of the American College of Surgeons with representatives of the AMA, AHA, ACP of September 30, 1950,* in *71-90 collaboration. Joint Commission on Accrediatation of Hospitals.* 1950, Archives of the American College of Surgeons: Chicago.
15. *Minutes of the meeting of the Board of Regents of October 22, 1950.* 1950, Archives of the American College of Surgeons: Chicago.
16. *Minutes of the meeting of the Board of Regents of October 21, 1950.* 1950, Archives of the American College of Surgeons: Chicago.
17. *Minutes of the meeting of the Board of Regents of October 27,1950.* 1950, Archives of the American College of Surgeons: Chicago.
18. *Minutes of the joint meeting of the American College of Surgeons with representatives of the AMA, AHA, ACP of November 19,1950, in collaboration Joint Commission on Accreditation of Hospitals. 1950.* 1950, Archives of the American College of Surgeons: Chicago.
19. *Minutes of the meeting of the Board of Regents of November 20, 1950.* 1950, Archives of the American College of Surgeons: Chicago.
20. *Minutes of the joint meeting of the American College of Surgeons with representatives of the AMA, AHA, ACP of March 4, 1951. In 71-90, collaboration, Joint Commission on Accreditation of Hospitals.* 1951, Archives of the American College of Surgeons: Chicago.

21. Brauer, C., *Champions of Quality in Health Care. A History of the Joint Commission on Accreditation of Healthcare Organizations.* 2001, Lyme, CT: Greenwich Publishing Group.

CHAPTER 13
The College Takes on Fee Splitting and Unethical Practices

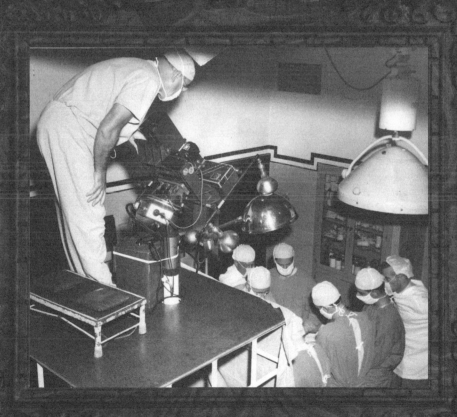

Floyd Ramsdell sets up his 3-D movie camera, San Francisco, 1951

When the College was founded, fee splitting was endemic among physicians and surgeons. In its most common form, the surgeon paid the referring doctor, almost always a general practitioner, a portion of his fee without the patient's knowledge. Obviously, this was an inducement for the practitioner to continue to refer patients to the surgeon. Ethical surgeons refused to split fees because the referral was not based on who was the best surgeon to care for the particular problem of the patient, but purely on financial gain, an immoral and unethical concept. The patient was, in effect, sold to the surgeon and bought by the surgeon.

In its more sophisticated, but still unethical forms, the referring physician would assist at the operation or before trained anesthesiologists were available, give the anesthetic, and the surgeon "kicked back" a portion of the fee, again without the patient's knowledge. Surgeons and referring physicians justified this because the referring physician was providing a service, but the College and ethical surgeons believed that the patient should be informed about who was providing what service, and each physician should bill the patient directly and separately for his services.

At the organizational meeting of the College in 1913 a motion was made and passed that each Fellow should pledge not to split fees. This dictum has been followed ever since.[1] Despite this, the practice was commonplace in many communities. If fee splitting was pervasive in a community or a particular hospital, surgeons who refused to split fees did not receive referrals. Young surgeons found it impossible to develop a practice in these circumstances, and were faced with capitulating or leaving. Either option favored the continuation of fee splitting in that community or hospital, which is why the practice continued unabated for decades throughout the country. The secret nature of the transaction led to concealment of fee splitting from the public and allowed the practice to continue.

Another ethical problem was itinerant surgery. At the invitation of the patient's general practitioner, a surgeon would come to his community hospital and operate on the patient, without necessarily seeing the patient beforehand. The postoperative care was left to the general practitioner. Sometimes the surgeon's fee was split with the patient's doctor. This was deemed unethical by the College and most surgeons because the surgeon had not established a doctor-patient relationship, and because the general practitioner was making the decision to operate. Most importantly, surgical care includes preoperative decision making and planning, the operation itself, and postoperative care in the hospital as well as outpatient follow up. By performing only the operation, the itinerant surgeon was abdicating a significant portion of his responsibilities to the patient. The participants in itinerant surgery claimed they were providing surgical services to those in communities who would otherwise be deprived of them.

Ghost surgery was closely related. When patients did not know or have contact with the surgeon who performed the operation, the surgeon was the "ghost." The College condemned this as unethical. A more current example was the practice of faculty members allowing residents to perform operations, with or without supervision, on patients who assumed the attending was doing the surgery.

The Pervasiveness of Fee Splitting

After Franklin Martin died in 1935, the College staff frequently received letters from Fellows complaining of fee splitting in their communities or hospitals. The staff routinely asked the correspondent to name the individuals and provide evidence that they were splitting fees.[2] This almost always ended the correspondence and was the reason the College was unsuccessful in stopping the practice, even among its Fellows. Proving allegations was almost impossible.

During the Great Depression, hospitals that were having financial problems expanded their medical staffs by appointing general practitioners to the courtesy staff, a category that gave them privileges to care for patients and perform surgery but not to participate in medical staff regulatory activities. This brought more patients into the hospital, but allowed untrained doctors to practice surgery and increased unethical activity, especially fee splitting. In two hospitals in Norfolk, Virginia, 85 percent of the medical staff had operating privileges.[1]

In 1938, MacEachern visited the New York Credentials Committee, which not only acknowledged that fee splitting was rampant there, but also wanted to legalize it, contending that it was impossible to stop.[3] Nevertheless, the College removed nine of eighteen New York hospitals from the provisionally approved or approved list between 1936 and 1938 for alleged fee splitting among their doctors and inadequate professional qualifications. Surprisingly, the hospitals did not challenge these accreditation decisions.

The American Board of Surgery (ABS), founded in 1937, included the following statement in its first booklet of information for candidates for board certification and in subsequent editions: "The Board, believing that the practice of fee splitting is pernicious, leading as it does to a traffic in human life, will reserve the right to inquire particularly into any candidate's practice in regard to this question." Whenever there was an issue of ethical standing, even on hearsay, ABS Secretary J Stewart Rodman informed the candidate that he did not meet the criteria for admission to the exam.[4]

The Executive Committee of the Board of Regents, meeting in September 1938, summoned four surgeons from Danville, Illinois, where fee splitting was rampant. Led by Chairman George Crile, they quizzed each of the four surgeons individually and determined that most of them were splitting fees with the family physician, who acted either as their assistant or as the anesthesiologist. The surgeons acknowledged that the family doctors were not good anesthetists. The committee members then met with the four individuals as a group and proposed that they stop the fee splitting practice and set up a program to train residents and interns, who could be used as assistants and anesthetists. Crile said they were trying to improve the situation in Danville for patients, and that if the four men would get together and change the way they practiced, the entire community might go that way.[5] A year later the Danville surgeons were still splitting fees.[6]

Before World War II, the College staff was convinced they could not control fee splitting by individuals. Furthermore, only approximately 50 percent of active surgeons were Fellows of the College. They believed the hospital standardization program could be used to pressure hospitals into eliminating fee splitters from their staffs. But this involved removing some of the most active surgeons, who were important to the hospital's bottom line. Another complication was that organizations, such as mining companies in West Virginia were hiring surgeons as full time employees, and no fee was generated.

A few universities were hiring full-time professors and collecting their fees to use for other purposes, which some believed was a variant of fee splitting.[7]

The practice continued in the private sector during World War II. In discussing a candidate for fellowship who was suspected of fee splitting, Regent Dallas Phemister said,

> The College has been absolutely spineless on the subject of fee splitting. I think it might be a good thing for a man like this to sue the College. If the evidence is as good as it seems to be that he is fee splitting, it would cure anyone else from challenging the stance of the Board of Regents on fee splitting.

Associate Director Bowman Crowell pointed out that there had been threats of lawsuits in the past, but no suit had ever been filed.[8]

The public did not view fee splitting as a major ethical issue. They held physicians in such high regard that neither they nor physicians discussed the cost of an operation, nor who was being paid, and how much, for the associated services such as referral, pre- and postoperative care, and anesthesia. They were content with paying the surgeon's fees and had no serious interest in knowing if or how the other physicians were paid. Lawmakers were sufficiently concerned to declare the practice illegal in 23 states by 1953. The Columbus (Ohio) Surgical Society was organized in 1945 by 57 surgeons with the primary purpose of eliminating fee splitting. They accomplished this by requiring an annual audit of their members financial accounts.[9] The Internal Revenue Service prosecuted Columbus physicians who deducted the cost of the split fees as business expenses, on the grounds that the payments were against public policy.[10]

Rebates for Glasses

Opticians frequently gave rebates to ophthalmologists after providing glasses and billing patients for them. As early as 1924, the Section on Ophthalmology of the American Medical Association (AMA) resolved that "the acceptance of commissions or considerations, either directly or indirectly, from opticians and optical houses, from the sale of glasses is absolutely contrary to all our standards of medical ethics, and is just as reprehensible as the splitting of fees."[11]

In 1948, the AMA took a strong stand on rebates for glasses. Every ophthalmologist in Chicago, including Fellows of the College, was cited for this except Dr. Derrick Vail, then chair of ophthalmology at Northwestern. It was rumored that they would be indicted. Although it was obvious that the College would have to expel these individuals, there is no record of such action.[12]

Several ophthalmology societies came together to deal with the ethical problems in their field. The College used their recommendations as a statement of ethics for ophthalmic surgeons. The statement emphasized that it was unethical for ophthalmologists to provide glasses for patients, to profit from the sale of glasses, to accept rebates from optical houses, to profit from an optician's services, or to split fees.[13,14] The ethical positions of the College and the AMA were firm, but there was no way to monitor or enforce the rules, so whether or not they changed behavior was unknown.

Graham Speaks Out

In November 1951, Evarts Graham, once the College's most severe critic, was elected Chairman of the Board of Regents, after which he addressed the Regents. He said that the College had done a solid job over the past 38 years.

> First, we have made the hospitals safer places for the performance of surgical operations and the care of surgical patients, and that also includes along with it the care of all patients, surgical or not. That, of course, in itself was a wonderful contribution, the like of which had never occurred before anywhere else in the world, and doesn't go on anywhere else in the world, even now, except in the North American Continent. The second big contribution was somewhat slow, but we are finally getting around to see that the people who were going to practice surgery in this country had certain qualifications and training, which would make them safe people for patients to have operate on them.

He went on to say,

> We are now confronted with a different kind of problem. We have good hospitals, and we have good young surgeons who can't get the surgery to do, because everywhere they go they are confronted with the horrible odor of fee splitting, and it seems to me that this business of fee splitting is a very essential and very important part of the tripod of improving American surgery. It is the third leg of the stool.

He continued,

> I think that the College ought to undertake a vigorous offensive campaign against fee splitting and not be content with signing pledges and not be content with calling up (before the Board of Regents) a guy like Shelton here, because he is suspected of fee splitting, but really to go at it in a big way at its source.

He said he had a lot of experience with fee splitting.

> Most of the Regents don't know it, but in my young cub days, I went to a small city in Iowa known as Mason City, Iowa. I found to my amazement, that fee splitting was rife there. I decided I would clean it up if it were possible to do so. And I did clean it up, I might say, in a period of two years. By going to the editors of the newspapers, writing editorials, unsigned, it is true. Writing and putting them in, speaking in the churches, talking to the women's clubs, talking to the Rotary Club and other luncheon clubs, and at the end of two years when I left to go into the army in World War I the place was clean.

Graham pointed out that the College had a public relations section, and that they should get busy and see to it that articles on the subject were published in the popular magazines like *Ladies Home Companion*, *Reader's Digest*, the *Saturday Evening Post*, and arrange radio skits,

> ...sob stuff: Mama would be here with us now if old Doc. Jones, who we trusted, hadn't sold her to a surgeon. It would probably cost us money, but it's more important than some of the things we're spending money on now. ... I would say that I am not so sure that I want to accept this high position here unless you men who constitute the Board of Regents are willing to go along with this program.[15]

Elected to the most powerful position in American surgery, Graham was determined to put an end to fee splitting, the evil that plagued him when he first entered practice. Now his colleagues could understand his anger and frustration over the College as a young man. He saw then that the College accepted fee splitters and looked the other way. This was his last chance to rid surgery of unethical practices.

The Regents Act

The Regents were energized by Graham's challenge and began the attack on fee splitting and other unethical practices by restating its "principles of financial relations in the professional care of the patient," a document that defined the various forms of fee splitting and declared them "dishonest and unethical."[16] Overcharging, ghost surgery, and rebates to physicians for technical services and appliances were also declared unethical. The document set forth billing procedures designed to prevent unethical practices, which ensured that patients would understand who performed each of the services they received. The charges from each surgeon or physician were to be provided to the patient in separate bills and paid by the patient to each surgeon or physician.[17]

Later, as some general practitioners and members of the House of Delegates of the AMA pushed for loopholes in the existing policies of the College and the AMA, the definitions of unjustified operations, ghost surgery, excessive fees, and fee splitting were made more specific.[18]

Likewise, principles of financial relations in the professional care of the patient were revised. The final document stated that in his relationship with patients, a Fellow of the ACS should inform the patient or a family member of the identities of the doctors who would collaborate in the care of the patient, and discuss, or have the surgeon's representative discuss, his fee with the patient or a member of the family before submitting a statement for his own services. In relations with professional colleagues, a Fellow should refuse to participate in, or countenance, any financial arrangement that would induce referral of a patient. He should refuse to permit a referring physician to collect his fee for him and refuse to collect the fees of other doctors collaborating in the care of patients.[19,20]

Acting on Graham's insistence that the College take the fee splitting problem to the public, and bolstered by the concurrence of Mr. Greer Williams, the College's newly hired director of public relations, the Regents decided to begin their campaign through the press.

At the Clinical Congress in New York City in September 1952, thirteen officials of the College and Regents held a press conference with the science writers who covered the Congress. Hawley and the Regents explained fee splitting and its variations, and how it put patients at risk for unnecessary surgery. They said the fee-splitting physician sent patients to the surgeon who gave them the biggest cut of the fee instead of referring to the surgeon with the most expertise. They declared that the practice of fee splitting and other unethical practices such as itinerant surgery, excessive fees, and ghost surgery were rampant throughout the country. Loyal Davis, the prominent head of surgery at Northwestern and a newly elected Regent, stated that fee splitting was prevalent and increasing in Chicago. They asked the public, doctors, and hospitals to help eliminate these "evils."[21,22] (Figure 13.1)

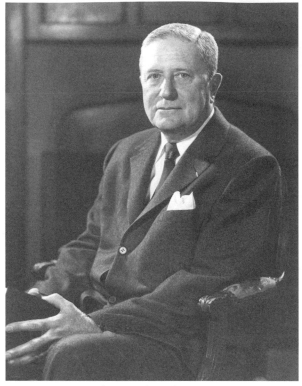

FIGURE 13.1 Dr. Loyal Davis, editor of *SG&O*; Regent; and ACS President, 1962–63.

The press sensationalized the fact that a group of the nation's leading surgeons criticized their profession in such strong terms. They took the announcement to mean that the College planned an organized crusade against the unethical practices of the medical profession. Stories appeared in at least 388 newspapers and the revelations engendered 36 editorials. Almost all of them were favorable to the College, but many asked how patients could avoid being victims of unethical practices and how the College planned to stop them.[23] Many popular and respected magazines requested interviews and more information from Greer Williams, the ACS Director of Public Relations. A few months later Paul Hawley gave a widely read and discussed interview to the *U.S. News and World Report* in which he stated that fee splitting was common and led to unnecessary surgery.[24]

Almost all physicians either read about the College's charges in newspapers and magazines or learned about them in hospital doctors' lounges or local and state medical society meetings. The College had not anticipated their vehement reaction. Those who did not split fees believed the College had publicly impugned them by painting the entire profession with a broad brush of unethical behavior. Hundreds of ethical doctors, believing their reputations had been sullied, sent angry letters and telegrams to the College. Many demanded that the College fire its director, Paul Hawley. The reaction to Loyal Davis' comments about fee splitting in Chicago was especially vitriolic; 159 members of the Chicago Medical Society, a constituent society of the AMA, signed a petition to revoke his membership. The society's executive council found him guilty of unethical conduct by a vote of 30 to 29.[23]

Davis was vigorously defended in person by College Regent Warren Cole, professor and chairman of the Department of Surgery at the University of Illinois and by 17 stories and editorials in Chicago newspapers.[23,25] Within a few months the Society dropped the charges, but simultaneously adopted a resolution stating in part that the "Chicago Medical Society deplores the unwarranted attack on and criticism of the medical profession by its own members and others."[26] Davis was chastised for exposing fee splitting, a practice condemned by the AMA and its constituent organizations, including the Chicago Medical Society. Obviously, the attitude of the Society was inconsistent with one of the gifts of the public to professions, namely, the privilege of self-regulation.

Members of the American Academy of General Practice were outraged at Hawley's exposition of unethical practices by physicians. Their president characterized him as a "temperamental old fellow" who has used "his high position with a great medical organization to give vent to his biased and distorted views."[27] He asserted that Hawley had frightened patients into refusing to have needed surgery. The Academy unanimously passed resolutions urging the AMA to take disciplinary actions against Hawley and the College. The resolution stated, "The American College of Surgeons, through its director and Regents, has attempted to arrogate unto itself powers which it does not possess and has held itself out as the palladium of medical virtue."[28] This organization of general practitioners, the other party in fee splitting with surgeons, was embarrassed. At the time, they were strongly advocating medical staff membership and surgical privileges for general practitioners and the adverse publicity did not help their cause. The House of Delegates of the AMA, which had a section on general practice, introduced resolutions to revoke Hawley's membership in the AMA, but they did not pass.

∾✝∾

The Iowa Problem

As the furor died down, groups of surgeons began to address fee splitting in their communities, several modeled after the example of the Columbus Surgical Society. The Iowa State Medical Society had adopted a resolution introduced by the American Academy of General Practice entitled "Elaboration of Medical Ethics," which basically supported fee splitting, a common practice in the state.[29] In March 1952, the Regents agreed that the document violated the policy of the College on fee splitting, and that there would be no Iowa Credentials Committee meeting in 1953, effectively blocking the applications for fellowship from the state.[30] The Central Credentials Committee, however, was authorized to admit six outstanding candidates from the University of Iowa School of Medicine after senior faculty protested.[31]

Regent Isidor Ravdin was appointed chair of a committee to investigate the Iowa situation.[32] He and others met with 14 Fellows in Des Moines and worked out a plan. Each Fellow in Iowa had to agree to submit his financial books and professional records for an audit to rule out fee splitting. Any Fellow unwilling to submit to an audit should resign from the College. Any Fellow who was unwilling to submit and would not resign voluntarily would be referred to the Board of Regents for expulsion from the College. All new applicants for fellowship must agree to submit to an audit of their financial books. The College would bear the expense of the audit of Fellows, of whom approximately one-third would be selected by lot.

A new credentials committee would be appointed to evaluate applicants for fellowship. The House of Delegates of the Iowa State Medical Society would be informed of the

College's action and the College would publicize the fact that the Fellows were taking positive action to restore the state to an ethical position in medical matters. Finally, no adverse action would be taken by the College against Fellows who had submitted combined bills in certain unusual insurance cases until the insurance companies agreed to pay more than one physician.[32]

Subsequently all but one of the 214 Fellows in Iowa consented to the inspection of their books, for which the cutoff date for accounts to be free of evidence of fee splitting was December 31, 1954.[33-35] None resigned.[36] The College hired Scoville, Wellington & Co, who audited one-third of the Fellows, beginning April 15, 1956.[37] The auditors looked for payments to physicians by the Fellow, payments to the Fellow by physicians, gifts or entertainment expenses by the Fellow to other physicians, their usual fees for appendectomy, hysterectomy, herniorrhaphy, and the condition of the Fellow's financial records. The selected Fellows were to make available to the auditor all financial records pertaining to his practice, including cash books, receipt books, and individual ledger cards for the period on and after January 1, 1955. A copy of his 1955 income tax return was also required. The Fellows would not be held accountable by the College for unethical practices prior to January 1, 1955.

Sixty-eight Fellows were audited, one refused, and one was on duty with the U.S. Navy. Fifty-four records were clean, and 14 Fellows had records that were suspect. Nine of these were paying general practitioners for assisting, three were being paid by the general practitioner, one was paying medical society dues for three other physicians, and one had excessive entertainment and business expense deductions. Seven had been paying referring physicians prior to January 1955, but then stopped. Further investigation of the 14 Fellows with evidence of dubious financial practices showed that nine of them had clean records and five had minor irregularities but were gradually complying with College policies. The lone surgeon who refused to be audited was scheduled for disciplinary action after consultation with Mr. Howe, the College's attorney.[38]

The second third of the Iowa Fellows, numbering 71, was then audited. All but five were clean. Three practices in Iowa complicated compliance with College policy: first, the refusal of certain insurance companies to pay separately each physician who participated in the care of the patient; second, the custom of reducing the surgeon's fee by 50 percent to permit the referring physician to bill the patient for his assistance at surgery and his postoperative care; and third, the refusal of a few old guard general practitioners to permit the surgeon to bill separately for the general practitioners' rural patients.[39]

The College's immutable stand forced the Iowa Fellows to eliminate their irregular and unethical practices and vindicated the decision of the Regents go public with the ethical problems. Those who took the brunt of the criticism by the profession, especially Hawley, Davis, and Board Chairman Graham, had reason to be proud of what they had done. In today's context, that the Iowa surgeons were willing to undergo these extensive audits is a remarkable valuation of their College fellowship.[38]

⋙ ✳ ⋘

Using the Iowa Solution

A group in Detroit organized the Detroit Surgical Society to eradicate fee splitting in Detroit.[40] The members affirmed their willingness to undergo financial audits. Although some members refused, the Society was effective and eventually disbanded because its goal had been achieved.[41,42]

As the success of forming local surgery organizations whose members disavowed fee splitting became known, societies sprung up in Fort Wayne, Indiana; Minneapolis, Minnesota;[43,44] Scranton and Lackawanna County, Pennsylvania;[36,45] and Hawaii.[46]

≈ ✳ ≈

Hospitals and Joint Commission

Throughout the war on unethical practices, the College leadership and practicing surgeons believed the newly formed Joint Commission should take a tough stand on ethics, and require accredited hospitals to enact policies and procedures that would preclude fee splitting, ghost surgery, excessive fees, and itinerant surgery. A Governor of the College, Dr. Edward Sprague of Newark, New Jersey, developed a set of medical staff rules that would obviate fee splitting, and asked the College to adopt them for use by hospitals. The Executive Committee declined to make recommendations to hospitals; instead, the College sent a copy of the Regents' "Statement on certain unethical practices" to the Joint Commission and the chairman of the governing board of each of its accredited hospitals.[29] This put pressure on hospital executives and medical staffs to deal with fee splitting in their institutions, and some took action.

Practicing surgeons pressured the College to educate the governing boards of hospitals about ethics and surgical privileges. Lack of support and interest by their boards often scuttled efforts to rid their hospitals of fee splitting. The College obtained the support of the American Hospital Association (AHA) and the Catholic Hospital Association for joint educational programs at selected meetings of these organizations.[43]

An example was Adelphi Hospital in Brooklyn, a well-known den of fee splitting, until a group of Fellows who practiced there took action. A former commissioner of the Joint Commission, who was hired as a consultant, induced the governing board and the medical staff to require a financial audit of every surgeon's records. The audit revealed that three members of the medical staff probably were splitting fees. The governing board and medical staff had agreed that fee splitters would be dismissed from the staff.[47]

The AMA responded to a hospital in Sitka, Alaska, where a proposed contract would have the hospital collect the fee for radiology services and split the fee fifty-fifty with the physician who requested the x-ray. The AMA clearly stated that this was unethical, and seemed to affirm the College's position on fee splitting, combined billing, and other such practices.[45]

≈ ✳ ≈

Health Insurance and Fee Splitting

A major problem for the College was the systems used by insurance companies to pay physicians and surgeons. Insurance companies usually sent the surgeon one check to cover the entire surgical benefit under the patient's contract. The surgeon then felt compelled to send a portion of the benefit to the anesthesiologist, the surgeon's assistant, and other physicians involved in the case, none of whom were eligible for separate reimbursement by the insurance company. Most often, one of these doctors was the referring physician. This practice of splitting fees was unethical; yet, there was no provision for the other members of the team to have access to a portion of the surgical benefit.

College officials asked insurance companies to send out two checks, one for the surgeon and one for the assistant, but insurance companies refused to do this except for Blue Cross and Blue Shield in Massachusetts. There, the assistant received 15 percent of the surgeon's fee, a practice that was unethical under College policy. Responding to pressure from the College and the AMA, several insurance companies were willing to issue two checks, but they were totally opposed to accepting more than one voucher because it fouled up their accounting system. Thus, only the surgeon could submit a bill, and the insurance company paid the second physician a portion of the surgical benefit, which was subtracted from the amount the surgeon received.

Compounding the problem was the large number of medical insurance plans, many of which were sponsored by medical societies, with more than 30 million subscribers. Hawley surveyed 74 Blue Shield plans and found large variations in how they paid physicians and surgeons for surgical services.[29,48] The College decided that when more than one physician participated in the surgical care, the patient should receive a report of the percentage of the payment that went to each physician involved. The College also asked insurance companies to establish uniform payment schedules for surgical assistants and for postoperative care and to make the payments directly to the physician, citing its policy on fee splitting and the AMA's principles of medical ethics, which precluded fee splitting. In the absence of computers, it was years before the insurance industry made this routine practice.[13,29]

The Regents invited Dr. James McCann, a Blue Shield official and a Fellow of the College, to meet with them in 1958. He explained why it was not possible for all Blue Shield plans to eliminate proration of fees in paying physicians. After hearing criticism from Hawley and Ravdin, he said,

> All sound physicians want abuses eliminated from practices, but
> Blue Shield should not be blamed for causing these abuses. Blue
> Shield is not a policeman; the medical society is the one responsible
> for discipline. Hospitals should be informed of those physicians
> who are practicing unethically and the hospitals forced to take
> action against them.[49]

After this meeting, the Regents set the policy that the College would take no action against Fellows and applicants who must practice proration because it was an established practice by Blue Shield plans in their area.[50] Their adaptation was an example of external forces imposing changes on society and the medical profession, which the College had no power to stop. This phenomenon would continue to frustrate the College and its Fellows throughout the second fifty years of its existence.

An ironic problem associated with fee splitting is that it helped to drive general practitioners to seek surgical privileges in hospitals. Receiving full payment for a surgical procedure without having to split the fee was obviously better than serving as the referring physician and receiving only a portion of the fee. It was during the College's drive against fee splitting that the American Academy of General Practice was pushing for surgical privileges for their membership.[51] The simplest way for general practitioners to rid themselves of the fee splitting problem was to do the operation themselves. Later, the College would take this issue to the public.

Clinics and Group Practices

As the public understanding of fee splitting grew, creative subterfuges to disguise it surfaced. In the Midwest, especially in Illinois and Ohio, groups of surgeons formed clinics and hired general practitioners as associate members of the clinics. Associate members were paid a salary or a commission based on how many patients they referred directly to the clinic or the number of patients that entered the clinic from their geographic area. The College prepared a statement condemning this practice, which was a cover for fee splitting.[52]

The Ses Clinic in Los Angeles was a group of general practitioners who asked the College if their practice was ethical. Surgeons had offices within walking distance and came to the clinic to see patients (at the invitation of the general practitioners). The surgeon operated on the patient, and sent the patient back to the group. He sent his own bill, and then submitted 40 percent of the amount collected to the clinic for its overhead. They discontinued this practice after learning from the College that is was unethical.

After the College said it was guilty of unethical practices, the Springfield Rural-Urban Clinic in Illinois reported that they discontinued their paid, part-time category of clinic membership for physicians, which effectively stopped their fee splitting.[31]

Not all of the arrangements for division of professional fees were deemed unethical by the College, yet to some they appeared to involve fee splitting. The Georgia credentials committee reviewed a candidate who was a member of the staff of the Emory University Clinic. His eligibility was questioned because of the financial relationship of the clinic to the university. The statement of organization of the clinic provided that each section of the partnership would pay a graduated percentage of its gross income to the university. The credentials committee had decided that the arrangement was unethical because it was the practice of medicine by a corporation, a practice the profession deemed unethical during the first half of the College's existence. The Regents wisely decided that what constitutes the practice of medicine by a corporation was determined by the laws of the state and by the principles of ethics of the AMA.[14]

Individual Fellows in Baltimore solicited the College to prevent the organization and operation of a private patient clinic by the Johns Hopkins University and Hospital, which was to serve private and semiprivate patients who came directly to the hospital. Their doctors would be the full-time staff of the medical school and hospital, and the clinic would set fees and bill the patients. Expenses would be deducted from the collections and the remainder transferred to the income accounts of the appropriate clinical departments of the school of medicine. The issue was put before the Board of Regents because it was a matter of practice of medicine by a corporation. The Board of Regents replied that the issue was not within their province.[51] Given that the majority of physicians now practice in groups, the arrangements that were thought to be unethical 50 years ago are now the norm and considered ethical. Nevertheless, in the context of the College's war against fee splitting, these university clinics clearly were splitting fees.

Issues with the AMA

From the beginning of the College's exposure of unethical practices to the public, its leaders wanted to work with the AMA, widely accepted as the organization that spoke for physicians in economic, ethical, and political matters. That the College went public on an ethical issue was a major departure for a specialty organization that had respected the AMA as the voice of medicine. The AMA's code of ethics proscribed fee splitting, so the College leaders felt their plans were in line with AMA policy. But many individual members of the AMA, as well as many of its constituent organizations, such as the Chicago Medical Society, were outraged that the College had usurped the prerogative of the AMA to speak out publically on a matter of medical ethics. In the wake of Hawley's *U.S. News and World Report* interview, 11 resolutions were introduced at a meeting of the AMA's House of Delegates, all condemning his public disclosure of fee splitting. The theme was that statements from a minority group such as the College did not represent the views of the profession; only the AMA had the right and authority to speak for the profession on ethical issues.[53]

This reaction spurred Greer Williams, Director of Public Relations, and Loyal Davis, Chairman of the Public Relations Committee, to ask the Regents if they were resolute in standing up against the criticism of the AMA. The Regents adopted a resolution affirming their right to speak for the profession on ethical matters without first seeking permission from the AMA or its affected constituent organizations and published it in the *Bulletin*. They also asked Board Chairman Graham to request the AMA to form a joint committee with the College to combat unethical practices.[31,40]

This was especially important because the constituent organizations of the AMA, such as local and state medical societies, were not required to adopt the AMA's Code of Ethics, and many of them had not done so. In addition, the Code of Ethics could be interpreted as having loopholes that conflicted with the College's hard line stance on fee splitting.

Regent Leland S McKittrick, of Boston, was a member of the AMA's Council on Medical Education and Hospitals, and eventually, its chairman. He was the obvious choice to chair the College's Committee to Collaborate with the AMA on Unethical Practices. McKittrick arranged a meeting with representatives of the AMA and the Joint Commission, a group that eventually agreed on definitions of unjustified operations, ghost surgery, fee splitting, and excessive fees.

Although the AMA code of ethics proscribed fee splitting, the payment of one physician by another for services rendered to a patient was not specifically prohibited. The primary example was when the surgeon paid the assistant for his services out of the insurance company's payment to the surgeon, a transaction prohibited by the College, which maintained that each physician must bill the patient separately for his services. The AMA contended that since the insurance company would not pay the assistant directly, it was appropriate for the surgeon to pay him out of the payment he received. Loyal Davis corresponded with the chairman of the board of trustees of the AMA, Dr. Hugh Hussey, and to the executive vice president, Dr. FJL Blasingame about this issue, but the AMA would not modify its position.[54] They agreed that both organizations were free to publicly advocate their positions.[55]

The College remained resolute in its condemnation of unethical practices. The awareness of the public made many doctors cautious about violating the College's principles. The Joint Commission required hospitals to have methods to prevent fee splitting in place. Groups of surgeons in communities pledged not to split fees. Given time, the practice became less common, although there were periodic charges of fee splitting in the Midwest, especially in Chicago.[56] By 1970 it was no longer an issue.

—✳—

Itinerant Surgery

The Hill-Burton Act of 1946 provided federal funds to achieve the goal of 4.5 beds per 1,000 persons in every county in the country. Hundreds of hospitals were built, many in rural communities that had no surgeons. This led to a practice called itinerant surgery, in which a local physician, usually a general practitioner, called on a surgeon from a larger community to operate on patients. The "itinerant" surgeon may or may not have seen the patient before the procedure, but almost always left the postoperative care to the general practitioner. Sometimes the itinerant surgeons split the fee with him. The College issued an official statement on itinerant surgery in 1960. Itinerant surgery was defined as:

> any surgical operation performed, except one upon the patient whose chances of recovery would be prejudiced by movement to another hospital, in which, because of the distance from the patient, the operating surgeon must delegate the exacting responsibility for postoperative care to another, who by training and experience is not fully qualified to undertake it.

There was a long explanation of this definition, which refuted various arguments that had been proposed to justify itinerant surgery. The primary reasoning was that postoperative care was as important as the operation itself, and in some cases more important.[19]

This statement was sent to all College chapters, Governors, and committee members, with instructions that Fellows who engaged in itinerant surgery should be disciplined and that applicants for fellowship who performed itinerant surgery should be denied fellowship.[57] The effectiveness of the College's stance was not measured, but increased access of patients to qualified surgeons in larger communities, public education, and a growing number of surgeons effectively diminished the practice. Recently, a growing shortage of general surgeons has created access problems in smaller communities, an issue dealt with in a later chapter.

—✳—

Medical Student Program on Ethics

The College invited a third or fourth year medical student from each of the 90 medical schools in the United States and Canada to attend Clinical Congresses of the College. The purpose was to educate the students about unethical medical practices during their formative years.[14]

A Significant Achievement

The College's fight against unethical practices was successful because of the serendipitous confluence of a few strong personalities, unafraid to speak out and unafraid of the personal consequences of doing so. One was Evarts Graham, whose early experience in a small Iowa community sensitized him to the evils of fee splitting and led him to know that it could be addressed and stopped. Another was Paul Hawley, whose life had been at risk numerous times in his long military career and who was not afraid of anything. Loyal Davis, always outspoken and opinionated, despised fee splitting and was willing to put his reputation in Chicago on the line by speaking out. Finally, Isidor Ravdin, the confident, swashbuckling surgeon, never felt vulnerable when dealing with ethical issues. Obviously, the other Regents and staff also displayed gumption and wisdom. Together, guided by moral courage, this group orchestrated one of the College's greatest achievements during its first hundred years.

REFERENCES

1. Stephenson, G.W., *American College of Surgeons at 75*. 1990, Chicago: American College of Surgeons.
2. *Minutes of the meeting of the Board of Regents of May 9, 10, 1936*. 1936, Archives of the American College of Surgeons: Chicago.
3. *Minutes of the meeting of the executive committee of January 9, 1938*. 1938, Archives of the American College of Surgeons: Chicago. p. 1-43.
4. Rodman, J.S., *History of the American Board of Surgery. 1937-1952*. 1956, Philadelphia: J.B. Lippincott Co.
5. *Minutes of the meeting of the xecutive Commitee of September 10, 1938*. 1938, Archives of the American College of Surgeons: Chicago.
6. *Minutes of the meeting of the Executive Committee of July 29, 1939*. 1939, Archives of the American College of Surgeons: Chicago.
7. *Minutes of the meeting of the Board of Regents of October 29, 1939*. 1939, Archives of the American College of Surgeons: Chicago.
8. *Minutes of the meeting of the Board of Regents of June 27, 1943*. 1943, Archives of the American College of Surgeons: Chicago.
9. *The Columbus Surgical Society. History.* Columbussurgicalsociety.com/about.html 2010.
10. Rodwin, M., *The organized American profession's response to financial conflicts of interest: 1890-1992*. The Milbank Quarterly, 1992. **70**: p. 703-741.
11. Snell, A. *Chairman's Address. Some principles of medical ethics and the practice of ophthalmology*. in *American Medical Association Section on Ophthalmology. 92nd annual session. June 4-6, 1941*. 1941.
12. *Minutes of the meeting of the Board of Regents of February 2, 1947*. 1947, Archives of the American College of Surgeons: Chicago.
13. *Minutes of the meeting of the Executive Committee of December 3, 1955*. 1955, Archives of the American College of Surgeons: Chicago.
14. *Minutes of the meeting of the Executive Committee of December 4, 5, 1955*. 1955, Archives of the American College of Surgeons: Chicago.
15. *Minutes of the meeting of the Board of Regents of November 3,4, 1951*. 1951, Archives of the American College of Surgeons: Chicago.
16. *Minutes of the meeting of the Board of Regents of April 15, 1952*. 1952, Archives of the American College of Surgeons: Chicago.
17. Hawley, P., *American College of Surgeons restates principles of financial relations*. Bulletin of the American College of Surgeons, 1952. **37**: p. 233-236.
18. *Minutes of the meeting of the Board of Regents of October 9, 1953*. 1953, Archives of the American College of Surgeons: Chicago.
19. *Minutes of the meeting of the Board of Regents of February 27,28, 2960*. 1960, Archives of the American College of Surgeons: Chicago.
20. *Minutes of the meeting of the Board of Regents of June 10,11, 1960*. 1960, Archives of the American College of Surgeons: Chicago.
21. *Surgeons rip fee splitting as "dishonest." On increase in Chicago, Dr. Davis says.*, in *Chicago Daily Tribune*. 1952: Chicago.
22. Lawrence, W., *Drive on split fees may be on TV, radio.*, in *New York TImes*. 1952: New York.
23. *About the Chicago Medical Society. Mission and history.* http:www.cmsdocs.org
24. *Too much unnecessary surgery. Interview with Dr. Paul Hawley.*, in *U.S. News and World Report*. 1953. p. 48-55.

25. Williams, G., *Fee-splitting. Public education to what? Exhib 5-d-i. In: Minutes of the meeting of the Board of Regents of April 4,5, 1953*. 1953, Archives of the American College of Surgeons: Chicago.

26. *Medical Board abandons probe of Loyal Davis.*, in *Chicago Daily Tribune*. March 11, 1953: Chicago.

27. *Family doctors protest.*, in *New York Times*. March 24, 1953: New York.

28. *Assail Chicago doctor's rap at fee splitting.*, in *Chicago Daily Tribune*. March 24, 1953: Chicago.

29. *Minutes of the meeting of the Board of Regents of February 19,20, 1955*. 1955, Archives of the American College of Surgeons: Chicago.

30. *Minutes of the meting of the Board of Regents of October 3,4,6, 1953*. 1953, Archives of the American College of Surgeons: Chicago.

31. *Minutes of the meeting of the Board of Regents of April 4,5, 1953*. 1953, Archives of the American College of Surgeons: Chicago.

32. M*inutes of the meeting of the Executive Committee of March 21, 1954*. 1954, Archives of the American College of Surgeons: Chicago.

33. *Minutes of the meeting of the Executive Committee of August 10, 1954*. 1954, Archives of the American College of Surgeons: Chicago.

34. *Minutes of the meeting of the Board of Regents of June 4,5, 1955*. 1955, Archives of the American College of Surgeons: Chicago.

35. *Minutes of the meeting of the Executive Committee of October 29, 1955*. 1955, Archives of the American College of Surgeons: Chicago.

36. *Minutes of the meeting of the Board of Regents of November 13,14,18, 1954*. 1954, Archives of the American College of Surgeons: Chicago.

37. *Minutes of the meeting of the Board of Regents of February 11,12, 1956*. 1956, Archives of the American College of Surgeons: Chicago.

38. *Minutes of the meeting of the Executive Committee of October 5, 1956*. 1956, Archives of the American College of Surgeons: Chicago.

39. *Minutes of the meeting of the Board of Regents of March 1,2, 1958*. 1958, Archives of the meeting of the Board of Regents of March 1,2, 1958: Chicago.

40. *Minutes of the meeting of the Executive Commttee of July 31, 1958*. 1953, Archives of the American College of Surgeons: Chicago.

41. *Minutes of the meeting of the Executive Committee of March 21, 1954*. 1954, Archives of the American College of Surgeons: Chicago.

42. *Personal communication Dr. Charles Lucas to David Nahrwold*. 2010.

43. *Minutes of the meeting of the Board of Regents of October 8,9, 1960*. 1960, Archives of the American College of Surgeons: Chicago.

44. *Minutes of the meeting of the Board of Regents of February 8,9, 1964*. 1964, Archives of the American College of Surgeons: Chicago.

45. *Minutes of the meeting of the Board of Regents of October 12,13, 1957*. 1957, Archives of the American College of Surgeons: Chicago.

46. *Minutes of the meeting of the Board of Regents of December 6,7, 1959*. 1959, Archives of the American College of Surgeons: Chicago.

47. *Minutes of the meeting of the Board of Regents of May 11,12, 1957*. 1957, Archives of the American College of Surgeons: Chicago.

48. *Minutes of the meeting of the Executive Committee of February 10, 1956*. 1956, Archives of the American College of Surgeons: Chicago.

49. *Minutes of the meeting of the Board of Regents of June 7,8, 1958*. 1958, Archives of the American College of Surgeons: Chicago.

50. *Minutes of the meeting of the Board of Regents of December 12, 13, 1958*. 1958, Archives of the American College of Surgeons: Chicago.

51. *Minutes of the meeting of the Board of Regents of February 3, 4, 1957.* 1957, Archives of the American College of Surgeons: Chicago.
52. *Minutes of the meeting of the Executive Committee of November 23, 1952.* 1952, Archives of the American College of Surgeons: Chicago.
53. Davis, L., *Fellowship of Surgeons. A History of the American College of Surgeons.* 1960, Chicago: American College of Surgeons.
54. *Minutes of the meeting of the Board of Regents of June 23,24, 1961.* 1961, Archives of the American College of Surgeons: Chicago.
55. *Minutes of the meeting of the Board of Regents of February 17,18, 1962.* 1962, Archives of the American College of Surgeons: Chicago.
56. *Minutes of the meeting of the Board of Regents of June 24, 25, 1966.* 1966, Archives of the American College of Surgeons: Chicago.
57. *Minutes of the meeting of the Board of Regents of December 4,5, 1960.* 1960, Archives of the American College of Surgeons: Chicago.

CHAPTER 14
Shaping Change and Adapting to Change

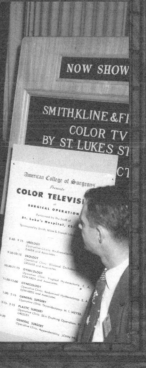

By 1960, specialization was flourishing. The College, which from its founding spoke for all of surgery, was having difficulty satisfying all surgical specialties, many of which had developed their own organizations. Another organization was formed to represent the specialty of general surgery, and the International College of Surgeons was challenging the American College of Surgeons (ACS) as the voice for surgery throughout the world. The specialties of oral surgery and otolaryngology were fighting with the profession of dentistry over who should perform operations on the mouth, lips, jaws, and neck in a classic turf battle. Vascular and pediatric surgery, spawned from general surgery, were on their way to becoming specialties by the end of the century. Finally, the College debated where the specialty of anesthesiology should fit within the structure of organized medicine.

OB/GYN Leaves the Nest

Members of the Advisory Council on Obstetrics and Gynecology were unhappy with the College. Its chairman, Dr. Donald G Tollefson of Los Angeles, wanted the College to influence the Joint Commission to place more emphasis on maternal and fetal medicine and less on the incidence of Cesarean section. He also wanted the Joint Commission on Accreditation of Hospitals to require that hospitals have an adequate blood bank, because hemorrhage was still a major cause of maternal death. The Joint Commission should also require hospitals to create departments of anesthesia for obstetrical services, and to standardize the care of the premature infants. Finally, he pointed out that although there was a session on gynecology at the Clinical Congress, there was none on obstetrics. He said, "We have 1,800 members who have paid dues, and they have no meetings." He recommended that there be two sessions in obstetrics and two in gynecology.[1] The Advisory Council, composed of leaders in the field, were chafing at being constrained by the College. They clearly knew that by itself the College could not standardize care of premature infants or create separate obstetrical anesthesia departments. Those were battles only obstetricians could wage successfully, and they wanted to do so.

In their discussion of Tollefson's complaints, Dr. Newell W Philpott, the OB/GYN Regent from McGill University, pointed out that there was a worldwide movement to separate OB/GYN from general surgery. In Great Britain they had broken apart completely. In Canada, where Philpott lived, there was friction between general surgeons and obstetricians/gynecologists as well. Several Regents said that gynecologic surgeons were not up to par, but if they had more time on the program, perhaps they would improve.

Chairman Allen decreed that the OB/GYN group would get time on the program for "fetal mortality." He and the Regents would inform the OB/GYN community that they could set up their separate Clinical Congress program as ophthalmology and otolaryngology had done.[2] The Regents had no expertise in the field so this was a simple solution; it had the unintended effect of putting even more distance between OB/GYN and the leadership of the College.

Some hospitals were refusing general surgeons privileges to perform gynecologic procedures. There were rumors that obstetricians and gynecologists were planning to form a college. Philpott was asked to chair a committee on relations with the American Academy of Obstetrics and Gynecology, in the hope that the College could improve its relationships with specialists in obstetrics and gynecology and stave off the movement to form a college.

Subsequently, Philpott reported that a committee had been formed to discuss changing the name of the Academy to a college, and that this had been discussed at great length within the specialty of OB/GYN. He said they had several complaints about the College, including that they had no representation on the Joint Commission and were ignored by the College's journal *Surgery, Gynecology, and Obstetrics*. During a two-year period, only eight percent of the articles were relevant to obstetrics or gynecology. They did not have adequate representation on the Clinical Congress programs, and fewer than 50 percent of the members of their Academy were Fellows of the American College of Surgeon, yet the number of obstetricians/gynecologists approached that of general surgeons.

In March 1954, Philpott recommended that the College make every effort to resist change. General surgeons were doing 60 percent of the gynecology in the country. He planned for his committee to meet with a group from the Academy to discuss the issues. He also recommended that he be replaced as a member of the Board of Regents by one of the dissenting gynecologists, a suggestion that was not accepted.[3]

In November, Philpott reported that there was "grave dissatisfaction" among OB/GYN specialists and strong agitation to form an American College of Obstetrics and Gynecology at the meeting of the American Academy of Obstetrics and Gynecology in December. This would set a precedent for further fragmentation of surgery. He recommended that the College negotiate with the Academy before its meeting on December 12 and that the College either create a semi-autonomous specialty section for obstetrics and gynecology or, if an OB/GYN college were formed, to push to create a federation of surgical colleges as a means to exert some control.[4] Philpott and the College were too late. In December 1954, the American Academy of Obstetrics and Gynecology morphed into the American College of Obstetricians and Gynecologists (ACOG).

In trying to placate the obstetricians/gynecologists, Paul Hawley recommended to the Joint Commission that Dr. John Brewer, chairman of obstetrics and gynecology at Northwestern, be appointed to represent the College on the Board of Commissioners at its next vacancy.[5] Not satisfied, ACOG asked to be a corporate member of the Joint Commission, but was denied. ACOG then appealed to the College for support, but the Regents declined to help.[6]

Continuing to make the point that their college was equivalent to the surgeons' college, ACOG leaders also applied to the College for membership on the tripartite OB/GYN residency review committee. The Board of Regents stated that the College did not have authority to grant this request. ACOG clearly wanted to displace the American College of Surgeons as a member of the tripartite committee.[7]

Regent Isidor Ravdin, representing the College, met with three representatives of the ACOG,

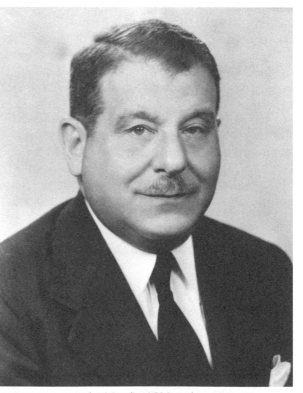

FIGURE 14.1 Dr. Isidor S Ravdin, ACS President, 1960–61.

including John Brewer. (Figure 14.1) They agreed that ACOG should not be a member of the Joint Commission at this time. The three representatives asked if the College would support ACOG for membership on the residency review committee if the American Board of Obstetrics and Gynecology changed its requirements for the training of gynecologists, which excluded general surgeons. They did not come to agreement on this. They did agree to consider Ravdin's insistence that a general surgeon should not have to give up his American Board of Surgery certificate before he could be certified by the American Board of Obstetrics and Gynecology.[8]

Representatives of the College, the American Board of Obstetrics and Gynecology, and the Council on Medical Education of the AMA met to discuss the request of the ACOG to be represented on the residency review committee for OB/GYN. They decided that the new organization was not of sufficient stature to be represented. The real reason was that they were resentful of ACOG's aggressiveness in trying to exclude general surgeons from practicing gynecology.[9]

The basic issue behind the ongoing skirmishes between ACOG and the College was that ACOG and its members did not believe general surgeons should practice gynecology. It was a turf battle. Eventually, general surgery residents received little, if any, instruction in gynecologic surgery and therefore were unable to include it in their practices. This effectively ended the battle between the organizations and the era in which general surgeons performed gynecologic surgery. It also marked the beginning of the separation of obstetrics and gynecology from the ACS, although one of the Regent's seats continues to be reserved for an obstetrician/gynecologist and the Advisory Council for Obstetrics and Gynecology continues to offer advice.

Who Does Oral Surgery?

The fragmentation of surgery was not limited to gynecology. Hawley received numerous requests from Fellows and hospitals for a statement from the College defining oral surgery. These were related to complaints that some dentists were performing cleft lip and palate repairs and even lymph node dissections of the neck for cancer. The Regents stated,

> No person should be permitted to perform surgery for which he has not had adequate training in a progressive, integrated and approved residency program. Surgery of the head and neck is specifically included in this proscription.

The Regents also believed that otolaryngologists were not adequately trained for major surgical procedures and should not do neck dissections and similar extensive surgery.[6]

The newly formed Society of Head and Neck Surgeons, which required American Board of Surgery (ABS) certification for membership, expressed concern to the College that otolaryngologists and dentists were performing head and neck surgery. They requested a statement that head and neck cases should be assigned to general surgery services and not to specialty services. The Society also requested that the College establish a Clinical Congress course on head and neck cancer, organized by general surgeons. A resolution from the Society of Maxillofacial Surgeons condemned the increasing encroachment by dental oral surgeons on the practice of medicine. To avoid involvement in a turf battle, the Regents took no action on these matters.[10]

The members of the Society of Head and Neck Surgeons, almost all general surgeons who specialized in head and neck surgery, reflected the commonplace view that otolaryngologists were not adequately trained for this subspecialty. Further evidence of this was that the Cancer Committee submitted a resolution that head and neck cancer surgery, other than that limited to the upper respiratory tract, was properly in the field of general surgery. The committee believed it was improper for another specialty group (otolaryngology) to be conducting discussions about head and neck surgery.

The Clinical Congress program committee declared that oral surgeons and otolaryngologists would not be placed on programs dealing with head and neck surgery. This was the beginning of a long period of rancor between the specialties of general surgery and otolaryngology about head and neck surgery, which eventually included surgery of the thyroid and parathyroid glands. Given that all surgical specialties were represented in the College, the fragmentation of surgery almost always left the College discredited by the specialty it did not support. For this reason, the Regents often refused to take a stand on turf issues.[11]

Relieved, the Regents congratulated Dr. Dean Lierle, the esteemed head of otolaryngology at the University of Iowa, when he reported that the American Board of Otolaryngology had increased its training requirements to at least four years, of which at least one year must be in general surgery and at least two years in otolaryngology. Furthermore, the board agreed that otolaryngologists wishing to do tumor surgery of the head and neck should have additional general surgery training beyond the required four years of training.[10]

The feature editor of the magazine *Harper's Bazaar* in the June 1960 issue recommended to its readers that their cosmetic surgery should be performed only by plastic surgeons certified by the American Board of Plastic Surgery. Several societies of otolaryngologists protested that they also were qualified to perform cosmetic surgery, and the College received official complaints from them and from Fellows who were otolaryngologists.

Dr. Frank McDowell, vice chairman of the American Board of Plastic Surgery, wrote Hawley that the board deplored the *Harper's* article, stating that it had no prior knowledge whatsoever of the publication of this "blatantly commercial article." Moreover, McDowell asked the College for its help and support in dealing with this "miserable situation." The College took no action, but this was the beginning of a long battle between plastic surgery and otolaryngology over cosmetic surgery, one that played out publicly at meetings of the American Board of Medical Specialties (ABMS), when otolaryngology sought approval for a certificate of special competence in facial plastic surgery.[12]

≈ ✳ ≈

Anesthesiologists in the College of Surgeons?

During the 1950s, many hospitals were attempting to recruit anesthesiologists as hospital employees. Anesthesia was a young specialty; there were only about 3,000 anesthesiologists in the country and only about 700 of them were board certified. The hospitals were motivated by a shortage of anesthesiologists, the need for supervision of nurse anesthetists, and the logistics of managing a busy operating suite schedule while meeting the requests of surgeons for their favorite anesthesiologists. Having a group of employed anesthesiologists obviated these problems and put the hospital in control of managing the operating suite. Many anesthesiologists preferred employment because it guaranteed an income, eliminated the expense of anesthesia machines and other equipment, allowed them to integrate nurse anesthetists into their practices, and obviated travelling from one hospital to another.

But reflecting the medical profession's aversion to taking a salary, and concerned that their specialty would be controlled by hospital administrators, the American Society of Anesthesiologists and the American Board of Anesthesiology declared that taking a salary was unethical. Newly trained anesthesiologists were told that they would not be admitted to the Society if they were salaried. To make matters worse for them, membership in the American Society of Anesthesiologists was required as part of the criteria for admission to the board certification examination. Young men faced the prospect of being banned from board certification if they were employed by hospitals.

The controversy over hiring of physicians by hospitals also involved pathologists and radiologists. Hospital employment was opposed by the AMA and concerned all physicians. The College was also concerned; after all, if hospitals could hire members of these specialties, they could also hire surgeons. Regent Harold Foss was appointed chairman of a committee to evaluate the possibility of a closer relationship between the College and the specialties of anesthesia, pathology, and radiology. The College might have wanted to lend its prestige and its considerable influence with the Joint Commission to help employed anesthesiologists oppose their certifying board and their most influential society. Furthermore, if the College decided to include anesthesiologists in its fellowship, it could exert considerable control over the specialty of anesthesia.

In 1951, Foss's committee recommended associate membership in the College for anesthesiologists. The committee had sought the advice of the eminent Harvard anesthesiologist Henry Beecher, who helped them develop requirements, including board certification, one year of internship and two years of full-time training in an approved anesthesia residency, four years of practice, and administration of 2,000 anesthetics. Hawley and others were concerned about unethical practices in anesthesia, including secret deals with anesthesia equipment manufacturers. He said that it would be best not to take anesthesiologists into the College because the College would be taking on their fight. Regent Cave moved that the matter be tabled, ending the discussion, but not the issue.[2]

Two years later the Regents heard a presentation by Dr. Lloyd Mousel of Seattle, an anesthesiologist, who described the attempt by the American Society of Anesthesiologists and the American Board of Anesthesiology to force him to accept their ideas of proper contractual relations with a hospital that employed him. After hearing this, the Regents passed a resolution that the Board of Regents of the ACS deplored the actions of the American Society of Anesthesiologists and the American Board of Anesthesiology, which was sent to these organizations.[13]

Dr. Henry Beecher, the eminent Harvard anesthesiologist, was invited to advise the Regents about admitting anesthesiologists to the College. He said there were many bad practices in anesthesia that violated the ethics of the medical profession. Evarts Graham said that the situation was almost intolerable and the College had an obligation to deal with it. He believed strongly that this was best done by admitting anesthesiologists to the College. Most of the Regents were reluctant, but Graham, Davis, and Ravdin were adamant about admitting them. Beecher thought that the College should admit a few carefully chosen men to fellowship and require that they sign a pledge, demonstrating their support for properly trained nurse anesthetists and free choice of the method of anesthesiologists' method of compensation. Davis prepared a pledge that also precluded "dishonest money seeking and commercialism," and required the signee "to refuse all secret money trades with consultants and practitioners, makers of anesthesia equipment and appliances, and to make my fees commensurate with the services I render, and to avoid discrediting associates..."[14]

Three months later the Regents approved Davis's pledge, and Ravdin presented a list of names of anesthesiologists recommended by both Henry Beecher and Dr. Robert Dripps, chairman of anesthesia and Ravdin's colleague at the University of Pennsylvania. After adding a few names to the list, the Regents decided to invite them to apply for fellowship. They agreed that applications from these men would be handled specially, but future applications would go through the regular procedure of application for fellowship.[15]

At the meeting of the Executive Committee of the Board in January 1955, however, Drs. Blalock and MacKenzie questioned the wisdom of admitting anesthesiologists. They pointed out that there was dissention and disagreement within the specialty itself, and the College would be forced to take sides. They also argued that very few anesthesiologists would be qualified for fellowship, making it difficult for those admitted to the College to have an impact on the ethics and practices in anesthesia. Finally, they believed that it would be difficult to justify two pledges for membership in one organization. Six months later the Regents voted to rescind their action.[16] Most of the Regents had not been enthusiastic during the discussions, and may have been too polite to voice objection to the aggressive tactics of Ravdin, Graham, and Davis. Of these, Graham was the most adamant, and a majority of the Regents may not have wanted to offend the old stalwart.

The Board of Governors was opposed to admitting anesthesiologists to the College, and formally resolved that the College remain an organization of general surgeons and surgical specialists. They recommended that proper attention be paid to the various surgical specialty groups to maintain this objective. To ensure attention to the specialties, the Governors recommended that the bylaws be changed to require one representative on the Board of Regents from each of the specialties of obstetrics and gynecology, ophthalmology, otolaryngology, urology, neurosurgery, orthopaedics, and anesthesiology. They recommended increasing the number of Regents by three. At the time they understood that anesthesiologists would be admitted to the College, so they provided a list of anesthesiologists for admission as requested by the Regents, even though they were opposed to admitting anesthesiologists.[11]

≈✻≈

American Board of Abdominal Surgery

College Fellows were solicited by the International Association of Surgical Clinics, located at 103 Park Avenue in New York City, which was attempting to form an American Board of Abdominal Surgery. Initial efforts by the College staff to obtain more information about the new board were unsuccessful, except to learn that the fancy Park Avenue location was simply a mailing address.[17] Later, they learned that the American Board of Abdominal Surgery requirements for training were four years of formal, progressive, surgical training in a hospital approved for surgical training by the Council of Medical Education and Hospitals of the AMA; or three years of formal training and a minimum of two years of acceptable surgical practice; or in lieu of formal training, 16 years of acceptable surgical practice. Perhaps because of the College's interest in this board, four of the nine Fellows of the College who were members of the Board of Governors of the American Board of Abdominal Surgery notified the College that they had resigned.[18] Those who had not resigned did so after receiving letters from the College asking them about their position on the board.

Soon thereafter, in October 1958, Dr. Blaise Alfano, executive secretary of the abdominal surgery board, officially requested that the College and the American Board of Surgery sponsor the board. The College declined and the ABS replied,

> the American Board of Surgery, believing that general surgery is a comprehensive field, does not encourage the establishment of separate boards within the province of general surgery and for this reason, respectfully declines to sponsor a board of abdominal surgery.[19]

Having been rejected by these potential sponsors, in 1959 the organizers formed the American Society of Abdominal Surgeons, which became the sponsor of the American Board of Abdominal Surgery.

Thereafter, the organizers made a bizarre attempt to obtain the sponsorship of the AMA.[20] This came to the attention of the College's Board of Governors at their meeting in October 1961. Dr. Henry Swann, a member of the Board of Governors representing the General Surgery Section of the AMA, recounted the meeting of the Section held during the AMA meeting in New York City in June 1961. He told the Governors the meeting was packed with individuals who did not usually attend, and who took over the proceedings, even preventing some regular attendees from entering the room. The slate of nominees for the officers of the section, composed of three distinguished members of the ACS, was disregarded, and a slate of surgeons who were not board certified was nominated from the floor and elected. Only one of them was a member of the ACS.

A resolution was passed that the Section on General Surgery would sponsor the American Board of Abdominal Surgery for approval by the ABMS, the umbrella organization for the certifying boards. Another resolution called for the Section to provide assistance to the board for approval by the Advisory Board and for approval by the Council on Medical Education and Hospitals of the AMA.[21]

After telling this story, Swann introduced a resolution to the Board of Governors that commanded the Board of Regents of the College to publish statements informing the fellowship that the American Board of Abdominal Surgery had no official status and that the Board of Governors strongly supported the position of the Board of Regents in disapproving the establishment of a board of abdominal surgery by any group not meeting the high standards of professional training and conduct that characterized the existing, recognized, specialty boards. This resolution was "unanimously adopted, with great enthusiasm, by the Board of Governors."[22]

The resolution of the Section on General Surgery was brought before its house of delegates, but the American Board of Abdominal Surgery failed to gain approval from the AMA.[23]

The American Board of Abdominal Surgery continued to certify abdominal surgeons at the time of the College's centennial, claiming approximately 2,700 diplomates.[24] The board did not achieve approval of the successor to the Advisory Board, the ABMS, the credential preferred by most hospitals and other health care organizations. The American Society of Abdominal Surgeons continues to hold an annual clinical congress and other educational activities.

International College of Surgeons

An enduring issue for the College was the International College of Surgeons. For many years, the College leadership believed that the International College had lower standards than the ACS and that this lowered the standards of surgery everywhere, counteracting the progress made by the College to elevate them. Board Chairman Allen thought the problem should be handled by keeping members of the International College off the ACS programs and by announcing that the ACS disapproved of its Fellows appearing on the programs of the International College. He noted that of 348 Fellows taken in at the International College meeting in Cleveland, 168 had been rejected by the American College of Surgeons.

Hawley announced to the Regents in 1951 that the International College was setting up its own certifying boards, which he said would have very low standards, but would be marketed to the public as meeting the same standards as the American specialty boards.[2]

A problem for the College was that the AMA supported the International College. Its president was a member, and Morris Fishbein, the outspoken editor of the AMA journal, was said to be a member as well. This precluded engaging the AMA in the fight against the International College.

The Regents agreed that a Fellow of the International College could not be a member of a committee of the College. Subsequently, when Fellows were recommended for committees, Miss Grimm checked them for membership in the International College and they were not even brought up for discussion if they were a member.[2, 25]

The problem for the College was complex. Of the 456 men initiated or advanced to the rank of "certified Fellows" of the International College in September 1951, 241 were Fellows of the ACS and 215 were not.[26] Seventy-five had been rejected for fellowship in the ACS because of inadequate training, an insufficient experience in major surgery, status as a general practitioner who did some surgery, or for ethical reasons.

Hawley pointed out that the public was unable to distinguish between the two organizations and the word "international" captured the public's attention. He was especially concerned that there would be a campaign to force hospitals to recognize "certification" by the International College as evidence of qualification for surgical privileges, even though there was usually no examination before the International College's board, and when one was given, in his opinion, it was not sufficiently rigorous.

Approximately 2,400 Fellows of the ACS were also Fellows of the International College of Surgeons. Some of them were malcontents who never received what they considered proper recognition by the ACS. Some of them disliked the full-time academic people that dominated the leadership of the College. Others joined to get a trip abroad every year or two that they could deduct from taxable income. Some plastic surgeons and urologists were unhappy with the College because they could not get into leadership positions. Most were simply "joiners," people who like to belong to organizations.[27]

In 1957, the leadership of the International College sent a letter to all young diplomates of the ABS, inviting them to join the International College and informing them that postgraduate courses in all the surgery specialties were offered through the International College at the University of Vienna, the University of Rome, and most of the other important surgical centers in the world. The Regents were angry and frustrated, but decided to take no action.[7] The problem for the Regents was that their own Fellows were joining the International College and participating in its activities, but there was nothing they could do about it. They seemed resigned to this until the opportunity to represent surgery within the World Health Organization (WHO) arose.

The International College of Surgeons had applied to be the surgical organization that WHO, an agency of the United Nations, would recognize to represent surgery throughout the world. The College designated Brig. Gen. Sam F Seeley, stationed in Europe as United States Army Consultant in Surgery, as the official representative of the College to a meeting of the World Health Organization. He was charged with preventing the International College from receiving the designation and obtaining it for the ACS. Both organizations were turned down, however, because neither was truly international. Seeley recommended that the College seek the designation by forming an international federation of surgical colleges.[28] The Regents agreed and engaged the Royal College of Surgeons of England in developing an organization that would eventually be expanded to include the other reputable surgery organizations of the world.[5]

Doctors Ravdin, Cole, Davis, and Hawley visited London in April 1956, where officials of the Royal College agreed that a federation of English speaking surgical societies should be formed. Scandinavian and Dutch societies would be considered later and other countries might be considered when their surgical standards were deemed adequate. They agreed that expenses of the Federation would be borne by the member organizations; the ACS invested approximately $5,000 to get it started.

Ravdin and Hawley met with representatives of English speaking colleges and societies throughout the world in London in May 1957. They agreed to form the International Federation of Surgical Colleges and Societies. The administrative details were left to Sir Harry Platt, of England's Royal College. The initial meeting of the Federation was held in conjunction with the College's 1958 sectional meeting in Stockholm, following which the College agreed to pay annual dues in the amount of ten cents for every Fellow, which came to approximately $2,250.[7, 10, 18]

In 1960, WHO officially designated the Federation of Surgical Colleges and Societies the surgical representative of the World Health Organization.[9] To the disappointment of the College leadership, the Federation did nothing to improve surgical standards in the next few years. The College gave the Federation manuals for the care of trauma patients and other manuals for distribution, but nothing was done.[29]

The Federation had difficulty determining its role in international surgery. The College, after funding an unsuccessful meeting in Oslo at which research papers were presented,[30] proposed that the Federation establish a clearinghouse that maintained a list of approved programs where surgeons from "backward countries" could obtain research or clinical training.[22, 31] The College invited representatives of the Federation to the Clinical Congress in Atlantic City in 1962 and entertained them and their wives.[32] The Federation established the clearinghouse and decided to create surgical missions to bring postgraduate training to hospitals and medical schools in developing countries.[31] But in the next three years there were no applicants, and John Paul North recommended that the College seek a graceful way to disengage from the Federation.[33]

Ravdin attended the Federation meeting in 1965 and reported that most of its members contributed very little money; some not at all. J EnglebertDunphy, and later, Jonathan Rhoads represented the College at the Federation and implemented a plan to solicit contributions from U.S. Fellows for its activities.[34-36]

Eventually, the Federation offices were moved from the Royal College to the ACS, but the activities remained at a low level and the College gradually withdrew from the leadership. After the turn of the century, the Federation began to focus its support on a young organization, the College of Surgeons of East, Central, and Southern Africa, which takes responsibility for surgical education and examinations. The International

Federation supports basic science education in these areas and provides a visiting professor for an annual surgical conference.

≈✦≈

The College and Change

The inexorable rise of specialization created problems for the College, because as specialties such as obstetrics and gynecology matured, they created their own organizations, certifying boards, and educational activities. In due course they also advocated for their specialties among those in elected offices. At its founding, the College had been the haven for all surgical specialists, but as the work of each specialty expanded and became more complex over the decades, it became impossible for one organization to meet the needs of all specialists. The leadership of the College had difficulty adapting to this reality and, as exemplified by the gradual shift away from the College by OB-GYN, the College leadership reacted with animosity, which created bitterness that did not dissipate quickly.

Specialization also created turf battles, and the prestige of the College led the warring parties to seek its help in negotiating peace. In this role, the collective wisdom of the College helped to shape the future of specialties and their success.

External challenges to the sole authority of the College such as the International College of Surgeons and the American Board of Abdominal Surgery caused the Regents to react acerbically. But as soon as it was apparent that these challenges did no real damage, the College ignored them. The claim that organizations with lower standards were harmful was not substantiated, and individuals who did not meet the high standards of the College have always managed to continue to practice in the United States. Other organizations that have lower standards do educate, and probably raise the standards of practice of their members. But the College, whose leaders have been fixated on the highest standards, has always been critical of organizations with lower standards. This moral and ethical rigidity continues to favorably influence the quality of surgical practice throughout the world.

The 1960s might be best characterized as the beginning of the end of widespread unethical practices, and the beginning of the adult period of the life of the College. The validation of the value of surgical ethics by the successful suppression of widespread unethical practices confirmed the indispensability of the College in the modern era of health care. Nevertheless, the reality of specialization and the inability to meet all the needs of surgery and surgeons demonstrated that the College could not, and cannot, solve all the problems that confront the surgical profession in spite of the expectations of many of its Fellows.

≈✦≈

REFERENCES

1. *Minutes of the meeting of the Board of Regents of October 22, 1950.* 1950, Archives of the American College of Surgeons: Chicago.
2. *Minutesof the meeting of the Board of Regents of April 13, 1951.* 1951, Archives of the American College of Surgeons: Chicago.
3. *Minutes of the meeting of the Executive Committee of March 21, 1954.* 1954, Archives of the American College of Surgeons: Chicago.
4. *Minutes of the meeting of the Board of Regents of November 13,14,18, 1954.* 1954, Archives of the American College of Surgeons: Chicago.
5. *Minutes of the meeting of the Executive Committee of June 3, 1955.* 1955, Archives of the American College of Surgeons: Chicago.
6. *Minutes of the meeting of the Executive Committee of February 10, 1956.* 1956, Archives of the American College of Surgeons: Chicago.
7. *Minutes of the meeting of the Board of Regents of May 11,12, 1957.* 1957, Archives of the American College of Surgeons: Chicago.
8. *Minutes of the meeting of the Board of Regents of October 10, 1958.* 1958, Archives of the American College of Surgeons: Chicago.
9. *Minutes of the meeting of the Board of Regents of March 7, 8, 1959.* 1959, Archives of the American College of Surgeons: Chicago.
10. *Minutes of the meeting of the Board of Regents of October 12,13, 1957.* 1957, Archives of the American College of Surgeons: Chicago.
11. *Minutes of the meeting of the Board of Regents of February 19,20, 1955.* 1955, Archives of the American College of Surgeons: Chicago.
12. *Minutes of the meeting of the Board of Regents of October 8,9, 1960.* 1960, Archives of the American College of Surgeons: Chicago.
13. *Minutes of the meeting of the Board of Regents of April 4,5, 1953.* 1953, Archives of the American College of Surgeons: Chicago.
14. *Minutes of the meeting of the Executive Committee of August 10, 1954.* 1954, Archives of the American College of Surgeons: Chicago.
15. *Minutes of the meeting of the Board of Regents of November 19, 1954.* 1954, Archives of the American Colege of Surgeons: Chicago.
16. *Minutes of the meeting of the Board of Regents of June 4,5, 1955.* 1955, Archives of the American College of Surgeons: Chicago.
17. *Minutes of the meeting of the Board of Regents of March 1,2, 1958.* 1958, Archives of the meeting of the Board of Regents of March 1,2, 1958: Chicago.
18. *Minutes of the meeting of the Board of Regents of October 4, 5, 1958.* 1958, Archives of the American College of Surgeons: Chicago.
19. *Minutes of the meeting of the Board of Regents of December 12, 13, 1958.* 1958, Archives of the American College of Surgeons: Chicago.
20. *Minutes of the meeting of the Board of Regents of Spetember 30, October 1, 1961.* 1961, Archives of the American College of Surgeons: Chicago.
21. *Letter from Blaise F. Alfano to the Section on General Surgery, AMA. In: Minutes of the meeting of the Board of Regents of September 30, October 1, 1961.* 1961, Archives of the American College of Surgeons: Chicago.
22. *Minutes of the meeting of the Board of Regents of October 6, 1961.* 1961, Archives of the American College of Surgeons: Chicago.
23. *Minutes of the meeting of the Board of Regents of October 13, 14, 1962.* 1962, Archives of the American College of Surgeons: Chicago.
24. *The American Society of Abdominal Surgeons website. http://abdominalsurg.org.*

25. *Minutes of the meeting of the Board of Regents of November 3,4, 1951.* 1951, Archives of the American College of Surgeons: Chicago.

26. *Minutes of the meeting of the Board of Regents of December 3, 1951.* 1951, Archives of the American College of Surgeons: Chicago.

27. *Minutes of the meeting of the Board of Regents of October 9, 1953.* 1953, Archives of the American College of Surgeons: Chicago.

28. *Minutes of the meeting of the Board of Regents of March 21, 1954.* 1954, Archives of the American College of Surgeons: Chicago.

29. *Minutes of the meeting of the Board of Regents of December 4,5, 1960.* 1960, Archives of the American College of Surgeons: Chicago.

30. *Minutes of the meeting of the Board of Regents of June 23,24, 1961.* 1961, Archives of the American College of Surgeons: Chicago.

31. *Minutes of the meeting of the Board of Regents of February 23, 24 1963.* 1963, Archives of the American College of Surgeons: Chicago.

32. *Minutes of the meeting of the Board of Regents of June 22, 23, 1962.* 1962, Archives of the American College of Surgeons: Chicago.

33. *Minutes of the meeting of the Board of Regents of June 13, 14, 1964.* 1964, Archives of the American College of Surgeons: Chicago.

34. *Minutes of the meeting of the Board of Regents of October 16, 17, 1965.* 1965, Archives of the American College of Surgeons: Chicago.

35. *Minutes of the meeting of the Board of Regents of June 24, 25, 1966.* 1966, Archives of the American College of Surgeons: Chicago.

36. *Minutes of the meeting of the Board of Regents of September 29, October 1, 1961.* 1967, Archives of the American College of Surgeons: Chicago.

CHAPTER 15
Taking Care
of the Fellows

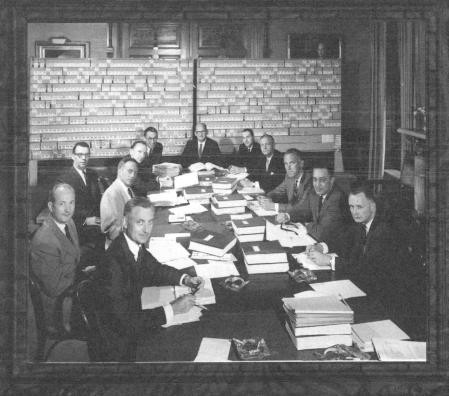

Director Paul Hawley wanted the College to disengage from the hospital standardization program because it consumed so much of the human and financial resources of the College, preventing it from meeting the needs of the fellowship, especially continuing education and professional development. Soon after the standardization program was passed on to the Joint Commission, Hawley and the Regents began to pay more attention to the fellowship.

Postgraduate courses were introduced at the Clinical Congress in Boston in 1950. The most popular were the vascular and fracture courses, and the pre- and postoperative care course was also very well attended. The nutrition course had the lowest attendance, so it would be combined with pre- and postoperative care.

More than 300 papers were submitted for the Surgical Forum, and 164 were selected for presentation. The success of the Forum reflected the burgeoning interest and activity in science and research after the war. The founder of the Forum, Regent Owen Wangensteen, always supporting young surgeons, suggested that the College provide scholarships in investigative surgery. The Regents were enthusiastic about this but did not act immediately. A volume of the Surgical Forum papers was available for ten dollars within four months of the presentations; a printing of 4,000 was ordered. The annual publication of the Forum papers has been eagerly anticipated by surgical investigators ever since. At its centennial, the College has adopted the practice of publishing them in a special issue of the *Journal of the American College of Surgeons*, making them available to the entire fellowship.

Regent Philpott observed the audience for the Martin Lecture at the Clinical Congress in 1949 and said it was mostly women. Because of this, he reasoned that the lecture should be on a general subject related to medicine, but a subject of general interest rather than a scientific subject, and that it should not be delivered by a surgeon. His recommendations were adopted.

The importance of exhibitors at the Clinical Congress was emphasized by Controller Edward Sandrok at a meeting of Regents. He said the exhibitors needed better access to the attendees or they would no longer pay the $50,000 that supported the College. The exhibits were often located in another hotel not frequented by the attendees.[1]

At this point the Clinical Congress was one of the largest conventions in the country, in the league with the AMA and large commercial organizations. The College was moving toward rotating Clinical Congress locations between Chicago, San Francisco, Los Angeles, and Atlantic City. But with this rotation the Fellows would tire of watching the same Fellows operate for the televised operative clinics sessions, the most popular sessions at the Clinical Congress. Hawley was enthusiastic about cinematography, or ciné, a new method to record events, including operations, on film using special lighting, lenses, and artistic techniques. He believed the use of ciné could replace the operative clinics and solve the problem. Ciné was later replaced by videography, the recording of events on digital media.[2]

❦

The Clinical Congress Program

Although a program committee reported to the Regents, the Regents devoted most of one of their four annual meetings to setting the program for the Clinical Congress. Often, they deliberated intensely for as much as an hour over one session, and occasionally tempers flared. In 1951, the distinguished anesthesiologist, Dr. Henry Beecher of the

Massachusetts General Hospital in Boston, had arranged a program on anesthesia for the Clinical Congress in San Francisco. Regent Alfred Blalock suggested it should be called "Metabolic Disturbances During Surgical Care," and a motion was made to approve this. Evarts Graham, the Midwesterner from Washington University in St. Louis, objected because he felt anesthesia was intruding into surgery, and because all the anesthesia program participants were Bostonians. When Allen tried to placate him, Graham said that he, Allen, was also from Boston, and that this would be noted by those west of the Mississippi (including Graham). The Regents went on to discuss other parts of the program, but Graham came back to "Metabolic Disturbances," criticizing Beecher and telling Allen that he was Chairman of the Board and should have discussed the problem with Beecher and solved it. Allen said they would have to rescind the motion to approve the program, but Graham, apparently cooling off and getting himself under control, said "We should deal with it later."

They then talked about participants in the gastrointestinal hemorrhage session. Wangensteen suggested Leon Goldman from San Francisco as a speaker, which prompted Graham to remind everyone that it was not the custom to load up the program with men from the city in which the meeting was held. "That does not mean you should load it up with Boston people, necessarily." They then settled on a person who Miss Grimm said was not a Fellow of the College, eliminating him, and then Graham suggested John Stewart from Buffalo. Graham said, "He is from the West; he is from Buffalo," meaning, of course, that he was west of Boston.

The Advisory Council for Orthopaedic Surgery suggested a man from St. Louis as a participant in the orthopaedic session. Graham said, "He is no longer in St Louis, thank God. He is one of the big bugs in the International College, and he is an unscrupulous fellow."[2]

While the Regents were making changes in the program that had been recommended for 1952, Loyal Davis moved that the program committee be "wiped out, and a new one appointed." This was done. Davis thought that the program committee should set up the program and the Regents should stay out of it. Graham agreed that the Regents were spending too much time on the program, but Allen persisted in wanting the Regents to go over the program committee's recommendations. Finally they agreed to appoint a new program committee with a Regent as chairman and a Governor as a member, and the remainder young surgeons. They then spent the rest of the morning in the nitty-gritty details of planning the program. Much of the time was spent deciding who was going to do what, and several Regents were at odds over the proposed selections.[3]

This propensity of the Regents to involve themselves in minutiae stemmed from the 15 years that the College had no Director, and the Regents were forced as a collective to function as the Director. This tendency has surfaced from time to time ever since. Perhaps it is the result of what some have called the controlling nature of surgeons or comes from the sense of surgeons that in caring for their patients they must be attentive to every detail.

Television and Motion Pictures Replace Operative Clinics

Review of the 1952 Clinical Congress revealed that only 3,280 tickets were issued for hospital operative clinics compared with 11,000 in Chicago in 1949 and 8,000 in Boston in 1950. On the first day of clinics, 19 of the 29 hospitals presenting them had no visitors. The program committee agreed to eliminate hospital operative clinics for the Chicago meeting in 1953 except those presented in connection with postgraduate courses. This effectively ended the hospital operative clinics. Franklin Martin had established them for surgeons and would-be surgeons to learn directly from experts, an activity that elevated the standard of surgical care during the course of 40 years.[4]

In contrast to the hospital operative clinics, the College staff reported a huge increase in the number of attendees at postgraduate courses during the same period, and more were added. The television clinics attracted phenomenal attendance, were well conducted, and stimulated enthusiastic compliments from the audience. Likewise, the motion picture programs played to capacity audiences and some people had to be turned away.[4] Martin's concept of learning by watching experts operate stayed alive and thrived with new technology.

Wangensteen pushed to have the Clinical Congress in Atlantic City, an attractive place with its boardwalk and beach. Evening entertainment was sparse in Atlantic City, however, so for the first Clinical Congress there in 1954 the College brought in a symphony orchestra program called the Voice of Firestone. It was a tremendous success, bringing in $5,000, which was put into the research scholarship fund.

Another problem in Atlantic City was that there were no suitable hospitals with surgical staffs that could perform operations for the ciné television program. Ravdin worked with the sponsor of ciné clinics, the pharmaceutical firm Smith, Kline, and French, to obtain approval from the Federal Communications Commission for a closed wire service from Philadelphia to Convention Hall in Atlantic City. The issue of itinerant surgery was so sensitive that to avoid accusations no surgeons from outside the Philadelphia area were invited to participate in the broadcast.[5] From the standpoint of attendance at scientific sessions, the Atlantic City Congress was the most successful ever.[6]

The growing complexity and size of the Clinical Congress led Loyal Davis to recommend that the College hire a full-time convention manager to handle housekeeping activities of the Clinical Congress and the sectional meetings, and relieve Mr. Sandrok and Mr. Shannon from these time-consuming duties. The Director was empowered to hire another person to help Sandrok, and this led to the establishment of a permanent position, currently held by Mr. Felix Niespodziewanski, who joined the College in 1990.[7]

The College staff regularly evaluated the Clinical Congress and reported to the program committee and the Regents. The Fellows were consistent in wanting the ciné television program to focus on more common, less complicated, surgical procedures. Hawley, never at a loss for an opinion, mused that surgeons attended the television programs to be entertained, rather than instructed.[8] This was accomplished by selecting surgeons who were popular and could engage the audience.

The motion picture programs at the Clinical Congresses would not have been possible without the generous financial support of Davis and Geck, later a division of American Cyanamid Company, and Ethicon, a Johnson and Johnson Company. Smith, Kline, and French Company supported the television programs that featured surgical procedures.

By 1950, the College had 1,200 approved films on file, and they were coming into the College at a rate of more than 100 per year. Dr. Charles Peustow, noted for his operation to relieve chronic pancreatitis, was chairman of the motion picture committee until 1951. He developed a new process for reviewing films, using individuals who were familiar with both the subject matter and the technical aspects of film making. The AMA also made medical motion pictures.[9] Dr. Hilger Jenkins of the University of Chicago, an innovator in the use of media for surgical education, chaired the ACS medical motion picture committee from 1952 to 1966, and introduced "spectacular problems in surgery," motion pictures that depicted the management of unique cases, such as resection of an enormous abdominal tumor. Ethicon donated $50,000 for a College film library that lent its collection to medical societies, hospitals, and other health care organizations for continuing medical education. Contemporary films, usually narrated by the author, were presented at the Clinical Congresses. In 1955, 133 films were shown. and Jenkins received the Distinguished Service Award for his contributions. (Figure 15.1)

The breadth of material presented at the Congress expanded greatly during the 1950s to include most of the common general surgical problems. For example, sessions at the 1961 Clinical Congress included regional perfusion for cancer, operative and postoperative cardiopulmonary crises, management of sepsis, surgery of duodenal ulcer, complications of cholecystectomy, diagnosis and management of diseases of the spleen, tumors of the colon, and the place of surgery in the treatment of thyroid disease. The postgraduate courses were pre- and postoperative care; gastrointestinal disease; diseases of the liver, biliary tract, and pancreas; cardiovascular surgery; injury of joints

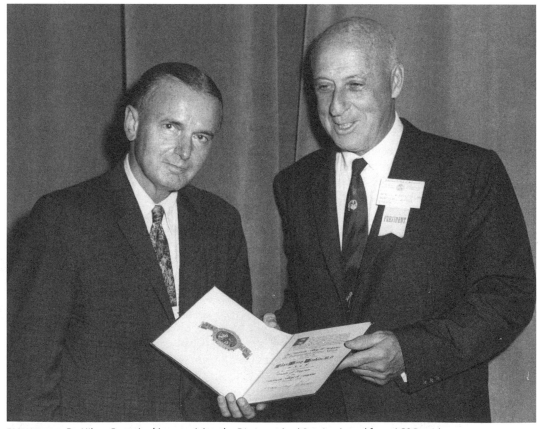

FIGURE 15.1 Dr. Hilger Perry Jenkins, receiving the Distinguished Service Award from ACS President Dr. Newell W Philpott.

of the upper extremity; gynecology and obstetrics; cancer; thoracic surgery; and recent advances in pediatric surgery.[10]

⋈

Sectional Meetings

The College also continued to hold three-day sectional meetings, usually four per year, in medium sized cities throughout the country. The third day was devoted exclusively to operative clinics. Attendance was good. In 1953, registration reached 6,432, double that of 1951.

Hawley held a sectional meeting in Panama in 1952 as a means of raising the stock of the College in Central and South America.[2] Of the 200 registrants, 59 came from the United States. This success led him to have another in São Paulo, Brazil in 1953.[11] In 1954, the sectional meetings were held in Charlotte, North Carolina; Reno, Nevada; Omaha, Nebraska; French Lick, Indiana; Montréal, Quebec; and London, England.

The College engaged the American Express Company to make arrangements for a Caribbean cruise in 1957 on the S.S. *Homeric*, a 20,000 ton, 100 percent air-conditioned, Italian ship capable of accommodating 600 passengers, with the primary stop in San Juan, Puerto Rico, for the sectional meeting.[12] Registration was 562, and this was the most successful of all the sectional meetings.[13] This spurred the staff to engage American Express for a cruise that included sectional meetings in Stockholm and Edinburgh, using the ship as the hotel for the participants.[13] Wealthy people were travelling throughout the world, and physicians were further incentivized by the ability to deduct some of the cost as educational expense, a welcome relief from the 91 percent marginal tax rate for the country's highest earners.

⋈

Fellowship Requirements

Dr. George Stephenson, Assistant Director, managed the fellowship application process. (Figure 15.2) He reminded the Regents of the requirement that applicants who graduated after January 1, 1938 and before January 1, 1944, must have had at least two years of residency. Many surgeons throughout the country had not met the requirement because they were inducted into military service. These surgeons, through no fault of their own, were ineligible for College fellowship or board certification, yet they had extensive surgical experience during the war. Stephenson was concerned that the same situation would pertain after the Korean War, when many men would not meet the current requirements of three years residency plus two years of preceptorship, or four years of residency. Allen, Blalock, and Hawley strongly agreed that the length of training requirements could not be compromised. They expressed no compassion for these surgeons, stating that they could enter residencies at VA hospitals after military service and be trained up to standards.

Stephenson also devised a new plan for processing applications. The Central Credentials Committee verified training and obtained the surgical list. The local committee then evaluated the candidates and the history review committee evaluated their case records.[2]

On Stephenson's recommendation the Regents abolished the senior candidate group, which was composed of individuals from the junior candidate group who had passed Part I of the American Board of Surgery (ABS) exam. The junior candidates received valuable supervision and guidance from local chapters of the College.

The Board of Regents Committee on Requirements for Fellowship included Drs. Daniel Elkin, Leland McKittrick, and Loyal Davis, who was the chairman. They established the policy that after July 1, 1956, all surgeons accepted by the College for fellowship should be qualified by examination of the surgical specialty boards.[14] A consequence of this was that the only training requirements of the College were those established by the respective boards. Fellowship

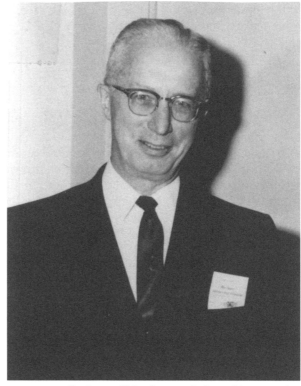

FIGURE 15.2 Dr. George W Stephenson, Assistant Director and later Associate Director of ACS.

in the Royal College of Physicians and Surgeons of Canada was accepted as qualified training, and the Central Credentials Committee would evaluate the training of applicants from foreign countries.[15] All applicants were required to practice their specialty for at least one year before their application would be evaluated. These have been the requirements through the centennial of the College.

As of 1953, there were 18,289 Fellows. Of these 9,737 were general surgeons. The next largest groups were 1,820 obstetricians/gynecologists, 1,065 urologists, and 1,021 orthopaedic surgeons.[14] Continuing a trend begun in the 1930s, 92 percent of the initiates were board certified by 1952.[16]

The College Develops Scholarships

Wangensteen, who previously had advocated for research fellowships sponsored by the College, was appointed chairman of the new Committee on Research Fellowships in 1952. The Committee required that the research fellow's institution give him or her a full-time faculty appointment and adequate facilities.[17] Wangensteen also developed one-year research scholarships for post-residency training and the Mead Johnson scholarship for research training during residency.[18, 19]

Wangensteen personally designed application forms and established the mechanics of reviewing applications, interviewing candidates, and selecting the awardees.[5] Charles O Finley, administrator of the College's disability insurance program, agreed to fund two research fellowships for 1957 at $20,000 each.[20] As of November 1957, the scholarship funds totaled $81,547, and nine individual scholarships were awarded. Finley had contributed a total of $40,000,[21] and Mead Johnson Company, manufacturer of nutritional products, a total of $18,000.[22]

Dr. William Drucker of Cleveland was awarded the first research scholarship. Many years later he served as Professor and Chairman of the Department of Surgery at the University of Toronto. Dr. John Landor of the University of Chicago received the research scholarship in 1959. The founding chief of general surgery at Robert Wood Johnson Medical School, he continued investigation throughout his academic career. The first Mead Johnson award was given to Dr. James Jude of Baltimore Maryland, a second-year resident. Jude, later a cardiothoracic surgeon, worked with Kouwenhoven and Knickerbocker to develop the technique of closed chest cardiac compression for cardiopulmonary resuscitation, the standard of care for the next 50 years.[23]

A Fellowship of Surgeons

Board Chairman Evarts Graham asked the Regents to authorize a history of the College, to be written by Director of Public Relations Mr. Greer Williams, with the assistance of Miss Eleanor K Grimm, who came out of retirement in Florida for the project. She gathered information by creating notebooks containing copies of relevant portions of the minutes of the Board of Regents, programs of various functions, letters, and her own notes, totaling approximately 2,000 pages.[24] By January 1, 1955, she had organized the raw material for the book in approximately 2,000 pages.[25] The expense for the book was estimated at $15,000.[26]

Greer Williams resigned from the College in 1954 without having written the book, and Dr. Loyal Davis agreed to write it.[22] Completed in 1959, *A Fellowship of Surgeons* was published by Charles C Thomas and Company of Springfield, Illinois, and later reprinted by the College.[27] The Regents decided to give a copy to each layperson who gave an aggregate of $500 to the building fund campaign, which was in progress.[28]

Davis's book has been the standard reference for the first 40 years of the College's history. His close association with the College for many of those years helped him bring out the personalities of the leaders and lent insight into the important decisions of the Regents. Miss Grimm's notebooks, a research tour de force, remain in the College Archives, available to scholars including the current authors, to whom they were invaluable.

Public Relations

Hawley believed that the public and the profession needed more exposure to the College. He hired Mr. Greer Williams in 1951 as the first director of public relations. Williams's first project was to publish the *Daily Clinical Bulletin*, a Clinical Congress daily newspaper that highlighted events and news. He also wanted to get more press and television coverage for the College and the Clinical Congress, so he invited reporters to attend and made officials of the College and presenters available to them.[29] Prodded by the Professional and Public Relations Committee, Williams encouraged freelance writers to prepare articles for lay magazines and newspapers, sent material to the deans of medical schools for distribution to medical students, and created a speakers bureau that supplied College chapters with speakers for their meetings.[5]

Within months of his hiring, the Regents declared war on fee splitting, and Williams was a central resource in managing the reaction of the public, which was positive, and of the profession, which was negative. He tended to be more philosophic than action-oriented on the fee splitting problem and some of the Regents were not enthusiastic about his approach. Assigned to write the history of the College, he was unable to get started on the project.

Williams resigned in June 1955, and was replaced by Mr. Robert Cunningham on a part-time basis.[12] He was guided by Loyal Davis, Chairman of the Professional and Public Relations Committee, who used the committee to introduce his plans for the College, most of which were eventually accepted by the Regents. Davis established the Distinguished Service Award, the College's highest award, and a committee to evaluate candidates, which granted the first award in 1957 to Dr. H Winnett Orr, the pioneering orthopaedic surgeon of Lincoln, Nebraska. He had donated his library of 2,600 medical books, many of them rare, to the College.[30]

Through Davis's work, the College film library was made available to county medical societies and other organizations. He also recommended that the College establish and maintain closer relations with the American Medical Association (AMA), so that problems common to both organizations could be discussed. Among the "problems" at the time were the aggressive American Academy of General Practice, which was pushing for hospital privileges for general practitioners, a definition of general practice, the proration of Blue Shield fees to surgeons and their assistants, and accreditation of hospitals.[31]

Loyal Davis and his committee oversaw the writing and production of a movie entitled "Hands We Trust," which portrayed the education and training of a surgeon who becomes a Fellow of the College.[8] Mr. Ronald Reagan, Davis's son-in-law, then a well-known Hollywood actor and later president of the United States, narrated the film.[16] The movie was shown nine times on television in 1962 to an audience estimated at 184,800 people, and 24 times before various medical and lay groups.[28]

South America

Hawley and Alton Ochsner were concerned about the large increase in Fellows in Central and South America. Very few of them had education and training matching that of U.S. Fellows. The fact that the College had Fellows in 59 countries around the world that had varying surgical standards was of concern to the Regents. Some believed that the College had the obligation to elevate the standard of surgery throughout the world, especially in Central and South America. They hoped that Fellows from these countries would elevate standards by participating in College educational activities. Others thought this was futile. An elephant in the room was the International College of Surgeons, always a thorn in the side of the College, which had lower standards for admission and to which many surgeons outside the U.S. were attracted, especially those who could not meet the training requirements of the College.[3]

During the 1950s, several committees and individuals were appointed to tour the Central and South American countries to evaluate the possibility of recruiting a few good young men into the College to serve as a nidus for improving the quality of candidates from those countries and elevating surgical standards there.[14, 17, 26, 32] Despite these efforts, no concrete results were achieved and the situation languished.

≈※≈

Reorganization

Evarts Graham completed his term as Chairman of the Board of Regents in 1954 and Isidor Ravdin was elected, but not before he made an emotional speech commending Graham for his yeoman's service to the College. Indeed, Graham had elevated the standards of education and training by linking College requirements to board certification, led the fight against unethical practices, and persistently held the College to the highest ethical standards, even in the face of criticism by the profession.

Ravdin thought that too much detail was brought before the Board of Regents, so he created standing committees related to Hawley's administrative organization of the College to replace the Board's outdated committee structure. The departments of the College were executive, organization and assembly, fellowship, professional services and accreditation, and business and finance.[8]

The new, corresponding standing committees were: 1. Liaison committees with the executive department, including the Executive Committee of the Board of Regents, the Committee on Professional and Public Relations, and the Committee on Professional Liaison; 2. The Liaison Committee for the Department of Organization and Assembly; 3. The Liaison Committee for the Department of Fellowship; 4. The Liaison Committee for the Department of Professional Services and Accreditation, which included the chairmen of the committees on cancer, trauma, nutrition and blood transfusions and allied problems; and 5. The Finance Committee.

The bylaws were changed to reflect the reorganization. The number of Regents was increased to 19. The President of the College served on the Board of Regents, bringing the total to 20. Vacancies on the Board of Regents would be filled by the Board of Governors. There would be a Central Committee on Credentials, as well as local credentials committees organized within cities, states, provinces, countries, or other areas. The members of these committees would be nominated by ballot of the Fellows in the respective area. The committees on credentials would act under the supervision of the Director and be subject to the control of the Board of Regents. Recommendations for admission to fellowship would be submitted to the Board of Regents for approval. Counseling committees would be organized within states, provinces, countries, or other areas. Counseling committees would submit to the nominating committee of the Fellows recommendations to fill vacancies on the Board of Governors within their respective areas, select advisory committees on local arrangements for sectional meetings, and assist the administrative officers of the College with local problems that may arise. They would act under supervision of the Director.

A five-person committee of the Board of Governors would make nominations for the officers of the Board of Governors and fill vacancies on the Board of Regents. They would also meet with and advise the nominating committee of Fellows. A five-person nominating committee of Fellows, appointed by the President of the College, the Chairman of the Board of Regents, and the Chairman of the Board of Governors acting jointly, would nominate the President, the First Vice President and the Second Vice President, and make nominations to fill vacancies on the Board of Governors.[33] These major organizational changes have remained in place.

After this reorganization the meetings of the Board of Regents became highly organized and efficient. The Executive Committee of the Board managed daily affairs and made decisions between Board meetings. The Board ratified Executive Committee decisions and occasionally modified them. The reorganization that Hawley and Ravdin conceived and implemented was a major achievement in the history of the College, one that served the College well and was not significantly altered until the reorganization of College departments in 2000.

A New Facility

In 1954, the College purchased the property on the south side of Erie Street for $170,000, so it then owned both sides of Erie Street between Wabash and Rush Streets in Chicago, setting the stage for Hawley's request for a new headquarters building to house its activities that were centered in the Nickerson Mansion, an exquisite structure designed as a home, not as an office building.[34]

The Building Committee, chaired by Loyal Davis, determined that the location of the College was superior to any other site in the Chicago area, and that the College should construct a building on the south side of Erie Street. With the concurrence of the Board of Governors, the Regents agreed.[8, 35] Davis selected the architectural firm of Skidmore, Owings, and Merrill to prepare plans and sketches.[16, 36]

The Finance Committee of the Board of Regents wrestled with paying for the new building. They decided to solicit contributions from the fellowship before imposing a dues increase. A letter sent out over Ravdin's signature requested a contribution of $500 from each Fellow, but this yielded only approximately $100,000.[28] More effective measures were needed. With the concurrence of the Board of Governors, the Regents raised dues from $40 to $50 and increased the initiation fee from $100 to $150.[36-38] When Contoller Sandrok pointed out that this would not cover the cost of the building, the Finance Committee and the Regents decided to impose an assessment of $200, payable over four years. Fellows who had already contributed $200 or more to the building fund voluntarily were excluded, and Canadian Fellows were given five years to pay up. New initiates had six years, so the campaign would end in 1968.[39] Sandrok had estimated that the campaign would yield a maximum of $3,953,500 by that time.[10]

Because there was nothing about assessments in the bylaws, Mr. Howe, the College's legal counsel, recommended and the Regents implement an addition to the bylaws that required Fellows to pay annual or other dues or assessments as may from time to time be determined by the Board of Regents. It was also added to the bylaws that the Board of Regents could terminate the membership of any Fellow, giving teeth to the assessment.[40]

Dr. Richard H Morris of Everett, Massachusetts, age 90, wrote Sandrok that as a retired Fellow he was not responsible for the building assessment, but he wanted Sandrok to know that he bequeathed $1,000 to the College upon his death.[41] Not all the Fellows were as generous, but many were as obstinate about the assessment. After a year, 5,580 of the 19,355 Fellows had not replied to the first bill for the assessment. Forty Fellows resigned, 175 retired, and 75 initiates cancelled their induction, all due to the assessment. Approximately 1,200 letters had been received relative to the assessment,

350 of which were critical of the Regents. Many Fellows said that they would not pay or might ultimately pay under protest.[42]

Groundbreaking ceremonies for the new building were held on October 2, 1961. Special spades were ordered and each officer present turned a shovel full of earth. The new building was to be eight stories high and made of reinforced concrete with a special finish on the exposed columns. Large tinted glass windows would occupy the spaces between the columns. The first floor was a library and reception area. The business, finance, and assembly departments were on the second floor and the Martin Memorial Foundation on the third floor. The fourth floor housed the executive offices. The fellowship and professional services departments were on the fifth floor. The sixth floor was for utilities. The lunchroom and expansion space were on the seventh floor, and the eighth

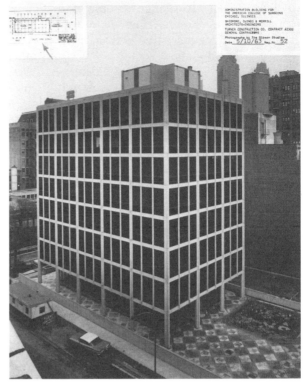

FIGURE 15.3 ACS headquarters at 55 E. Erie Street, Chicago.

floor was for the Board of Regents. Johnson and Johnson paid for furnishing the library on the first floor, and Ethicon furnished the Regents room on the eighth floor.[43]

The building was occupied in mid-1963, about two years after construction began. The work of the employees was greatly facilitated by the modern structure, and visitors to the College, especially representatives of other organizations, were impressed by it.[44] (Figure 15.3)

Of the 22,054 Fellows assessed, 47 were delinquent for three years or more. A handful of the most unyielding were expelled from the College.[45] Total disbursements for the building were $3,192,100 and building fund receipts were $3,866,400. The excess would be used through the years for maintenance and repairs.[46] Mindful of the anger over the assessment, in 1970 the Regents established a building replacement fund with annual contributions of $20,000 from College funds.[47]

⋙✳⋘

Hawley's Legacy

Paul Hawley gave the College exactly what it needed. With a household name among physicians because of his military service, his leadership in establishing academic VA hospitals, and his efforts to merge Blue Cross and Blue Shield, the profession listened to what he had to say, and say he did. In speeches, articles, and interviews he railed against fee splitting and other unethical practices, the poorly organized insurance industry, and government involvement in health care. His effectiveness was enhanced by the fortuitous convergence of some of the College's most effective leaders in its history: Evarts Graham, Arthur Allen, Isidor Ravdin, and Loyal Davis. Together, they suppressed the fee splitting cancer that had eaten away at the College's reputation since its founding.

Equally important was the new attention they paid to the Fellows of the College through unprecedented innovation: A Clinical Congress markedly improved by spectacular learning experiences using closed circuit television, cinematography, and motion pictures, an expanded Surgical Forum, scholarships for young surgical investigators, sectional meetings in the form of cruises to interesting destinations, a public relations department that informed the public and the profession of the good work of the College, a reorganization that improved the efficiency of the College staff and its committees, and finally, a beautiful new building in a desirable location from which the College would accomplish its mission for almost four decades.

REFERENCES

1. *Minutes of the meeting of the Board of Regents of November 20, 1950.* 1950, Archives of the American College of Surgeons: Chicago.
2. *Minutesof the meeting of the Board of Regents of April 13, 1951.* 1951, Archives of the American College of Surgeons: Chicago.
3. *Minutes of the meeting of the Board of Regents of December 3, 1951.* 1951, Archives of the American College of Surgeons: Chicago.
4. *Minutes of the meeting of the Executive Committee of November 23, 1952.* 1952, Archives of the American College of Surgeons: Chicago.
5. *Minutes of the meeting of the Executive Committee of March 21, 1954.* 1954, Archives of the American College of Surgeons: Chicago.
6. *Minutes of the meeting of the Board of Regents of November 19, 1954.* 1954, Archives of the American Colege of Surgeons: Chicago.
7. *Minutes of the meeting of the Executive Committee of June 3, 1955.* 1955, Archives of the American College of Surgeons: Chicago.
8. *Minutes of the meeting of the Board of Regents of March 1,2, 1958.* 1958, Archives of the meeting of the Board of Regents of March 1,2, 1958: Chicago.
9. *Minutes of the meeting of the Board of Regents of October 22, 1950.* 1950, Archives of the American College of Surgeons: Chicago.
10. *Minutes of the meeting of the Board of Regents of October 14, 1960.* 1960, Archives of the American College of Surgeons: Chicago.
11. *Minutes of the meeting of the Board of Regents of April 14, 1952.* 1952, Archives of the American College of Surgeons: Chicago.
12. *Minutes of the meeting of the Board of Regents of June 4,5, 1955.* 1955, Archives of the american College of Surgeons: Chicago.
13. *Minutesof the meeting of the Board of Regents of February 3, 4, 1957.* 1957, Archives of the American College of Surgeons: Chicago.
14. *Minutes of the meting of the Board of Regents of October 3,4,6, 1953.* 1953, Archives of the American College of Surgeons: Chicago.
15. *Minutes of the meeting of the Board of Regents of October 9, 1953.* 1953, Archives of the American College of Surgeons: Chicago.
16. *Minutes of the meeting of the Board of Regents of December 12, 13, 1958.* 1958, Archives of the American College of Surgeons: Chicago.
17. *Minutes of the meeting of the Board of Regents of April 15, 1952.* 1952, Archives of the American College of Surgeons: Chicago.
18. *Minutes of the meeting of the Board of Regents of March 21, 1954.* 1954, Archives of the American College of Surgeons: Chicago.
19. *Minutes of the meeting of the Executive Committee of December 4, 5, 1955.* 1955, Archives of the American College of Surgeons: Chicago.
20. *Minutes of the meeting of the Board of Regents of October 6, 7, 1956.* 1956, Archives of the American College of Surgeons: Chicago.
21. *Minutes of the meeting of the Board of Regents of October 29-31, 1955.* 1955, Archives of the American College of Surgeons: Chicago.
22. *Minutes of the meeting of the Board of Regents of December 7, 1957.* 1957, Archives of the American College of Surgeons: Chicago.
23. Kouwenhoven, W., Jude, JR, Knickerbocker, GG., *Closed-chest cardiac massage.* JAMA, 1960. **173**: p. 1064-1067.
24. *Minutes of the meeting of the Board of Regents of November 13,14,18, 1954.* 1954, Archives of the American College of Surgeons: Chicago.

25. *Minutes of the meeting of the Executive Commttee of July 31, 1958.* 1953, Archives of the American College of Surgeons: Chicago.

26. *Minutes of the meeting of the Board of Regents of April 4,5, 1953.* 1953, Archives of the American College of Surgeons: Chicago.

27. Davis, L., *Fellowship of Surgeons. A History of the American College of Surgeons.* 1988, Chicago: American College of Surgeons.

28. *Minutes of the meeting of the Board of Regents of February 27,28, 2960.* 1960, Archives of the American College of Surgeons: Chicago.

29. *Minutes of the meeting of the Board of Regents of November 3,4, 1951.* 1951, Archives of the American College of Surgeons: Chicago.

30. *Minutes of the meeting of the Board of Regents of May 11,12, 1957.* 1957, Archives of the American College of Surgeons: Chicago.

31. *Minutes of the meeting of the Executive Committee of December 3, 1955.* 1955, Archives of the American College of Surgeons: Chicago.

32. *Minutes of the meeting of the Board of Regents of February 19,20, 1955.* 1955, Archives of the American College of Surgeons: Chicago.

33. *Minutes of the meeting of the Board of Regents of February 11,12, 1956.* 1956, Archives of the American College of Surgeons: Chicago.

34. *Minutes of the meeting of the Board of Regents of June 9, 10, 1956.* 1956, Archives of the American College of Surgeons: Chicago.

35. *Minutes of the meeting of the Board of Regents of October 12,13, 1957.* 1957, Archives of the American College of Surgeons: Chicago.

36. *Minutes of the meeting of the Board of Regents of March 7, 8, 1959.* 1959, Archives of the American College of Surgeons: Chicago.

37. *Minutes of the meeting of the Board of Regents of October 2, 1959.* 1959, Archives of the American College of Surgeons: Chicago.

38. *Minutes of the meeting of the Board of Regents of December 6,7, 1959.* 1959, Archives of the American College of Surgeons: Chicago.

39. *Minutes of the meeting of the Board of Regents of June 10,11, 1960.* 1960, Archives of the American College of Surgeons: Chicago.

40. *Minutes of the meeting of the Board of Regents of October 8,9, 1960.* 1960, Archives of the American College of Surgeons: Chicago.

41. *Minutes of the meeting of the Board of Regents of December 4,5, 1960.* 1960, Archives of the American College of Surgeons: Chicago.

42. *Minutes of the meeting of the Board of Regents of March 4, 5, 1961.* 1961, Archives of the American College of Surgeons: Chicago.

43. *Minutes of the meeting of the Board of Regents of Spetember 30, October 1, 1961.* 1961, Archives of the American College of Surgeons: Chicago.

44. *Minutes of the meeting of the Board of Regents of November 1, 1963.* 1963, Archives of the American College of Surgeons: Chicago.

45. *Minutes of the meeting of the Board of Regents of October 3-5, 1969.* 1969, Archives of the American College of Surgeons: Chicago.

46. *Minutes of the meeting of the Board of Regents of June 18, 19, 1965.* 1965, Archives of the American College of Surgeons: Chicago.

47. *Minutes of the meeting of the Board of Regents of February 6-8, 1970.* 1970, Archives of the American College of Surgeons: Chicago.

CHAPTER 16
The North Era.
Calm and Quiet

Paul Hawley, "The Director," retired on January 31, 1961. He was boisterous, fun-loving, and often in hot water. Isidor Ravdin, at the end of his six-year term as Chairman of the Board of Regents and responsible for selecting the next Director, understood that the College needed a less hectic atmosphere and a less controversial Director. Ravdin himself had to contend with Hawley's excesses even while giving him full support. John Paul North, a tall, quiet, thoughtful surgeon who had little apparent desire for fame, had been a Fellow in Ravdin's laboratory after graduating from the University of Pennsylvania School of Medicine and completing his surgical training under Eldridge Eliason there. (Figure 16.1)

North then taught surgery at the medical school under Ravdin, who was chairman of the department while in private practice in Philadelphia. At the outbreak of World War II, North joined the University of Pennsylvania's 20th

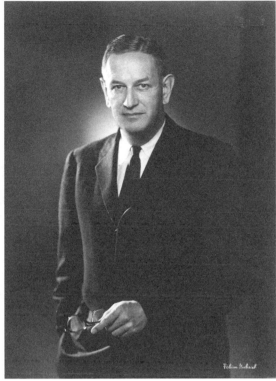

FIGURE 16.1 Dr. John Paul North, Director, 1961–69.

General Hospital, under the command of Colonel, and later Brigadier General, IS Ravdin, as chief of the surgical service.[1] After the war, he became chief of surgery at the Dallas VA Hospital and clinical professor of surgery at its affiliated University of Texas Southwestern Medical School. Ravdin knew that North, his mentee, would lead the College with competence and dignity, and he convinced the Regents to name him as the College's fourth Director as of February 1, 1961. Soon thereafter, Loyal Davis was elected Chairman of the Board of Regents.

The Education Programs— Improvement and Innovation

One of North's first initiatives was to assess and improve the education programs of the College. He found that 21 percent of all doctors of medicine who registered for the Clinical Congress in 1960 and 16 percent of the registrants for the postgraduate courses were not Fellows of the College.[2] North believed that these poorly qualified doctors were attending the Clinical Congress to learn surgery and surgical care in order to perform surgery, which North believed would lower surgical standards, but the Regents resolved to continue to make the education programs of the College open to all physicians.[2]

North also found that approximately 9,500 Fellows lived within 500 miles of the New York-Philadelphia-Baltimore area; while within a similar range of Memphis there were 3,200; of Dallas 1,900; and of Denver only 1,000. Thereafter, sectional meetings were restricted to cities within easy reach of Fellows. One four-day sectional meeting was held each year; the remainder were three-day meetings.

"Meet the Professor" sessions were introduced at the Clinical Congress in 1964; they were an instant hit.[3] Regent William Longmire, who graced the College with his calm demeanor and wisdom, noting that the Surgical Forum presentations were restricted to young surgeons, developed a peer-reviewed "papers session" for senior Fellows that continues to be popular.[4] (Figure 16.2)

North arranged for the Audio-Digest Foundation, a subsidiary of the California Medical Society, to tape sessions at the Clinical Congress and sectional meetings. The cassette tapes were sold by subscription, giving Fellows and others the opportunity to obtain continuing medical education

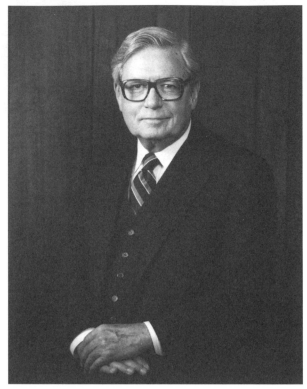

FIGURE 16.2 Dr. William P Longmire Jr, ACS President 1972–73.

in their automobiles or in the privacy of their homes or offices using cassette players, the standard technology for playing music at the time.[5]

Another of North's innovations was Hotelevision, a closed circuit service that was shown on hotel room television sets to provide Fellows with information about Clinical Congress sessions, their location, and speakers.[6, 7]

≈✳≈

SESAP

The National Advisory Commission on Health Manpower, appointed by the President, had three concerns about the health care system: first, the rapid rise in the cost of health care had not been accompanied by a corresponding increase in life expectancy; second, there was a gap between current medical knowledge and its use in practice; third, physicians needed an incentive to use the educational opportunities available to them. Periodic re-licensure based on continuing education or a compulsory examination would provide that incentive, and soon states were implementing this recommendation.

A committee of the Board of Governors discussed the problem of continuing medical education, a significant concern of the government. The committee noted that only about 5,000 of the 29,000 Fellows of the College attended the Clinical Congress, suggesting that the fellowship was not taking advantage of available educational opportunities.

A poll showed that College Fellows favored a voluntary self-assessment examination that would count as continuing education for relicensure.[5] The College's Committee on

Continuing Education was impressed with the popular self-evaluation program of the American College of Physicians (ACP), and with the support of the American Board of Surgery (ABS), recommended a similar examination for general surgery.[8] The Committee developed a 700-question, ten-hour, open-book examination drawn from 2,500 questions prepared by examination committees.[7] The answers were graded and the results reported confidentially to the surgeon, who was also given a syllabus for study.

The first version of the Surgical Education and Self-Assessment Program (SESAP) was made available in 1971. SESAP eventually was issued in an electronic version, and became one of the College's most popular educational resources. At the time of the College's centennial, it was linked to the ABS's maintenance of certification program. Fellows received credit for using it as a self-assessment tool because it prepared them to successfully complete their recertification examinations.

≈ ✳ ≈

North Brings Important Change

North established the "think session" at Regents' meetings, a time reserved for Regents to voice thoughts that could not easily be expressed during the transaction of routine business. Later, many organizations adopted this technique. North quietly went about fixing many chronic problems, almost always with creative, although not spectacular, solutions. The state and provincial judiciary and counseling committees were replaced by advisory and counseling committees. The advisory committees were to assist the central judiciary committee and the administrative officers of the College in the investigation of facts with respect to disciplinary matters, submit to the nominating committee of Fellows recommendations to fill vacancies at-large on the Board of Governors, assist the officers and Regents with respect to local problems, and perform such other functions and duties as might be delegated to them by the Board of Regents.[9]

Another important innovation was creation of the Liaison Committee on the Structure of Standing Committees, chaired by Regent William Longmire. The committee took on the problems of committee members serving until they retired or died, insufficient representation of specialties, and lack of common standards between committees. The recommendations became known as the "Longmire Rules":

> (1) The structure of the various committees shall, insofar as possible, be uniform. (2) Each committee shall have adequate representation from the various surgical specialties. (3) The tenure of all members shall be limited.

Longmire's committee defined active, senior, and liaison members of committees and established a limit of three, three-year terms. The mechanisms for choosing officers of committees and the composition of executive committees were also delineated. These policies greatly improved the operation of the College and are still known as the "Longmire Rules" in honor of their architect.[10] North also established a communications department, bringing together several information and editorial units of the College.[11]

Portraits, Large and Small

With the move into the new Erie Street building, Regent Reed Nesbit was commissioned to investigate where the painted portraits of the presidents of the College, then at the Murphy Memorial, should be hung. He reported that "the Murphy" could not accommodate more portraits of the customary large size, and there had been no plan to hang them in the new building. "Perhaps this manner of commemorating our illustrious leaders has become anachronistic," he said, and recommended that presidents, chairs of the Board of Regents, and chairs of the Board of Governors be memorialized henceforth by 8-inch by 10-inch photographs.[9]

As might be expected, the leaders who had envisioned their portraits hanging in the Murphy Auditorium were not enthusiastic about his recommendation. Regents Merrill Foote and Willard Parsons, who spoke up in favor of continuing painted portraits, were immediately dispatched to study the matter.[4] They found space for 14 additional portraits in the Rare Book Room by taking down a moose head, and a total of 55 additional spaces in the Murphy by moving bronze plaques around and repositioning some portraits.[12] Edith Davis continued the tradition of donating portraits of presidents to the College in 1962, when she sent John Paul North a portrait of her husband Loyal, painted by the noted William Draper, whose painting of President Kennedy hangs in the National Gallery.[13]

This settled the issue until the late 1960s, when fewer donations of portraits were received and the Regents decided that if an oil portrait was not donated, the College would pay for a color photograph of the individual, to be hung in the College headquarters.[14, 15]

The Planning Commission Focuses on Finances

As the health care environment became more complex, the Regents responded by creating a planning commission to guide the College in its future activities. The commission's report in 1963 was based on extemporaneous interviews with a large number of Fellows from every conceivable activity and locality. The Fellows were pleased that the College continued to take strong positions on fee splitting and hospital accreditation, and that its annual scientific sessions had improved markedly with the ongoing development of the Surgical Forum and postgraduate courses.

But the commission noted that the College had not addressed the problem that many foreign medical graduates, who had residency training in the United States, were unable to become Fellows of the College. They could not attain board certification, a requirement for fellowship. The boards had the policy of requiring two years of practice before admission to their examinations, but after completing their training and going home, many foreign medical graduates could not regain entry into the States.[12] Another area of College responsibility that was languishing was the inspection of residency programs.

Solutions to problems such as these required large amounts of staff time and money for staff travel. Although the fellowship thought the College was doing well, the rapidity of change in surgical practice and the increasing involvement of the federal government left many problems unaddressed. Furthermore, there was no formal mechanism through which the College could deal with the government on issues affecting patients or the well-being of its Fellows.

Regents Wade and Parsons emphasized the need for more staff and better salaries. The Franklin H Martin Memorial Foundation, which owned *Surgery, Gynecology, and Obstetrics,* was contributing $150,000 to $200,000 annually to the College, but significant increases were unlikely.[16] The members of the planning commission agreed that more money was needed and increasing dues would be necessary.[17] Nevertheless, commission member Dr. Jonathan Rhoads, Ravdin's personal surgeon and his successor as chair of surgery at the University of Pennsylvania, suggested that the Director be given some leeway in spending additional money if there would be a pressing need for funds in the following year.

As the decade of the 1960s wore on, the College's financial situation grew worse. Deficits were projected for 1968 and 1969. Jonathan Rhoads led the finance committee to engage independent investment counsel to review the management of College funds. They recommended that Northern Trust Company continue as custodian of the pooled investment account, valued at $3.9 million, but that Butcher & Sherrerd of Philadelphia be appointed as investment advisor and broker. Northern Trust was to be instructed to carry out Butcher & Sherrerd's investment decisions. They were authorized to sell and reinvest up to 25 percent of the portfolio in each calendar year, thus increasing the aggressiveness of the investment strategy.[18] The Regents, wanting to make more money off the investments, approved this and a dues increase to $90 in 1970, which increased the College's income by $700,000 and eliminated the deficit.[19]

⤳ ✳ ⤲

The Library, Now a Liability

With the imperative to reduce expenses, the Library committee evaluated the facilities and services of the library, which included 38,000 volumes of books and bound journals and 675,000 reprints. Eight librarians lent books to any requesting physician by mail, prepared bibliographies on request, sent at least three reprints to anyone requesting information on a clinical topic, and prepared packets of information on medical topics for nurses, technicians, insurance companies, and lawyers, as well as physicians. The library also maintained a staff that translated articles into English from French, German, Italian, Spanish, Portuguese, Polish, and Russian.

The consensus was that the College could no longer afford to maintain this library and its services, but should establish a collection of books, pamphlets, instruments, and other material relating to American surgery that were of historical importance.[20] Eventually, the staff was reduced to three, the collection of reprints was given to the Texas Medical Association,[21] and the books and journals were distributed to seven new medical schools.[13, 22]

This led to the retirement of Miss Marguerite Prime, who had been the College's librarian for 38 years and one of its most stalwart and loyal managers. She and many others were motivated by the belief that their daily work was for the benefit of surgical patients, which indeed it was. Miss Prime treasured the gift of a silver tray engraved with the names of Drs. Isidor Ravdin, Owen Wangensteen, and Paul Hawley.[23]

The Board of Governors

The 1967 meeting of the Board of Governors was its largest in history, with 151 Governors and 28 chapter presidents or their representatives present as guests. This indicated the great interest of surgeons in the issues of the day, especially the intervention of the federal government in health care. The Governors felt a strong obligation to bring the opinions and concerns of practicing surgeons to bear on the College's activities. They complained, however, that they had no way to force the Regents to deal with the reports they sent them, nor did the Regents have a process for examining the reports of the Governors and taking or not taking action. The Regents often dealt with the most important Governors' reports by forming a committee of Regents to study the same problem. Not surprisingly, they usually arrived at the same conclusions and recommendations and, of course, everything was delayed because of this cumbersome process.[6]

The Regents agreed that they did not adequately address the work of the Governors. They decided in 1968 to solve this by inviting the Chairman, Vice Chairman, and Secretary of the Board of Governors to attend all future meetings of the Board of Regents.[15] This was a major step forward, for it has allowed these officers to participate in discussions and established a direct two-way communication between the Governors and the Regents.

Founding the Council of Medical Specialty Societies

In 1964, Dr. J Englebert Dunphy, president of the College, was asked by the president of the American College of Obstetricians and Gynecologists (ACOG) to meet with him and the president of the American College of Physicians (ACP) for an informal discussion about the formation of an interdisciplinary council.[24] The meeting went well. The purposes would be to promote communication among the specialty organizations, to share administrative experiences and seek mutually advantageous solutions to problems, and to promote advances in medical education through joint programming and providing broader perspectives on patient care.[25]

At their 1965 meeting, as the legislation proposing Medicare was being debated, the representatives of the three organizations, then called the Tri-College Council, passed the following resolution:

The sense of the meeting was that there was an acute necessity for the viewpoints of the specialists composing the ACP, ACOG, and the ACS to explore the possibility of developing lines of communication with the AMA in the hope that a more uniform, representative opinion on pending legislation be available to the public. The Council suggests to the staffs of the three organizations that informal communication within the limits of staff authority be started at once with the staff of the AMA.

The representatives called for each of their organizations to be more active politically, and for the AMA to increase its political activity. Obviously, they were hoping that a combined effort that included the AMA would have more clout with the government.[26]

The Association of American Medical Colleges (AAMC) and the American Hospital Association (AHA) were not adverse to the government employment of physicians, which the AMA opposed. But the Tri-College Council did not believe the AMA was effective in its defense of private practice. They accused the AMA of not using the best talent of the specialist groups in its leadership, and they asserted that recent legislation enacted by Congress (Medicare) indicated that the AMA had not kept up with public opinion and must find new leadership. They opposed the long apprenticeship in county and state society activities that was required before attaining top leadership in the AMA and which deterred specialists. The group suggested that the system of populating the scientific sections of the AMA House of Delegates be abandoned and that some specialty colleges and societies be invited to nominate individuals directly. The AMA representatives present said this would be impossible because it would require a bylaws change that the House of Delegates would not support.[11]

The Tri-College Council was effective in negotiating favorable regulations for residency training with the Social Security Administration under the Medicare program. Believing that it would acquire even more clout by including more specialty societies, the Council convinced its parents to include the American Academy of Pediatrics and the American Psychiatric Association in its membership.[27] The Tri College Council changed its name to the Council of Medical Specialty Societies (CMSS) in 1967.[6]

At the CMSS meeting on January 8, 1969, plans were made to invite into membership those specialty societies representing all the primary certifying boards. A few problems were encountered in determining which specialty society was the primary representative, but eventually the goal was accomplished.[5,8] Several subspecialty societies were added beginning in 2005. The current goal of CMSS is to provide a forum for collaboration to influence policy, medical education, and accreditation from a broad, cross-specialty perspective.[28]

Formation of the CMSS was an important event in the history of organized medicine because it signaled the permanence of specialty medicine, and provided a strong political and professional voice for a large body of physicians who felt disenfranchised by the AMA. CMSS also brought together organizations that by themselves were not sufficiently strong to have an impact in professional and political affairs. John Paul North's successor, Dr. C Rollins Hanlon, would lead the organization in this effort.

Working with the AMA Interspecialty Committee

The AMA, to which almost all physicians had traditionally belonged, understood that the interests of the growing number of specialties and subspecialties were causing them to create their own specialty organizations, and even to band together into broader specialty groups, such as the CMSS. Eventually, specialists would no longer depend solely on the AMA to represent them. Concomitantly, general practitioners were pressuring the AMA to support their efforts to create their own certifying board. Specialists, feeling that the AMA was an organization for the general practitioner and those without training who called themselves specialists, were demanding a stronger voice within the AMA. The AMA responded to this threat to its membership and political clout by forming the interspecialty committee, which in 1967 consisted of representatives of 15 specialties,

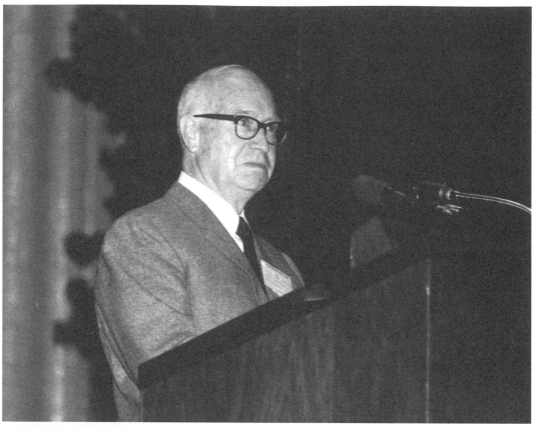

FIGURE 16.3 Dr. Howard Mahorner, ACS President-Elect, in 1969.

including the College. The College appointed long-time AMA leader Regent Howard Mahorner of New Orleans, who would be the AMA's president in 1970, to represent the College. (Figure 16.3)

The interspecialty committee served as a forum for the exchange of information and as a unifying influence on the profession. For example, in December 1966, representatives from 11 national societies listened to informal presentations and participated in discussions with officials from the Department of Health, Education, and Welfare (HEW), the U.S. Public Health Service, the Social Security Administration, HEW Division of Welfare, and the Defense Department. They learned of amendments to the Medicare law that included podiatrists in the Medicare program, coverage of 1,300,000 totally disabled persons under 65 years of age, and broader provisions for maternal and child care and for mental health. The HEW Division of Welfare announced that by 1975 every state must have a plan to provide quality medical care for all who are medically indigent (Medicaid). The plans must be comprehensive and include dental care, drugs, availability of consultation, transportation of patients to sources of care, and utilization reviews similar to in-hospital care. The participants were astonished at this vast expansion of the influence of government in health care.

In response to concern about the physician supply for the war in Vietnam, Defense Department officials said that 15,000 physicians were on duty with the military with an annual turnover rate of 4,500. They anticipated that by 1967 the Berry Plan, which deferred doctors until their specialty training was completed, and military residency programs would meet most of the requirements for specialists. They said that about

3,000 interns would be available for the draft, and a draft of physicians from practice may be necessary. There was a shortage of nurses available for overseas duty.[6]

The specialties, including the College, appreciated the information they received through the interspecialty committee, but the committee had no authority to implement anything. It was simply a discussion group. The real authority lay with the House of Delegates, which excluded the voices of specialty societies. Mahorner, after consulting with John Paul North, introduced a resolution at the interspecialty committee meeting in 1968 that would allow interspecialty committee representatives to nominate individuals for the House of Delegates. Separately, the CMSS made the same request.[14] This engendered long discussion that was "very close and pointed." Dr. George Logan, a pediatric representative, pointed out that the CMSS was an alternate organization if the specialties could not be represented in the AMA, and this angered some of the AMA representatives. They said Mahorner's proposal would require a bylaws change, which was not in the cards. Later, the House of Delegates turned down his proposal.[18]

Mahorner was able to get the interspecialty committee to pass on to the AMA the request that application blanks for medical staff membership contain a statement that the applicant would agree not to engage in fee splitting.[15] The response from the House of Delegates was: "Resolved, that the AMA reemphasize its desire that the Joint Commission continue to require that all medical staff members of a hospital comply with the principles of medical ethics and the appropriate licensing laws of their state for the accreditation of any hospital." Although the AMA opposed fee splitting, it believed that a surgeon who paid his assistant was not splitting fees, whereas the College believed he or she was. Therefore, the AMA would not support the wording of the College's statement.[29]

Members of the interspecialty committee decried the domination of hospital boards by laypersons and their consequent domination of medical staffs. Responding to AMA pressure, the Joint Commission included a statement in its standards that "physicians who are members of the medical staff, where legally permissible shall be eligible and should be included in the membership of the hospital governing bodies in the same manner as are all knowledgeable and effective individuals."[30]

The interspecialty committee gave the specialties access to the AMA, but no real authority within it. Specialists felt they were underrepresented in the House of Delegates, where authority resided. This continued to be an issue. In the 1960s the AMA made its Washington, DC, office available to the specialty societies, and many of them took advantage of this courtesy to obtain information about government activities in health care. The specialty colleges and societies had moved into the political arena to the extent that they gathered relevant information and discussed the issues, but they did not yet have the resources or the modus operandi for what later came to be known as advocacy. Almost all advocacy in Washington for the profession continued to flow through the AMA.

Premature Publicity

The first successful kidney transplant was performed in 1954, and became commonplace soon thereafter. The first successful liver, heart, and pancreas transplants were done in the 1960s. Repair of intracardiac defects began in the 1950s, followed by valve replacements and coronary artery bypass grafting in the 1960s. Hospitals, medical schools, and sometimes surgeons were quick to seize on the public relations opportunities afforded by these astonishing surgical feats. The College Committee on Public Relations prepared a statement on premature publicity related to organ transplants, noting that medical centers hired public relations experts to get news out, but long-term results were not provided in these news stories. The statement asked surgeons to seriously consider the wisdom of their announcements, and if they felt it was wise, they should prepare the press with an honest appraisal of the procedure and the potential problems for the long term.[31]

The publicity surrounding the world's first heart transplant by Christiaan Barnard in Cape Town, South Africa, in 1967 led the College to establish a committee on premature publicity, whose name intimated its agenda. The Regents approved a statement derived from the committee's recommendations, the essence of which was that immediate publicity surrounding the performance of new surgical procedures is not in the best interest of patients. They asserted that the surgeon had the final responsibility for avoiding and preventing unwise publicity.

The Regents also made a statement on human experimentation and the public disclosure of results after noted heart surgeon Dr. Denton Cooley implanted an artificial heart in Mr. Haskell Karp in 1969, followed by transplantation of a donor heart that kept him alive for 30 hours.[30] Noting that increased activity in organ transplantation and the use of artificial organs had compounded the complexity of the ethical problems in the relations with communications media, the Regents said that animal studies were required as an essential prelude to using new techniques in humans.

Guidelines established by the National Institutes of Health and the Medical Research Council in Canada included that the procedure to be carried out must be fully described, with risks and mechanisms for protecting the patient; that the risks to the subject would be allayed by the potential benefit; that the patient did not abdicate rights by consenting to participate; and that continuing surveillance had to be guaranteed. Release of results should be by an authority responsible for governing the trials. Institutional committees should set the standards for protocols.

Because of allegations surrounding Cooley's acquisition of the artificial heart, which had been developed under Dr. Michael DeBakey's supervision, and because he willingly participated in the publicity surrounding the case, Cooley was put on College probation for one year in June 1970,[7] and he received a stern letter from Chairman of the Board of Regents William Longmire. The probation was lifted in June 1971.[32]

Some might believe that reprimanding one of the world's most distinguished and celebrated cardiovascular surgeons was evidence of the College's strong moral and ethical foundation. Others might agree with Cooley, that he was simply doing everything possible for his patient.

The College Versus Oral Surgeon Dentists

The College staff had received complaints about dentists who were performing oral surgery. They found that facial injuries were assigned to armed forces dentists in Vietnam and on the hospital ship *Hope*. Dentists were performing head and neck surgery as part of their assignment, apparently because there was a lack of medical personnel. Dental surgeons requested departmental status in Charity Hospital in New Orleans to perform major surgery described as exclusively theirs: the mandible, tongue, dental gingiva, and facial wounds. The surgical service would be responsible for the workup and medical care of the patient but have no involvement in the surgery. If the patient had a complication the surgical service was to be notified and take responsibility for it.

In 1964, the Joint Commission issued a bulletin that gave broad approval to dental-oral surgeons. It said, "The practice of dentistry in its surgical specialty deals with diagnosis, the surgical and adjunctive treatment of diseases, injuries, and defects of the human jaws and contiguous structures."

Under protest by the College the statement was revised a year later:

> All dental or oral surgical procedures undertaken in the operating room by dentists shall be under the overall supervision of the surgeon in chief of the hospital. This principle permits the organization of an oral surgery service within the surgical department.

The Regents responded with their own statement, which was widely distributed:

> Pursuant to its ideals for optimum care of surgical patients, the Board of Regents of the American College of Surgeons affirms that major surgery involves total medical and surgical care of the patient. In order to provide such optimum surgical care, those who perform major surgical procedures should be doctors of medicine with adequate graduate education in surgery.[5]

Immediately after distribution of the Regents' statement, the American Dental Association, the American Society of Oral Surgeons, and the American Association of Dental Schools demanded an opportunity to present their position to the Board of Regents. In a written statement they criticized the College for releasing its statement without any consultation with their organizations. They pointed out that both the Joint Commission and the AHA approved of dentists on medical staffs, to be appointed in the same manner and subject to the same restrictions as physicians. They asserted that no group of surgeons had ever been able to agree on a definition of minor versus major surgery. They also pointed out that specialists in oral surgery must complete three years of advanced education in one of 129 hospital training programs to qualify for certification by the American Board of Oral Surgery. They also reminded the Board of Regents that each licensing district in the United States provided for the examination and licensure of dentists to perform all preventive, restorative, and surgical procedures necessary to maintain the oral health of the patient. Therefore, they said, the dentist who performs surgical procedures has the legal authority to do so.[29]

A small group of Regents was delegated to meet with representatives of the dental organizations and after several acrimonious meetings, all the organizations eventually agreed that the revised statement of the Joint Commission would prevail.[29] The Regents were successful in obtaining agreement that all specialties involved in surgery of the head, neck and oral cavity should work progressively toward the team approach in the care of patients. The responsible surgeon or captain of the team holds the final responsibility for the care of patients and that individual must be a doctor of medicine.[19]

Rejecting Overtures

John Paul North reported that Dr. Aldo Parentela, Executive Secretary of the International College of Surgeons (ICS) visited him about a closer relationship between the two colleges. The ICS had 12,500 members worldwide, about half of which were in the United States. Approximately 85 percent of those also were Fellows of the ACS and 90 percent were board certified. The requirements for admission to their fellowship included satisfactory completion of approved internship and surgical residency or the equivalent.

Their plan was to strengthen their foreign sections; Parentela had an impressive collection of letters from ministries of health expressing interest in the objectives of the International College, and they furnished the names of outstanding surgeons in their countries.

Dr. Parentela proposed that the two colleges jointly sponsor and finance visits to the United States by distinguished surgeons from Europe for lectures and clinics, issue a public statement that cordial relations now exist between the College and the ICS, encourage ACS Fellows to participate in ICS activities, and designate an official representative of the ACS on the advisory council of the ICS. He proposed that eventually the ICS would concentrate its activities in its foreign sections, and the ACS would concentrate its activities in the United States and Canada. North brought the proposals to the Board of Regents, which summarily declined to accept them.[33]

Two years later Parentela proposed to the College the creation of a new, unique world association of surgeons. He wanted to combine the International College of Surgeons, the International Society of Surgeons (Societe Internationale de Chirurgie), and the American College of Surgeons into a single organization called the World Association of Surgeons. He envisioned an international postgraduate school of surgery, an international institute of surgical research, a surgical journal, and other activities. The Board of Regents ordered the director to communicate the College's lack of interest in such a proposal, especially in light of the existence of the International Federation of Surgical Colleges.[8]

The Cold War

At the Regents' first meeting after the Cuban Missile Crisis, during the height of the Cold War, Assistant Director George Stephenson expressed concern about the growing number of applicants from other countries, some of whom had political ideologies that were not democratic, and others who were identified with organizations unsympathetic to the United States. Stephenson said there was some precedent for the Board of Regents to be concerned about this.

Years ago, an applicant who was said to have been 'on the wrong side' in the Spanish Revolution was denied fellowship. Those who are Fellows in Latin American countries who have been our strongest supporters have refused to endorse applications when they know that the individuals in question were of a political faith that made them unsympathetic to this country. However no formal expression of opinion on this matter by the Regents can be found in the College's records.[34]

Stephenson continued, "If the Regents were to take a firm stand and deny applicants who lean toward communism or are known to be unsympathetic to this country, it would be logical for them to take the same attitude toward any of our Fellows who were similarly disposed."[34]

The Regents instituted the adoption of a policy for information of the credentials committees, that applicants should be selected from individuals who are well disposed toward the United States and its institutions, and that applicants who are inimical to the United States should be considered to be not suitable for fellowship.

This statement was not to be publicized, but was to serve as a guide for the Central Credentials Committee.[34] There is no record of whether or not it was ever used, but it was an accurate reflection of the country's antipathy toward communism in the 1960s.

Strategic Planning

Regent Robert Zollinger suggested to the Regents a small, strong committee to evaluate where the College of Surgeons should go in the years to come. He said, "We must be engineered to meet the future head on." Momentous change was occurring, much of it precipitated by the unpopular war in Vietnam. Students were rioting and rejecting authority, underprivileged people were demanding services and respect, those in authority were abused and denigrated, parents lost control of their children, and the core values of institutions and associations were challenged.

The Chairman of the Board of Regents, Preston Wade, appointed a special committee consisting of the Executive Committee plus other College officials to meet in special session in July 1966 to explore and define the immediate and long-range policies and objectives of the College.[27] The committee developed a list of 50 recommendations, many of which were minor suggestions for improving the Clinical Congress and the internal operations of the College. The major recommendations related to the increased role of the federal government in health care. The Regents believed that the College should become more involved in government affairs, but the recommendations did not specify how. A "committee on surgical services" was created to keep abreast of socioeconomic developments and recommend policies that would constructively improve the care of the surgical patient. The graduate education committee was instructed to study the effect of Medicare on the quality of surgical residency programs.

The Board of Regents was asked to re-examine the 1958 proposal of the Board of Governors that hospitals include medical staff members on hospital governing boards. After obtaining the recommendations of a commission he appointed to determine how to attack heart disease, cancer, and stroke, President Lyndon Johnson succeeded in getting legislation to create regional medical programs to fund research for these diseases, recruit scientists to study them, and provide funding of $340,000,000 over three years. The Regents wanted the College to take advantage of the government support to strengthen or supplement the programs of the College, such as the activities of the commission on cancer. Finally, noting that because Medicare would increase the demand for medical services, exacerbating the shortage of nurses and allied health personnel, the Regents wanted the College to deal with this problem. The net result of the exercise was an enumeration of the issues and problems, the recognition that the College should do something, but no specific action plans.

Sensing that the College was not keeping up with government involvement in health care and that the College was no longer a strong influence in undergraduate or graduate medical education, the planning committee also recommended a committee to search for the successor to John Paul North. The search committee, chaired by Dr. Jonathan Rhodes, consisted of Drs. William Longmire, Howard Mahorner, Preston Wade, and Robert Zollinger.[35]

In mid-1968, Board of Regents Chairman Dr. Jonathan Rhoads, known for his great intelligence and wisdom, appointed Dr. William Longmire, Vice Chairman of the Board, to chair a steering committee for another Regent's planning conference, to be held in January 1969. Rhoads was concerned about the drifting of the College. He knew that a new Director would be appointed in 1969, and that Longmire

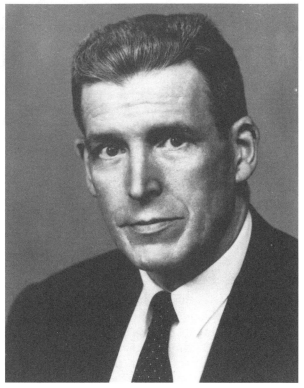

FIGURE 16.4 Dr. Jonathan E Rhoads, ACS President, 1971–72.

would probably be elected Chairman of the Board in October 1969. The plans formulated at the conference in January would set the agenda for the new Director, with the support and advice of future Board Chairman Longmire, who led the planning process. (Figure 16.4)

During the January 1969 planning conference, the participants focused on the position of the College concerning health care activities of the federal government, problems between the College and the surgical specialties, the international role of the College, continuing education, and surgical training.[33] Having seen to it that the strategic priorities of the new Director and his Board Chairman were in place, Rhoads, as chair of the search committee, now only needed to find a Director capable of dealing with these issues and working closely and happily with Longmire—and what more obvious choice than the brilliant C Rollins "Rollo" Hanlon, Longmire's medical school classmate at Hopkins and one of his best friends.

North succeeded in calming down the College after Hawley. He quietly went about improving the internal operations of the College, establishing databases for its operations, expanding the education program, reducing expenses, and representing the College with dignity.

REFERENCES

1. North, J., *The 20th General Hospital - I.S.Ravdin, Commanding General*. Surgery 1964. **56**: p. 614-623.
2. *Minutes of the meeting of the Board of Regents of March 4, 5, 1961*. 1961, Archives of the American College of Surgeons: Chicago.
3. *Minutes of the meeting of the Board of Regents of June 18, 19, 1965*. 1965, Archives of the American College of Surgeons: Chicago.
4. *Minutes of the meeting of the Board of Regents of October 6, 1961*. 1961, Archives of the American College of Surgeons: Chicago.
5. *Minutes of the meeting of the Board of Regents of June 2, 7-9, 1969*. 1969, Archives of the American College of Surgeons: Chicago.
6. *Minutes of the meeting of the Board of Regents of February 3-6, 1967*. 1967, Archives of the American College of Surgeons: Chicago.
7. *Minutes of the meeting of the Board of Regents of June 12-14, 1970*. 1970, Archives of the American College of Surgeons: Chicago.
8. *Minutes of the meeting of the Board of Regents of February 6-8, 1970*. 1970, Archives of the American College of Surgeons: Chicago.
9. *Minutes of the meeting of the Board of Regents of June 23,24, 1961*. 1961, Archives of the American College of Surgeons: Chicago.
10. *Minutes of the meeting of the Board of Regents of October 9, 1964*. 1964, Archives of the American College of Surgeons: Chicago.
11. *Minutes of the meeting of the Board of Regents of February 5, 6, 1966*. 1966, Archives of the American College of Surgeons: Chicago.
12. *Minutes of the meeting of the Board of Regents of June 22, 23, 1962*. 1962, Archives of the American College of Surgeons: Chicago.
13. *Minutes of the meeting of the Board of Regents of June 15,16, 1963*. 1963, Archives of the American College of Surgeons: Chicago.
14. *Minutes of the meeting of the Board of Regents of September 29, October 1, 1961*. 1967, Archives of the American College of Surgeons: Chicago.
15. *Minutes of the meeitng of the Board of Regents of February 2-4, 1968*. 1968, Archives of the American College of Surgeons: Chicago.
16. *Minutes of the meeting of the Board of Regents of October 8,9, 1960*. 1960, Archives of the American College of Surgeons: Chicago.
17. *Minutes of the meeting of the Board of Regents of November 1, 1963*. 1963, Archives of the American College of Surgeons: Chicago.
18. *Minutes of the meeting of the American College of Surgeons of June 7-9, 1968*. 1968, Archives of the American College of Surgeons: Chicago.
19. *Minutes of the meeting of the Board of Regents of October 10, 1969*. 1969, Archives of the American College of Surgeons: Chicago.
20. *Minutes of the meeting of the Board of Regents of February 3, 4, 1957*. 1957, Archives of the American College of Surgeons: Chicago.
21. *Minutes of the meeting of the Board of Regents of December 7, 1957*. 1957, Archives of the American College of Surgeons: Chicago.
22. *Minutes of the meeting of the Board of Regents of February 8,9, 1964*. 1964, Archives of the American College of Surgeons: Chicago.
23. *Minutes of the meeting of the Board of Regents of February 27,28, 29, 1960*. 1960, Archives of the American College of Surgeons: Chicago.
24. *Minutes of the meeting of the Board of Regents of October 3,4, 1964*. 1964, Archives of the American College of Surgeons: Chicago.

25. *Minutes of the meeting of the Board of Regents of February 6, 7, 1965.* 1965, Archives of the American College of Surgeons: Chicago.

26. *Minutes of the meeting of the Board of Regents of October 16, 17, 1965.* 1965, Archives of the American College of Surgeons: Chicago.

27. *Minutes of the meeting of the Board of Regents of June 24, 25, 1966.* 1966, Archives of the American College of Surgeons: Chicago.

28. *About the Chicago Medical Society. Mission and history.*

29. *Minutes of the meeting of the Board of Regents of June 13-15, 1969.* 1969, Archives of the American College of Surgeons: Chicago.

30. *Minutes of the meeting of the Board of Regents of October 3-5, 1969.* 1969, Archives of the American College of Surgeons: Chicago.

31. *Minutes of the meeting of the Board of Regents of June 13, 14, 1964.* 1964, Archives of the American College of Surgeons: Chicago.

32. *Minutes of the meeitng of the Board of Regents of June 11-13, 1971.* 1971, Archives of the American College of Surgeons: Chicago.

33. *Minutes of the meeting of the Board of Regents of October 11-13, 1968.* 1968, Archives of the American College of Surgeons: Chicago.

34. *Minutes of the meeting of the Board of Regents of February 23, 24 1963.* 1963, Archives of the American College of Surgeons: Chicago.

35. *Minutes of the meeting of the Board of Regents of October 6-9, 1966.* 1966, Archives of the American College of Surgeons: Chicago.

CHAPTER 17
The College Wakes Up

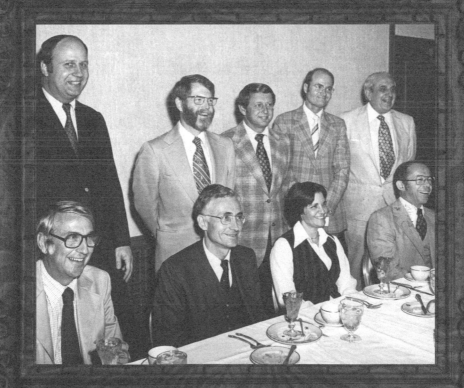

Dr. C Rollins Hanlon, known affectionately to almost everyone as "Rollo," was the professor and chairman of surgery at St. Louis University. He had been involved with the College as a Governor, and was surprised to be elected a Regent in 1967. A year later, during the Regents' meetings at the Clinical Congress in San Francisco, he was invited to a breakfast meeting by Regent John Brewer, the chief of OB/GYN at Northwestern University. While Hanlon was settling in with his breakfast, someone asked, "We wondered if you would be interested in becoming the Director of the College." Hanlon remembered being so surprised that he almost choked on his orange juice.[1] (Figure 17.1)

That the Regents selected him was not a surprise. He was one of the leading cardiac surgeons in the country. In 1950, while at Johns Hopkins, he developed, with Alfred Blalock, the Blalock-Hanlon operation, in which an

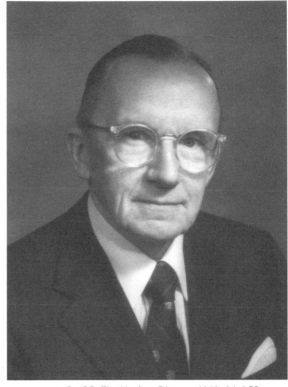

FIGURE 17.1 Dr. C Rollins Hanlon, Director 1969–86; ACS President, 1987–88.

opening is made between the two upper chambers of the heart to relieve the symptoms of transposition of the great vessels, a fatal congenital cardiac anomaly. But he was a leader as well. He had established St. Louis University as a major research and clinical center for the study and treatment of cardiac conditions. His attitudes and actions throughout his personal and professional lives were the products of rigorous intellectual discourse and exceptionally strong moral and ethical values, attributes that were apparent throughout his early career and were especially obvious during his tenure as Director of the College and later as an unpaid executive consultant. They had been honed, in part, during his undergraduate education at Loyola University Maryland and his chairmanship at St. Louis University, both Jesuit institutions. As a Regent, Hanlon had participated in the January 1969 planning conference; he knew what the strategic plan was and eagerly embraced it.

One of Hanlon's first projects was to review all the past official statements of the College; from them he derived principles, which he then collated in a document called *Statements on Principles*. This exercise provided Hanlon with the ethical foundation on which he based his conduct of the organization's affairs. Included are statements about fee splitting, practicing within the limits of a specialty, the surgeon's responsibility for preoperative diagnosis and care, the selection and performance of the operation, and postoperative surgical care. There also is proscription of itinerant surgery and on-the-job training. Moral and ethical fitness is advocated as is scientific honesty and placing the welfare of the patient above all else;[2] these principles were originally published in 1974 and have been revised periodically, most recently in 2008. They are available online at the American College of Surgeons (ACS) website.[3] Throughout his association with the College, Hanlon believed strongly that its purpose was to promote the ethical and competent practice of surgery.

When Hanlon was appointed director in 1969, the College was a large organization of complex interrelationships and operations. Its staff of approximately120 participated in the meetings and other activities of 102 standing and ad hoc committees and subcommittees, 64 credentials committees, 56 state and provincial (Canadian) advisory committees, 65 U.S. and nine foreign chapters, and nine specialty advisory councils. In addition, through designated representatives, the College maintained relationships with 27 other organizations such as the AMA, specialty societies, and certifying boards. Representatives of 21 other organizations served as members of 30 College committees.[4] The College had become a complex organization that demanded an astute manager, and Hanlon filled the bill.

During the 1960s, the unpopular war in Vietnam, the debate over civil rights, and the assassinations of President John F Kennedy, his brother Senator Robert Kennedy, and the Reverend Martin Luther King led to widespread unrest and demonstrations throughout the country, especially on college campuses. In 1970, students were gunned down by National Guardsmen at Kent State University. Immediately, almost 500 colleges and universities closed temporarily to avoid the possibility of violence. Five days later, 100,000 citizens marched in Washington, DC, to protest the war. A few months later the physics building at the University of Wisconsin was bombed, killing a graduate student. Young people were rejecting the country's political system and the authority of their elders, institutions, and parents. Some of them simply dropped out of mainstream society, reveling in the music of Joan Baez, the Grateful Dead and others, while adopting the dress and unkempt appearance that identified them as "hippies."

Medical students and residents were not hippies, but many of them adopted the long hair, beards, and unconventional dress of their generation. This was a problem for their professors, who tended to be strait-laced and rigid. Beards stuck out from surgical masks, allegedly creating an infection hazard, and patients did not appreciate being examined by young doctors in jeans and t-shirts. Rules about dress and comportment were set forth, broken, negotiated, and compromised. Several medical school deans were barricaded in their offices for refusing to yield to the demands of students, such as the creation of a student lounge. Eventually, there was accommodation on both sides, aided by the gradual withdrawal of troops from Vietnam, the end of the draft, and the official end of the war in 1975.

College leaders, many of whom were professors, had learned to avoid conflict by being manifestly attentive to the needs of medical students, residents, and young surgical faculty. This, and the desire to elevate surgical research, led the Regents to create scholarships for the research activities of surgical trainees from College funds, the first of which was awarded to Gary H Stevens, who was deemed the best of 26 applicants in 1969.[5] By 1980, the College was granting two scholarships of up to $15,000 per year for two years, and the Schering Company sponsored three scholarships for one year, each at $5,000.[6] The Loyal Davis Traveling Surgical Scholarship was funded in 1983 by a $250,000 gift from business tycoon Armand Hammer and his foundation, announced at a memorial service for Davis in the Murphy Auditorium attended by Davis's son-in-law and daughter, President and Mrs. Ronald Reagan.[7]

The Regents also reactivated the tradition of inviting medical students to the Clinical Congress as guests of the College.[8] By 1979, 30 students were invited, each of whom received $100 to defray expenses.[9]

Sensing that young surgeons in the College also needed more attention, the Regents appointed an ad hoc committee of young surgeons (which they defined as age 45 or younger) to study "relationships with young surgeons."[5] The committee was to determine how the College could be more helpful in the development of young surgeons and was to seek ways in which young surgeons could play a more meaningful role in College affairs.[10]

The committee noted that the average age of the Regents was about 60, that the Governors were not much younger, and that the primary problem was the communications between 19 members of the Board of Regents and the 7,000 young surgeons elected to the College in the previous five years.[11]

The committee requested that young surgeons be represented on all committees of the College, that a minimum of two Regents should be young surgeons, and that the governors should reflect the age distribution of the fellowship. Although these recommendations were ignored at first, the Regents agreed that a meeting of young surgeons, one from each College chapter, should be held annually in Chicago to teach them more about the College and current socioeconomic issues, and to arrange workshops in which they could express their views.[12, 13] This and a young surgeons panel discussion at the Clinical Congress soon became popular annual events.[14] The Regents were so pleased that they changed the name of the ad hoc committee to the Young Surgeons Committee and designated it as a standing committee.

Most importantly, the Regents agreed that a member of the committee should sit in an *ex officio* capacity during meetings of the Board of Regents and the Board of Governors. Ever since, many representatives of young surgeons have expressed their opinions at Regents' and Governors' meetings, participated in discussions, and influenced decisions.[8]

Another major change was made to bring younger men into the College and to provide continuity between membership in the candidate group and the award of fellowship.[15]

At Hanlon's first Clinical Congress as director, 1,379 surgeons, culled from 1,554 applicants, were admitted to fellowship. A majority of those not recommended by credentials committees were ophthalmologists who dispensed glasses, contrary to College policy. Other reasons were itinerant surgery, volunteering information on malpractice suits, or performing an insufficient number of major cases.[15] Almost 93 percent were board certified, a substantial improvement in just ten years. But because of the long training and the universal requirement for military service, the average initiate was approximately 37 years old, allowing for tenure in the College of only about 30 years. The Board of Regents voted to drop the requirement for seven years of training, which included one year of internship and, instead, permitted an individual to apply after completing graduate training and one year of practice. The College was responding effectively to the needs of young surgeons.

Young surgeons were not the only Fellows who wanted a stronger voice in the College. The Governors had a long history of not understanding, or misunderstanding, their own role in the College, in part because the College had not clarified it and in part because the Governors mistakenly thought they were part of the College's governance system. As government involvement in the health system grew, the Governors became more restive, anxious to goad the College into resisting even more intrusion, real and imagined. Hanlon recognized that the Governors, properly channeled, could bring the leadership of the College into a closer relationship with the fellowship and become a potent force for grass roots support of College positions on socioeconomic and other issues. He published an article in the *Bulletin* entitled "The Role of Governors and Chapter Officers," noting that under the bylaws the management and control of the business and professional affairs of the College is vested in the Board of Regents, and that the Governors are to act as a liaison between the Board of Regents and the Fellows, and as a clearinghouse for the Regents on assigned subjects and on local problems. Hanlon specified their duty to attend the Board of Governors' annual meeting, the sectional meetings, and the annual convocation at the Clinical Congress.[12]

Clarification of their role and the presence of the Chairman, Vice Chairman, and Secretary of the Board of Governors at all meetings of the Board of Regents had a salutary effect. By 1977, the Governors committee on functions and purposes of the Board of

Governors recommended that each Governor submit an annual report to the chairman of the Board of Governors and that Governors regularly attend chapter meetings and participate in chapter activities, thus putting them in regular contact with the Fellows in their area. Chapters and specialty societies looked to their Governors as sources of the latest information from the College and as vehicles for expressing their concerns and recommendations to the leadership of the College.

Beginning in 1978, each Governor submitted a written report to the chairman of the Board of Governors enumerating the concerns of the Fellows in his area, and any recommendations they had.[16] The chairman and the College staff analyzed the reports and generated a list of the top ten concerns of the fellowship, and this was presented to the Regents. The three top concerns in 1978 were the high premiums for professional liability insurance and the proliferation of lawsuits; the requirements for second opinions by Medicare and private insurers, implemented because of the public's concern about unnecessary surgery; and mandatory continuing education required for state licensure and hospital medical staff membership, in response to allegations that the knowledge of many physicians was out of date.[17]

The Regents responded to the concern about professional liability by renewing promotion of the College's patient safety manual, providing professional and public education, and monitoring developments related to professional liability. This plan guided the professional liability activities of the College for many years thereafter.[7]

The chairman of the Board of Governors and College staff wrote a response to the report of the Governors that described how the College was tackling the concerns of the fellowship. Both the annual report of the Governors and the response were published in the *Bulletin*, an effective way to inform the fellowship about the problems their colleagues were facing and how the College was addressing them. The annual reports eventually became cornerstones for the agendas of the Board of Governors, the College staff, and the Regents.[18]

≈⊰✳⊱≈

Continuing Medical Education (CME)

One of Hanlon's wisest moves was to hire Dr. Edwin H Gerrish as director of the assembly department. He was trained in pediatric surgery at Western Reserve University and stayed on the faculty briefly, but left to practice in Maybridge, South Dakota, as the only surgeon within a 100 mile radius, taking care of people with a wide range of surgical problems. A garrulous individual and an avid outdoorsman, Ed Gerrish related well to practicing surgeons, and their needs were reflected in his management of the Clinical Congress and other educational activities. His persona contrasted with the academic orientation of Rollo Hanlon, and the two of them made the fellowship feel that the College had something for everyone.

Because of declining attendance and financial problems the sectional meetings were phased out in favor of a spring meeting in a large city, the first of which was in New York City in 1973.[10, 19] As general surgeons became more restive about the disproportionate decline in their reimbursement from Medicare and the shrinkage of their surgical repertoire owing to the new, less invasive technologies used by gastroenterologists and interventional radiologists, the College decided to devote the spring meeting to general surgeons. A very popular feature was the town hall meeting, in which attendees could sound off about their problems (mostly socioeconomic) and receive answers from College officials.[20] Courses on vascular surgery and the new technique of fiberoptic sigmoidoscopy were filled to capacity.[21, 22]

Gerrish surveyed the fellowship about the Clinical Congress and learned that 60 percent had attended the previous four Congresses. Of the 52 percent that attended the live closed circuit telecasts, fewer than half said they were of high value, but more than half used films from the College's motion picture library, mostly for teaching.[12] Because of declining attendance and lack of sponsorship, the telecasts were discontinued in 1976.[23] Before performing new operations or modifications of existing operations, surgeons need to see them performed by an expert. The television program of the College served this need admirably, but the advancements in cinematography made available a wide range of teaching films that were not only shown at the Clinical Congress and sectional meetings, but were also accessible to surgeons year-round through the College's film library.

Gerrish, Hanlon, and the Regents, knowing of the interest of surgeons and their spouses in international travel, arranged a meeting with the Royal College of Surgeons of England in 1979,[24] and another with the French Academy of Surgery and the French Association of Surgery in 1981.[25] Tour packages after the meetings were subscribed by many attendees, and Gerrish noted that at the meeting with the French, "The unlimited supply of wine at the reception and the banquet helped almost everyone overlook the mediocre buffet dinner and the high cost of $80 per person."[26] These events accentuated the fellowship that grows among those committed to the ethical and competent practice of surgery, a fellowship that members of the College have noted when discussing the Clinical Congress.

The large number of organizations that offered a huge array of continuing education activities for doctors raised questions about the standards and quality of continuing medical education (CME). Simultaneously, CME was becoming mandatory for state licensure, hospital medical staff credentialing, professional society membership, and board certification. Through its Council on Medical Education, the AMA designated state medical societies as accreditors of regional CME programs, and in 1968 initiated the Physician's Recognition Award, given to physicians who participated in 150 hours or more of CME during a three-year period.

The AMA facilitated development of the liaison committee on continuing medical education (LCCME), which, in 1977, assumed the accreditation function previously carried out by the AMA Council on Medical Education. Five organizations agreed to serve as sponsoring organizations for the LCCME. They were the American Hospital Association (AHA), the American Medical Association (AMA), the American Board of Medical Specialties (ABMS), the Association of American Medical Colleges (AAMC), and the Council of Medical Specialty Societies (CMSS).[23] Although the AMA later withdrew from the LCCME temporarily, it was reconstituted as the Accreditation Council on Continuing Medical Education (ACCME) with the Federation of State Medical Boards and the Association for Hospital Medical Education as additional sponsors. Currently, the ACCME accredits state medical societies and other organizations that meet its standards, including the College, to confer CME accreditation and the designation of credit for qualified CME activities.

The ABMS responded to the public and governmental concern that doctors' knowledge was out of date with the standard that its member boards required recertification. The American Board of Surgery (ABS) began to issue time-limited certificates to its new diplomates in 1986. After 10 years the certificate expired, but could be renewed by passing a recertification exam.[17] Most, but not all, of the surgical specialty boards adopted time-limited certification. Implicit in recertification was the assumption that diplomates of the boards would engage in continuing education.

The International Department

The Regents asked Hanlon to develop an international department of the College that would concentrate on activities in the Western hemisphere but maintain enthusiasm for attracting well-trained surgeons from other countries.[27] Hanlon engaged the retired chair of neurological surgery at the University of Chicago, Dr. Joseph P Evans, to study surgical services in Colombia and serve as a liaison officer.[13, 29] Subsequently, he was named the College's assistant director for international liaison. For the next decade Evans cemented relationships with Latin American surgeons; he had the first version of the Surgical Education and Self-Assessment Program, or SESAP I, and various College manuals translated into Spanish, and supported medical school graduates in obtaining training in the United States.[29, 30] He pushed the College to increase the number of international guest scholarships to five, two of which were designated for Latin American surgeons. Before retiring he organized a workshop on principles of administration for Latin American surgery department chairmen. Dr. Evans opened the door to the modern relationship between Latin American surgeons and the College, for which he was given the College's Distinguished Service Award, its highest award.[31]

Medicare and Medicaid Begin
To Influence the Agenda

John Paul North had brought calm and quiet to the College after Hawley's boisterous term. The Clinical Congress was an outstanding educational and fellowship experience for the nation's surgeons, the Board functioned smoothly, and the staff finally had sufficient space in a modern building in the heart of Chicago to work efficiently and happily. The Social Security Act of 1965, which created Medicare and Medicaid, broke this tranquility, but it was not yet obvious that Medicare would draw the government into almost all aspects of health care. Hanlon participated in a planning meeting of the Regents a few months before he began as Director, where the consensus was that the College should join with the AMA to keep the financing and delivery of health care in the private sector, where it then resided. In the meantime, the College should make its views known in Washington on all health care policies, but not establish a Washington office, lest such a move be "misinterpreted" by the AMA, which was speaking for the profession.

A project spurred by government's increasing interest in health care and in physician manpower was the Study on Surgical Services in the United States, a massive, joint effort of the College and the American Surgical Association (ASA) to develop reliable and detailed data on the delivery of surgical care. Dr. George Zuidema, chairman of surgery at Johns Hopkins, chaired the five-year study and Dr. Francis D Moore, surgeon-in-chief of the Peter Bent Brigham Hospital, was vice chairman. The manpower data captured the most attention, suggesting that a modest reduction in the number of surgical trainees was warranted. This recommendation was gradually implemented by the residency review committee for surgery, which imposed higher standards on programs, and by the reduced federal support for graduate medical education.

The College staff used a powerful new computer to implement a longitudinal study of surgical residents, tracking them throughout their training and using the results for information on manpower in surgery and its specialties. In 1982, there were 1,656 initiates, of whom 40 percent were general surgeons and 60 percent were in other specialties, the largest of which were urology (179), otolaryngology (147), orthopaedic surgery (133), and ophthalmic surgery (127). Only 719 of the total had been members of the candidate group. The total number of individuals in the candidate group in 1982 was 7,136.[32]

The College database showed that the average general surgeon was 52.5 years old, lived in a metropolitan area of between 50,000 and 5 million residents, took five weeks of vacation per year, and spent 44 hours per week in practice. The cost of an initial office visit was $25, an appendectomy or hernia repair $550, a cholecystectomy $865, and sigmoidoscopy $54. The average professional liability insurance premium was $9,142.[32]

Research was flourishing because of the largess of the National Institutes of Health, which provided investigators with unprecedented funding through research grants, more than $1.1 billion in 1970, up from $400 million ten years earlier. Interest in the Surgical Forum remained high; between 900 and 1,000 abstracts were submitted annually.

The animals used for research were not always cared for appropriately, leading to criticism by the public and the formation of animal rights groups dedicated to shutting down all research using animals. Accreditation of animal facilities by the American Association for Accreditation of Laboratory Animal Care, which the College supported financially, was required by the National Institutes of Health beginning in 1970.[8] This ensured humane care and treatment of animals used for research, but the general public was still concerned, and the goal of animal rights groups has been to eliminate research using animals. In 1985, 80 bills to restrict the use of animals in research were introduced in 21 states.[33] Both enacted and threatened legislation led institutions and their investigators to use research methods that did not require animals and using animals only when absolutely necessary, a desired outcome of the public's concern.

Changes in Surgical Practice

Although the advent of cardiac surgery was a spectacular development after World War II, the practice of medicine and surgery changed more fundamentally during the 1970s and 1980s. Leading hospitals created units in which their sickest patients were housed together, many of them immediately after major cardiac, neurologic, or thoracic surgery. They were the first intensive care units, which were later populated by experts who used newly invented respirators, external defibrillators, and continuous intubation to radically redesign care of the critically ill. This spawned the new specialty of critical care medicine, approved for certificates of special competence in the fields of surgery, internal medicine, obstetrics and gynecology, anesthesia, and pediatrics.[34]

Doctors John L Ford, a surgeon, and Wallace A Reed, an anesthesiologist, opened the first freestanding ambulatory surgical facility, called a surgicenter, in Phoenix in 1970. Immediately, issues of safety arose, but they reported treating 5,200 patients in 18 months without a single death or emergency transfer to a conventional hospital.[13] Dr. Merlin DuVal, a surgeon who was assistant secretary for health and scientific affairs of the Department of Health, Education, and Welfare, wrote Hanlon to warn that if surgical procedures were moved outside the hospital, the cost of care given in the hospital would increase, thereby increasing overall health care costs which were already "out of sight."[35]

Nevertheless, the ambulatory surgery movement flourished, especially when Blue Cross and Blue Shield and other insurance carriers approved reimbursement for services provided without admission to a hospital. A major impetus was the opportunity for surgeons and other procedure-oriented specialists, such as gastroenterologists, to own ambulatory surgery facilities and derive income from facility fees as well as professional fees. The widespread and enthusiastic response of patients to avoiding hospitalization and the convenience for surgeons and patients alike established ambulatory surgery as the preferred method for many procedures in every procedural specialty.

Later, Blue Cross and Blue Shield pushed to require that certain procedures be done on an ambulatory basis, but the College insisted that this was not mandatory, and that surgical judgment based on patient age, anesthetic risk, and other factors might suggest that a given procedure should be done in a hospital.[26] Encouraged by the College, the Joint Commission developed an accreditation process for ambulatory surgery facilities, but the Accreditation Association for Ambulatory Health Care became the dominant accrediting body.

Another new method of practice was the health maintenance organization, or HMO. Patients were enrolled by insurance companies or other entities into their HMO, which hired physicians and surgeons of all specialties to care for them. Because primary care physicians served as "gatekeepers" for the access of patients to specialists, HMOs were thought to be more cost effective than traditional practice models. Specialty organizations complained that HMOs denied patients the right to select their physicians.[7, 26] Stimulated by the massive infusion of federal funds for planning and development, these programs covered approximately 8 million persons in 1973.[36] The College issued a policy statement decrying the practice of using the names of popular HMO physicians to recruit patients, and urged HMOs to adhere to the code of medical ethics of the AMA.

The culture of the profession was changing too. Advertising, especially for cosmetic surgery, previously deemed unethical and unprofessional, became so common that the bylaws of the College, which had made "solicitation of patients" a basis for disciplinary action, were changed to provide that "communications to the public" could not be deceptive.[37]

The use of new technology forced a new look at some of the College's most enduring principles. Patients treated for urinary calculi with the Dornier lithotripter, introduced in 1984, were usually charged an all-inclusive fee by the entity that owned the lithotripter. The fee was split between the institution and the several involved physicians including urologists.[38] This generated charges of fee splitting. The central judiciary committee developed a policy that the amount each physician would receive had to be identified on the statement.[20]

The financial relationships in HMOs also raised concerns about fee splitting.[39] The College kept its policy banning fee splitting; instead, the bylaws were changed to allow Fellows to participate in HMOs and independent practice associations, where there might be "discounting" of fees.[40]

Some surgeons did not appear to practice what had always been called surgery. The Regents were concerned about applicants for fellowship whose practices did not fit into existing categories, including critical care specialists and ophthalmologists who used lasers almost exclusively. After debate and advice from the appropriate advisory councils, these individuals were deemed surgeons and eligible for fellowship.[22]

Because almost half of all surgery was performed by general practitioners, the communications department of the College began a campaign to advocate "surgery by surgeons."[41] Other initiatives included radio and television public service announcements on hazards of diving, roller skating safety, skin cancer, outpatient surgery, and others.[21]

The attitude of allopathic physicians toward osteopathic physicians was also changing. The Regents were sympathetic with the suggestion of the AMA trustees that graduates of schools of osteopathy should be brought into the mainstream of medical practice. But the Regents could not support this until it was determined that schools of osteopathy meet the standards for medical schools approved by the Council on Medical Education of the AMA and the AAMC. The position of the Regents was that osteopaths not be admitted to residency programs approved by the College.[31] Over objections by the Board of Regents, both the American Board of Surgery and the American Board of Plastic Surgery began to accept graduates of schools of osteopathy for examination and certification in their specialties.[18, 40] Concomitantly, residency programs were admitting graduates of osteopathic schools for training.

≈※≈

Specialization

Specialization continued unabated during Hanlon's tenure. This phenomenon probably resulted in better health care for the public, but it created problems for the College and organized medicine. The American Board of Medical Specialties approved a certificate of special competence in vascular surgery in 1982,[21] and a certificate of special competence in hand surgery was proposed by the American Boards of Surgery, Orthopaedic Surgery, and Plastic Surgery.[32] The American Board of Obstetrics and Gynecology formed divisions of gynecologic oncology, maternal-fetal medicine, and reproductive endocrinology, each of which had a certificate of special competence.[32]

A major problem for the College was to keep specialty surgeons as members, to make them feel a part of the organization, and to recruit young specialists as members. An obvious way to keep in touch with surgical specialists was through their specialty organizations, and the Regents agreed that the advisory councils for the surgical specialties were convenient vehicles for two-way communication. But this required rethinking how advisory council members were appointed. They needed to be in the leadership of the specialty societies to communicate the issues facing the specialties and to bring information from the College to the societies. Advisory Council members who were also specialty society governors would be familiar with the issues of the College and could communicate them to members of the specialty societies and the College chapters.

After several proposals by the Regents that Hanlon believed were unworkable,[42] the long-range planning committee, under the chairmanship of Dr. David Sabiston, recommended that each Advisory Council be composed of three members appointed by the specialty societies, one member from the specialty certifying board, and three members from the Board of Governors. The specialty society representatives would be from the largest and most representative societies, as determined by the Advisory Council. Each Advisory Council would have a representative to the College program committee and to the Surgical Forum committee. (Figure 17.2)

Each council would select a chairman, and the 11 (later 12) chairmen would meet annually and select a chairman who would attend all meetings of the Board of Regents. The chairman of each Council would make an annual report that included the activities of the specialty board, the committees of specialty societies, and matters of concern to the specialty. The terms of office were fixed so that representatives would

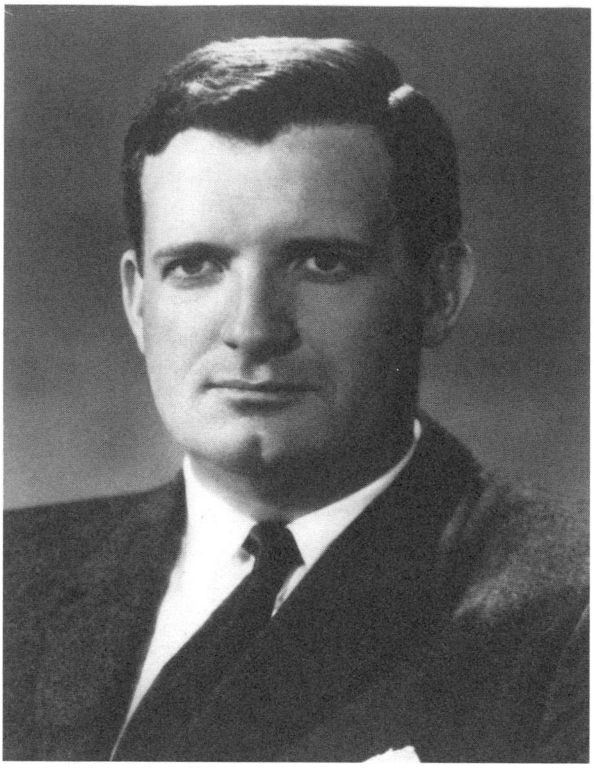

FIGURE 17.2 Dr. David C Sabiston Jr., ACS President, 1985–86.

have sufficient time on the Board of Governors or the certifying board to ensure their optimal representation.[9] The Advisory Councils were general surgery (created in 1970),[10] urology, thoracic surgery, plastic and maxillofacial surgery, pediatric surgery, otorhinolaryngology, orthopaedic surgery, ophthalmic surgery, neurological surgery, and gynecology and obstetrics. Vascular surgery was added in 1980. Sabiston's recommendation was approved, and this basic structure and modus operandi remains in place.[35, 50]

A typical example of the interaction between the advisory council chairmen and the Regents arose in February 1982. The distinguished chair of urology at Northwestern University, Dr. John Grayhack, noted that the American Urological Association lectureship at the Clinical Congress was established to bring speakers who would open new horizons and bring new ideas to the profession, or espouse a social philosophy that differed from those commonly held. He complained that speakers nominated by the urology advisory council had not been accepted by some of the Regents. He requested that the mechanisms by which speakers were chosen and approached be reevaluated.[44]

Although some of the issues between specialties and the College could be solved and others could not, the working relationship between the Advisory Councils and the Regents improved communications and established a mutual respect that has helped to promote discourse and prevent dissidence.

Nevertheless, the number of surgical specialists who attended College meetings gradually declined, so that at the 1980 spring meeting in Toronto, only 43 ophthalmologists attended, despite an excellent course on ophthalmologic trauma. Later, specialty postgraduate courses were omitted from the spring meeting because of low attendance.[25]

The College Withdraws from the AMA

When Hanlon took over the College directorship the financial ramifications of the 1965 Medicare and Medicaid legislation were becoming apparent. Costs were escalating because physician and hospital payments were based on their usual and customary charges. Providers learned quickly that as they increased their fees, Medicare increased its payments. Congress realized that constraints on Medicare expenditures would be necessary, and with input from health care economists and other experts, were struggling to determine how to do this. Many legislative proposals designed to slow the rate of Medicare spending were put forth. In 1970, for example, there were 29 bills classified as health legislation.

The problem for the College was how to keep current with information and how to influence the debates. At the Board of Regents planning session a few months before Hanlon took office, the Regents and officers rejected the notion of creating a Washington office, believing that their standing policy of letting the AMA speak for the profession in socioeconomic matters should be honored.

The AMA had expressed its concern over the fragmentation of the voice of medicine in meetings of specialty society representatives, attended by Dr. Hanlon and members of his executive team. The AMA leaders complained that four specialty societies already had their principal offices in Washington in 1970, and others were planning to establish offices there. The AMA was trying to make information and advice on government matters available to specialty societies.[45] Its office in Washington monitored legislation and the AMA encouraged specialty societies to work with it and through it. The larger specialty societies, including the College, met with the Washington office of the AMA regularly.[2]

While the College was trying to align itself and cooperate with the AMA on legislative matters, the AMA was diminishing the role of specialty societies, including the College, in its governance. Nevertheless, the College and the AMA were aligned in their support for the Bennett Professional Standards Review Organization (PSRO) bill, which established peer review organizations throughout the country to review the necessity and quality of care provided by physicians to Medicare and Medicaid beneficiaries. Both organizations supported the designation of family practice, general internal medicine, and obstetrics and gynecology as primary care specialties, and several cost containment measures, including peer review. The government punctuated its interest in primary care by providing medical schools with incentives to emphasize the training of primary care physicians.[46]

Dr. James Sammons, the AMA executive vice president, described in *American Medical News* as "flamboyant, emphatic, and bluntly pragmatic,"[47] decried the decline in AMA membership. Specialists were not renewing their memberships or not joining. He announced plans to make the AMA an organization of organizations, including specialty societies, which would have representation in the House of Delegates in proportion to the number of their members.[17] The interspecialty council of the AMA, later called the Interspecialty Advisory Council, gradually disintegrated as its clout was diminished.

Dr. John Beal, who succeeded Loyal Davis as chairman of surgery at Northwestern, resigned as the College representative to the house of delegates, complaining that the AMA was not working for the College.[25] The interests of the AMA and the College were diverging, and in 1980 the Regents took the bold step of not nominating another delegate to the AMA House of Delegates, tantamount to pulling out of the AMA.[48] This was a tipping point for the College, because it signaled the resolve of its leadership that fidelity to the fellowship was more important than a relationship to the country's most powerful physician organization. Standing up to the AMA was a major event in 1980, and one that shocked the fellowship as well as the AMA.

As the Regents contemplated this move, the College finally established its own Washington office.[49] Hanlon and the Regents had concluded that when the interests of the Fellows were not congruent with those of other organizations, such as the AAMC or the AMA, the Fellows needed to be represented by the College, and they resolved to do so. At first, the Washington office was viewed as an extension of the College's department of surgical practice, established in 1974 under Mr. James Haug to gather and disseminate data, some of which was published annually as the widely appreciated *Socio-Economic Factbook for Surgery*. The office was established with a staff of two, who were not registered as lobbyists, and concentrated on regulatory, rather than legislative matters.[50]

Graduate Medical Education

Hanlon wanted to position the College to influence discussion and debate over graduate and continuing medical education standards and their implementation. The College was a founding member of the tripartite council and therefore a prominent member of its successor, the Council of Medical Specialty Societies (CMSS). During Hanlon's tenure, the CMSS supported the establishment of the Liaison Committee on Graduate Medical Education (LCGME) and was one of its sponsors.

Although the College appointed members of the residency review committee for surgery (RRC-s), it could not influence broad policy decisions through these individuals. The College's ability to influence the important debates and discussions of the LCGME was through the CMSS, which had authority to approve decisions of the LCGME, and more importantly, veto authority to disapprove them. The early days of the LCGME were fraught with fights between the sponsors (aptly called parents) over the relationship between the LCGME and the residency review committees, the method of financing the organization, and the proposal of the AAMC to put medical schools, rather than hospitals, in control of graduate medical education. There were many more debates over lesser issues. Hanlon was a leader in the CMSS because of his brilliance, his careful preparation for meetings, and his ability to articulate reasonable solutions to problems. He was elected the CMSS president for a two-year term beginning in 1975.

In order to be influential in these organizations, Hanlon felt it necessary to become a leader, which inevitably led to his becoming an officer or a resource for the organization. This multiplied his duties enormously. He was managing the College, and simultaneously managing another complex organization, the CMSS, made even more complex because of the extraordinary difficulties in achieving rapid consensus, or even consensus at all. Hanlon dutifully reported the problems existing in these organizations and his efforts to help resolve them. The Regents, as indicated by their lack of discussion after his reports, did not seem to appreciate the significance or the extent of what he was doing. They did believe, however, that he was doing an excellent job.[51]

Hanlon had Dr. Theodore Cooper, his former student and, more recently, assistant secretary of health, speak to the Board of Regents in 1977. Cooper recommended that the College develop written policies on unnecessary surgery, specialization, economic issues in health care, and technology and technology transfer. He urged the College to begin a more active dialogue with high level public representatives on these issues. A special task force appointed to investigate this met with the chairman of Washington's National Business Group on Health, which was the health core of the Business Roundtable, and reiterated Cooper's recommendations. The business group felt that this concept was unusual and practical, and they encouraged the College to pursue it. They recommended Mr. Arthur Wood, the recently retired chief executive officer of the Sears Corporation as a resource person.

The College representatives also met with Mr. John Gardner, former secretary of the Department of Health, Education, and Welfare and, more recently, involved with the citizens lobbying group Common Cause. He was enthusiastic about the possibility of Mr. Wood as a potential chairman of the group. Mr. Gardner was disassociating from Common Cause, but was too busy to work with the College.[52] Mr. Wood also declined.

Hanlon had difficulty finding a chairman for the proposed lay advisory board, and as time progressed the Regents began to cool on the idea.[17] The subject was raised again five years later as a proposal for lay representation on the Board of Regents.[7] They discussed having lay representation either on the Board or as lay advisors, but decided not to pursue it.[22] Ignoring the recommendation of Dr. Cooper and the enthusiasm of major business leaders for the concept undoubtedly had consequences for the College in the long term. For 100 years the Regents have been unwilling to share governance of the College with anyone but surgeons.

Remarkably, Hanlon addressed all the issues laid out for the new Director, as then unnamed, at the Regent's planning conference in January 1969. He addressed surgical education and training, the need for representation in Washington, the problems with surgical specialties, and the international role of the College.

Hanlon had brought the College into the mainstream of what was happening to health care and the profession. Early in his tenure, because of the Regents' aversion to establishing a Washington office and because the College had lost its voice in graduate medical education, he had to work through other organizations. To be effective, he had to become a leader in those organizations. He did so by hard work and thorough preparation.

Throughout his tenure he generated the respect and admiration of all those involved. In an environment populated by America's elite medical leaders, "Rollo" was a better thinker, a harder worker, better prepared, and more principled than most. He met the challenges of his tenure with an excellent sense for the most efficacious strategic directions. But the College's biggest challenges were yet to come, for the long arm of the federal government was reaching into the pockets of physicians and surgeons, and they did not like it.

REFERENCES

1. Hanlon, C., *Personal interview. March 22, 1977.* 1977, Archives of the American College of Surgeons: Chicago.
2. *Minutes of the meeting of the Board of Regents of October 9-11, 1970.* 1970, Archives of the American College of Surgeons: Chicago.
3. *Statement on Priciples. American College of Surgeons.* 2011.
4. Stephenson, G., *Activities of the American College of Surgeons - Relations with other organizations.* 1969: Phoenix.
5. *Minutes of the meeting of the Board of Regents of October 10, 1969.* 1969, Archives of the American College of Surgeons: Chicago.
6. *Minutes of the meeting of the Board of Regents of October 24, 1980.* 1980, Archives of the American College of Surgeons: Chicago.
7. *Minutes of the meeting of the Board of Regents of February 4-6, 1983.* 1983, Archives of the American College of Surgeons: Chicago.
8. *Minutes of the meeting of the Board of Regents of February 4-6, 1972.* 1972, Archives of the American College of Surgeons: Chicago.
9. *Minutes of the meeting of the Board of Regents of February 2-4. 1979.* 1979, Archives of the American College of Surgeons: Chicago.
10. *Minutes of the meeting of the Board of Regents of June 12-14, 1970.* 1970, Archives of the American College of Surgeons: Chicago.
11. *Letter from William R. Drucker to Jonathan E. Rhoads, October 9, 1969.* 1969, Archives of the American College of Surgeons: Chicago.
12. *Minutes of the meeitng of the Board of Regents of June 11-13, 1971.* 1971, Archives of the American College of Surgeons: Chicago.
13. *Minutes of the meeting of the Board of Regents of October 15-17, 1971.* 1971, Archives of the American College of Surgeons: Chicago.
14. *Minutes of the meeitng of the Board of Regents of June 8-10, 1973.* 1973, Archives of the American College of Surgeons: Chicago.
15. *Minutes of the meeting of the Board of Regents of October 3-5, 1969.* 1969, Archives of the American College of Surgeons: Chicago.
16. *Minutes of the meeting of the Board of Regents of October 21, 1977.* 1977, Archives of the American College of Surgeons: Chicago.
17. *Minutes of the meeting of the Board of Regents of October 13-15, 1978.* 1978, Archives of the American College of Surgeons: Chicago.
18. *Minutes of the meeting of the Board of Regents of October 14-16, 1983.* 1983, Archives of the American College of Surgeons: Chicago.
19. *Minutes of the meeting of the Board of Regents of February 2-4, 1972.* 1972, Archives of the American College of Surgeons: Chicago.
20. *Minutes of the meeting of the Board of Regents of February 7-9, 1986.* 1986, Archives of the American College of Surgeons.: Chicago.
21. *Minutes of the meeting of the Board of Regents of June 10-13, 1982.* 1982, Archives of the American College of Surgeons: Chicago.
22. *Minutes of the meeting of the Board of Regents of June 10-12, 1983.* 1983, Archives of the American College of Surgeons: Chicago.
23. *Minutes of the meeting of the Board of Regents of February 10-13, 1977.* 1977, Archives of the American College of Surgeons: Chicago.
24. *Minutes of the meeting of the Board of Regents of June 3-5, 1977.* 1977, Archives of the American Colllege of Surgeons: Chicago.

25. *Minutes of the meeting of the Board of Regents of June 13-15, 1980.* 1980, Archives of the American College of Surgeons: Chicago.

26. *Minutes of the meeting of the Board of Regents of June 5-7, 1981.* 1981, Archives of the American College of Surgeons: Chicago.

27. *Minutes of the meeting of the Board of Regents of February 5-7, 1971.* 1971, Archives of the American College of Surgeons: Chicago.

28. *Minutes of the meeting of the Board of Regents of October 22, 1971.* 1971, Archives of the American College of Surgeons: Chicago.

29. *Minutes of the meeting of the Board of Regents of June 7-9, 1974.* 1974, Archives of the American College of Surgeons: Chicago.

30. *Minutes of the meeting of the Board of Regents of October 19-21, 1979.* 1979, Archives of the American College of Surgeons: Chicago.

31. Davis, L., *Fellowship of Surgeons. A History of the American College of Surgeons.* 1960, Chicago: American College of Surgeons.

32. *Minutes of the meeting of the Board of Regents of October 22-24, 1982.* 1982, Archives of the American College of Surgeons: Chicago.

33. *Minutes of the meeting of the Board of Regents of October 11-13, 1985.* 1985, Archives of the American College of Surgeons: Chicago.

34. *ABMS Maintenance of Certification. Ten Years Strong and Growing.* 2010: Chicago. p. 28-29.

35. *Letter from Merlin DuVal to C. Rollins Hanlon of April 4, 1972. In minutes of the meeting of the Board of Regents of June 9-11, 1972.* 1972, Archives of the American College of Surgeons: Chicago.

36. *Minutes of the meeting of the Board of Regents of October 12-14, 1973.* 1973, Archives of the American College of Surgeons: Chicago.

37. *Minutes of the meeting of the Board of Regents of June 8, 9, 1990.* 1990, Archives of the American College of Surgeons: Chicago.

38. *Minutes of the meeting of the Board of Regents of February 2-4, 1984.* 1984, Archives of the American College of Surgeons: Chicago.

39. *Minutes of the meeting of the Board of Regents of February 1-3, 1985.* 1985, Archive of the American College of Surgeons: Chicago.

40. *Minutes of the meeting of the Board of Regents of June 14, 15, 1985.* 1985, Archives of the American College of Surgeons: Chicago.

41. *Minutes of the meeting of the Board of Regents of October 17-19, 1980.* 1980, Archives of the American College of Surgeons: Chicago.

42. *Minutes of the meeting of the Board of Regents of June 9-11, 1978.* 1978, Archives of the American College of Surgeons: Chcago.

43. *Minutes of the meeting of the Board of Regents of June 8-10, 1979.* 1979, Archives of the American College of Surgeons: Chicago.

44. *Minutes of the meeting of the Board of Regents of February 5-7, 1982.* 1982, Archives of the American College of Surgeons: Chicago.

45. *Minutes of the meeting of the Board of Regents of February 6-8, 1970.* 1970, Archives of the American College of Surgeons: Chicago.

46. *Minutes of the meeting of the Board of Regents of June 9-11, 1972.* 1972, Archives of the American College of Surgeons.: Chicago.

47. Petty, R., *Political gains, grassroots problems.*, in *American Medical News.* 1980, American Medical Association: Chicago.

48. Hanlon, C., *Report of relations with the American Medical Association. In minutes of the meeting of the Board of Regents of October 17-19, 1980.* 1980, Archives of the American College of Surgeons: Chicago.

49. *Minutes of the meeting of the Board of Regents of February 1-3, 1980.* 1980, Archives of the American College of Surgeons: Chicago.

50. Hanlon, C., *The Washington Office. In Director's Memos.* 1986, Chicago: American College of Surgeons.

51. *Minutes of the meeting of the Board of Regents of June 6-8, 1975.* 1975, Archives of the American College of Surgeons: Chicago.

52. *Minutes of the meeting of the American College of Surgeons of February 3-5, 1978.* 1978, Archives of the American College of Surgeons: Chicago.

CHAPTER 18
Medicare and Physician Reimbursement Take Center Stage

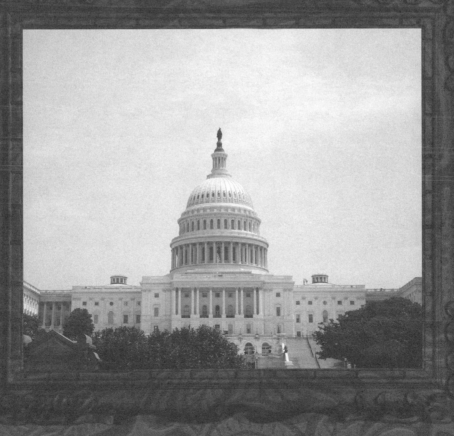

By the early 1980s, it was clear that Medicare costs were out of control. Health care expenditures were 5.9 percent of the gross domestic product (GDP) in 1965 and 10.5 percent in 1982. The medical professional societies were unsure of what to do.

In 1981, the American Society of Internal Medicine (ASIM) released a statement that the cognitive functions of physicians should be reimbursed at the same level as surgical skill functions. The suggestion was made that the increased payment for cognitive functions could be funded by a decrease in payment for procedures.[1] The surgical community was incensed. That the internists were pushing for better reimbursement was not surprising, but that they would imply that surgeons were not "cognitive" was demeaning. Surgeons made diagnoses, wrestled with decisions whether or not an operation would solve the problem, made difficult decisions during the course of an operation, and used cognitive functions extensively to care for patients postoperatively. The Regents delegated C Rollins Hanlon to speak with the president of the ASIM about this.[2] Evidently Hanlon represented the views of surgeons with temperance, for he described the visit as "a pleasant, informal, two-hour review of the subject of cognitive services in medicine."[1]

Surgeons were also sensitized by the proposal that physician payments could be incorporated prospectively into the diagnosis-related groups (DRG) system to be implemented for payments to hospitals. The American Medical Association (AMA) was advocating for an indemnity system in which physicians would be paid a fixed amount rather than a calculated proportion of their usual and customary fee. They could then bill the patient for the remainder of their fee. There were numerous proposals in Congress to pay physicians for Medicare services from a fee schedule established by the government.

Mr. James Haug, director of the department of socioeconomic affairs, told the Regents that they needed to decide which payment system they wanted, convene the specialty societies to find common ground, and ask the leadership to meet with Congressmen to advocate for the College's position.[3] Their response was to appoint a Regental committee on physician reimbursement. Later, they created an advisory council to the Regental committee, consisting of one representative from each surgical specialty.[4]

The committee met with specialty representatives and with Health Care Financing Administration (HCFA) administrator Dr. Carolyne K Davis, former dean of the School of Nursing and associate vice president for academic affairs at the University of Michigan. Any new payment system would be implemented by HCFA, and the committee wanted Dr. Davis to know that the College was willing to work with HCFA to develop a new system. They agreed that the payment system needed reform and discussed constructive approaches to modification of the system.[4]

Experts had been impressed with the work of Harvard economist William Hsiao, PhD, who proposed a payment system called the resource-based relative value scale (RBRVS). Hsiao's scheme was based on the costs of a physician's time and expense in performing a medical service.[5] In a move to provide leadership to the entire profession, Drs. Hanlon; W Gerald Austen, chairman of the department of surgery at Harvard; David C Sabiston, chairman of the department of surgery at Duke University; and David C Utz, the Mayo Clinic urologist (who later performed a prostatectomy on President Reagan), met with the leadership of the American College of Physicians (ACP) and agreed to present to their respective boards a plan to study the relative value system for payment of physicians under Medicare.[6]

In June 1984, the College and the ACP decided to submit a proposal to HCFA for a grant to develop a single relative value system for medicine and surgery. But the Federal Trade Commission (FTC) informed them that medical organizations could not develop relative value studies even if done under contract to HCFA. The FTC asserted that if the

Colleges produced a relative value scale and provided it to their Fellows, it could easily be converted to a fee schedule, which would be illegal price fixing.

Nevertheless, the AMA announced a plan to submit a proposal to HCFA to develop a relative value study. The Institute of Medicine of the National Academy of Sciences also scheduled a study to examine various approaches to setting values on physicians' services. Despite the FTC ruling, the College continued its participation in the activities of these organizations to influence them and to participate in any final negotiations with HCFA.[7]

Through the Deficit Reduction Act of 1984, the Reagan administration imposed a 15-month freeze, until September 1985, on Medicare Part B physician payments, leaving reimbursement for Medicare services at the July 1983 levels. The law also provided that physicians who accepted assignment could increase charges during the freeze, but they would not receive increased reimbursement. After the freeze, however, the increased charges would be used to update the usual and customary fee calculations.

Physicians who practiced in groups were required to accept assignment. The fees of physicians who did not accept assignment were monitored by HCFA. If their fees were knowingly and willingly increased, the government could incur assessments of up to double the charges that were in violation plus fines of up to $2,000 per violation and/or exclusion from the Medicare program for up to five years. This threat of legal action and fines angered physicians, but led most of them to participate.

The law also stated that from then on Medicare would pay 80 percent of what it deemed a reasonable charge and patients would be responsible for a deductible and a 20 percent copayment.[7] The provisions in the law stunned the medical profession. Suddenly, it seemed, the federal government decided to regulate a significant proportion physician incomes. Furthermore, physicians were intimidated into accepting assignment from Medicare beneficiaries, which many doctors believed was the first step in making themselves employees of the federal government.

HCFA set April 15, 1985, as a deadline for receiving proposals for physician reimbursement projects. Hanlon was told by HCFA administrator Dr. Carolyne Davis that HCFA wanted to fund a project that would produce a relative value study. This was a problem for the ACP/ACS joint effort because of the antitrust threat of the FTC and their estimate of three years to complete the task. Meanwhile, a project undertaken at the Boston University Health Policy Institute by a surgeon, Dr. Richard H Egdahl, piqued the interest of the American College of Surgeons (ACS) and ACP. Egdahl was developing a complexity and severity index of physician services that was based on skill, risk, judgment, time, and stress. The ACP and the ACS endorsed his proposal, which was submitted to HCFA on April 15, 1985.[8]

The College and the ACP continued to work on a system for physician reimbursement. Surgical specialty societies were asked to form relativity of services committees and identify procedures that constituted 75 percent of the services their specialties provided to Medicare patients.[9]

In August 1985, HCFA announced that it accepted the proposal submitted by William Hsiao, PhD of the Harvard University School of Public Health to develop a resource-based relative value study for physician services. The AMA was to serve as a subcontractor for the project and had agreed to provide advice, data, and nominations of medical experts. In making this selection, HCFA rejected Richard Egdahl's proposal. Hsiao's RBRVS for a medical service was based on the time involved, the complexity of selected high-volume/high-cost procedures, the opportunity cost of specialty training, and practice costs, including the cost of malpractice insurance.[10]

The College was ambivalent about participating with the AMA in developing the RBRVS through the Hsiao contract.[10] The fact that Hsiao got the contract did not necessarily mean that his system would be put into law by Congress. The ACP/ACS joint project on physician reimbursement was still active. The College leadership publicly emphasized that physician reimbursement was a major issue for the fellowship and that the College was committed to working on it vigorously in close relationship with the ACP and the surgical specialties. A list of members of the Board of Regents of the ACP was given to the College's Regents so that they could contact them and reinforce the need for the two colleges to work together.[11] The College was aligning itself with the surgical specialties and the ACP, rather than the AMA.

Because the imposition of a new physician reimbursement system for Medicare would involve legislation, the Regents decided to obtain help from a Washington, DC, consulting and lobbying firm, Health Policy Alternatives, which they retained for one year.[11] The Regent's executive committee and staff met with leaders of the ACP and agreed that the two colleges would identify procedures and study variations of fees for these procedures. They hoped to develop criteria and factors that would legitimatize differences in fees. The College also hosted a meeting with surgical specialty representatives where information was exchanged about what everybody was doing.[12]

President Ronald Reagan signed into law the Consolidated Omnibus Budget Reconciliation Act (COBRA) in April 1986. It extended, through December 1986, the freeze on Medicare payments to physicians who did not accept assignment, and it increased Medicare payments to participating physicians by one percent. The law created an 11-member Physician Payment Review Commission (PPRC) to make recommendations to Congress regarding the reimbursement of physicians under Medicare, and mandated the secretary of Health and Human Services to develop a relative value scale for Medicare reimbursement of physicians by July 1, 1987. Mayo Clinic surgeon Dr. Oliver H Beahrs, who later operated on Nancy Reagan, was appointed to the PPRC.[13]

Health Policy Alternatives, led by Mr. Glenn Markus, developed a written plan for the College to deal with legislative action on physician payment reform. The plan recommended a relative value scale in each state to account for variations in fees, practice costs, and professional liability insurance costs. The plan specified when surgical assistants could be used.[13]

Meanwhile, work on the Hsiao/AMA project to develop a resource-based relative value scale for physician services continued, and was scheduled for completion in July 1988.[13]

As if to prepare for the coming battle, James Haug and his two associates in the Washington office registered as lobbyists, signaling that in dealing with the government, the College was stepping away from its traditional reticence. The Markus plan set the agenda for the next director, Dr. Paul A Ebert. Rollo Hanlon, his job finished, was elected to the office of president elect of the College. It was a fitting honor and reward for this principled man who pulled the College off the path to irrelevance and made it once again a force for surgery and surgical patients.

⊱✳⊰

The New Director Goes to Washington

The search committee, chaired by Board Chairman Oliver Beahrs, recommended Dr. Paul A Ebert as Hanlon's successor. Ebert, who trained under Alfred Blalock at Hopkins, was chairman of surgery of the University of California at San Francisco, and was one of the country's leading pediatric cardiac surgeons. He practiced and advocated early correction of cardiac anomalies, which soon became standard practice. His impressive academic credentials belied his extraordinary accomplishments in his hometown of Columbus, Ohio, where as an undergraduate at Ohio State he was a consensus All-American baseball pitcher and also received All-American honors in basketball. He gave up a professional baseball career to attend medical school at The Ohio State University. (Figure 18.1)

Ebert quickly established himself as the surgical leader in Washington. He met with the staffs of the important congressional health-related committees and hosted meetings with the surgical specialty societies, successfully creating an informal coalition for which the College could speak. At these meetings the concept of the RBRVS and its implications for surgery were discussed. He supplied the PPRC, at their request, with data that Haug and his staff had gathered. The affable, modest, six-foot-four surgeon-athlete quickly became known in Washington as an honest, reasonable, and helpful representative of the surgical community. Ebert noted later that the

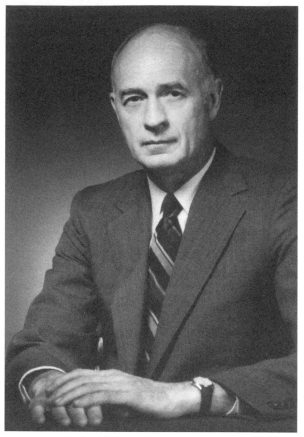

FIGURE 18.1 Dr. Paul A Ebert, Director, 1986–98.

College did not have a political action committee (PAC) and was a 501(c)(3) organization, so Washington insiders did not feel they owed anything to the College. When they needed support for legislation that would not disadvantage surgeons, Ebert supplied it. Later, he said, you could probably get assistance from that individual or group.[14]

The Sixth Omnibus Reconciliation Act of 1986 increased physician fees by 3.2 percent, but the prevailing charges for non-participating physicians was set at 96 percent of the amount allowed for participating physicians. Limits were imposed on maximum allowable charges for nonparticipating physicians, and incentives were provided for physicians to participate in Medicare. In general, physicians were being forced into Medicare, and forced into taking assignment. To control costs, it was essential to have almost all physicians in the program.[15]

In 1987, reimbursement for procedures that were deemed "overpriced" by HCFA were reduced by 2 percent. Payments to anesthesiologists for supervision of certified registered nurse anesthetists were also reduced. A fee schedule for radiology services was established. An RBRVS for pathology services was to be developed by April 1989. A host of other measures was directed toward saving money by reducing physician compensation in specific areas.[16]

With the escalating reduction of physician reimbursement and the looming AMA/Hsiao report, Ebert decided that the College needed a greater presence in Washington. A small office building at 1640 Wisconsin Avenue in Georgetown was purchased to house the five Washington office employees and to provide rental income.[17] The Washington activity of the College intensified. Ebert testified numerous times before Congress and met with the staff and individuals from several congressional and senate committees and with Paul Ginsburg PhD, executive director of the PPRC, from whom the Congress was receiving advice.[17]

≈ ✳ ≈

RBRVS Is on the Table

The long-awaited AMA/Hsiao report was released in September 1988. Ebert's testimony before the PPRC in November 1988 summarized the College's position. He said that the major conceptual objection to the AMA/Hsiao project or to any approach to set relative values based solely on so-called resource inputs is that it completely ignores the value of physician services to patients as a basis for establishing the relative value for those services. The College believed that a service of greater diagnostic or therapeutic value generally should be valued more than a less helpful service, even in cases where both involve the same amount of professional time or other so-called input costs. Patients would be expected to value superior quality services more than those of lesser quality. The Harvard project ignored each of these considerations. Ebert also pointed out the numerous assumptions, statistical estimates, and extrapolations that formed the basis of the project, as well as the small number of physicians interviewed for time and intensity, and the use of a relatively small number of services. He warned that sharp reductions in payment levels would reduce the willingness of many physicians to sign Medicare participation agreements or to accept assignment under the program.

Ebert emphasized that the volume of physician services was the key determinant of total Medicare spending. Physicians determined the frequency with which they see patients and the number and frequency of imaging and laboratory studies. The AMA/Hsiao project did not consider volume. Therefore, it would tend to encourage more services, the appropriateness of which might be suspect. Ebert believed that criteria should be developed to make judgments about the frequency, volume, and effectiveness of surgical services and evaluation and management services.[18] Here was a surgeon showing how Medicare might reduce its expenses. The PPRC and others in Washington were impressed. The College would use this goodwill in its efforts to protect the incomes of surgeons.

Many other physician groups expressed concerns about the AMA/Hsiao study, including the use of invalid data as the basis for extrapolation, the failure to take severity of illness into account, inadequate consideration of the cost of professional liability insurance, the failure to account for the quality and therapeutic value of services performed, inadequate consideration of geographical variation, and reliance on current procedural terminology (CPT) codes, which needed major revisions.[18]

In another effort to reduce costs, HCFA authorized two Preferred Provider Organization (PPO) demonstration projects. Medicare patients could enroll voluntarily in the PPO, whose physicians were required to accept assignment for all patients and to conform with the PPO's utilization review requirements.[19] The utilization review concept, in which organizations set standards for utilization of medical services such as the length of stay after operations, was implemented by hospitals to save money after HCFA began paying hospitals fixed amounts for cases that fell into diagnosis-related groups (DRGs). The shorter the hospital stay, the more money the hospital made.

At their meeting in February 1989, the Regents approved a Medicare payment reform plan that had been developed in consultation with the surgical specialty societies and

Health Policy Alternatives. The plan consisted of four elements: An increased emphasis on the development, dissemination, and application of practice guidelines; a national expenditure target for surgical services meant to control the volume of those services; a blended fee schedule with improved measurements of the supply-side or resource cost inputs, and important demand-side considerations; and financial protections for Medicare beneficiaries through fundamental changes in the Medicare assignment program. The fee schedule would be effective in 1991 and the volume targets in 1994.[20]

Dr. Ebert, several Regents, College staff, and their consultants met with key members of Congress and their staffs as well as HCFA, PPRC and other relevant groups to discuss the plan.

They also explained it at several meetings with specialty societies.[20]

Ebert announced the plan at a press conference in Washington on February 7. On the next day Dr. W Gerald Austen, Vice Chairman of the Board of Regents, advocated for the College's plan before the PPRC, with Ebert at his side. Between February 7 and June 8, 1989, Ebert made 19 trips to Washington for meetings with officials, staff of committees, or testimony advocating for the plan.[20] (Figure 18.2)

The separate volume performance standards for surgery were controversial. The AMA opposed the College's plan and sent a critique to all medical and surgical specialty societies. The AMA's House of Delegates went on record as favoring the AMA/Hsiao RBRVS method for establishing a Medicare fee schedule.

President Reagan's 1990 budget proposed significant reductions in Medicare payment levels for surgical services. It also proposed a three-year update policy under which there would be no Medicare economic index increase in prevailing charges for non-primary care services in 1990, and only a 1 percent increase in both 1991 and 1992. The reduction in physician reimbursement was continuing unabated.

Cost was not the only concern of the government. HCFA's annual 1987 Medicare hospital mortality data showed that 3.2 percent, or 188, of the nation's nearly 6,000 short term, acute care hospitals had mortality rates exceeding the expected range. This was an increase in mortality rates over the 1986 values. Quality of care was becoming a major issue for the public and for payers. In response, HCFA authorized professional standards review organizations to deny Medicare payments to hospitals and to physicians that delivered substandard hospital inpatient care.[20]

Yielding to the recommendations of the PPRC,[20] Congress passed the Omnibus Reconciliation Act of 1989 (OBRA 1989), which established a Medicare fee schedule based on a RBRVS, to be implemented over five years, beginning in 1992. The relative value was to include a geographically-adjusted estimate of the work required to provide the service,

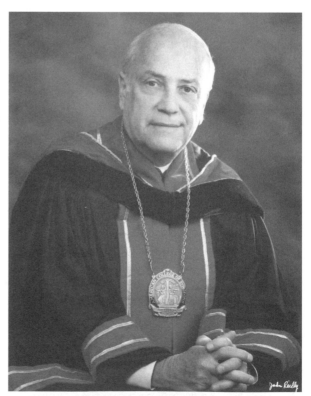

FIGURE 18.2 Dr. W Gerald Austen, ACS President, 1992–93.

measured in terms of physician time and the intensity of the work, the practice costs associated with providing the service, and professional liability expenses. A "conversion factor" was a multiplier that converted these values to the full allowable Medicare rate for a given service. Thus, the actual amount paid for a service could be adjusted by changing the conversion factor. OBRA 1989 required that the RBRVS be budget neutral, so HCFA could adjust the conversion factor annually to achieve budget neutrality.

Specialty payment differentials were eliminated in 1992. Each year Congress would establish the acceptable rate of growth for physician expenditures, called the Medicare volume performance standard (MVPS), to begin in 1992. Limits on the amount physicians could bill patients after receiving the Medicare payments (balance billing) was phased in over three years, from 125 percent in 1991 down to 115 percent in 1993 and thereafter. All physicians were required to accept assignment for Medicaid patients.

OBRA 1989 was landmark legislation for the medical profession because, for the first time in history, compensation for a significant proportion of their practices would be established by a fee schedule under complete control of the federal government. Subsequently, the only recourse for doctors to modify the fee structure was through the political process, a distasteful prospect for a profession that had been given the privilege of self-regulation since the country was founded.

To add to the problem, private insurers tended to follow the lead of Medicare in establishing their reimbursement policies. Nevertheless, given that RBRVS was inevitable, the inclusion of the volume performance standard and the requirement for physicians to accept assignment for Medicaid patients were victories for the College.

The fee schedule required a listing of every conceivable service provided by physicians. This was done using the AMA publication, *Current Procedural Terminology*, in which numerical code numbers were assigned to physician services. The accuracy and completeness of this publication were suspect, so the PPRC and the AMA teamed up to refine and expand the codes in *Current Procedural Terminology (CPT), Fourth Edition*.[21]

The rapid progression of science and technology brings a continuous stream of new procedures and services and modifications of old ones. Because of their linkage to physician compensation, the processes and procedures for revisions and modifications of the CPT manual had been issues since the Medicare fee schedule was adopted, and since private insurers established fee schedules based on the CPT. The AMA created the relative value update committee (RUC), which was an advisory committee to HCFA. The RUC, populated by representatives of the major specialties, uses physician input to recommend relative values for new or revised CPT codes.

In 1991, HCFA instituted a global surgical fee policy for Medicare. All preoperative visits after the decision to operate was made, all usual and necessary intraoperative services, and all postoperative visits up to 90 days after the date of operation were included in the surgical fee. Not included in the global fee was the initial evaluation or consultation by the surgeon to determine the need for operation.[22] Most surgeons had voluntarily used the global fee concept so the College did not protest.

The Medicare fee schedule was to take effect on January 1, 1992 and would be phased in completely by 1996. Ebert was successful in persuading HCFA to establish a separate MVPS for surgery, effective in 1993. He pointed out to Dr. Gail Wilensky, head of HCFA, that if the data were available, the College could keep surgeons from exceeding the MVPS and therefore save HCFA money. The purpose of the MVPS was to incentivize physicians to resist increasing the volume of services they provide. If the volume increased, the conversion factor would be decreased to maintain budget neutrality, and physician payments would decrease; if the volume stayed under the MVPS, the conversion factor would be increased, and physician payments would increase. Ebert had confidence that ethically grounded surgeons would not begin to perform unnecessary operations in order to increase their incomes under Medicare. Staff from HCFA met with staff of the College on numerous occasions thereafter to work on this. The College also hosted a meeting of surgical specialty society representatives to discuss the fee schedule.

Ebert and the College staff proposed that HCFA supply the College with data on surgical volume performance. The College would then make it available to surgical specialty organizations and to the College's chapters, which would establish volume assessment and review committees. The College also agreed to respond to specific requests from HCFA to carry out focused studies of volume related issues in particular regions or locales. Initially, the Medicare volume assessment plan of the College would focus on significant variations in the surgical services and procedures. The College would use peer pressure and peer education to bring about change, inasmuch as it had no authority over the activities of individual physicians.[23]

Assistants at Surgery

Obtaining a separate MVPS for surgery was not the only challenge Ebert and the College faced from HCFA. Throughout the late 1980s and early 1990s, HCFA tried to eliminate Medicare payments for physician assistants at surgery. The College staff and HCFA had an ongoing battle over which surgical procedures required a surgical assistant, so the College and the surgical specialty societies prepared lists of procedures that required assistants.[20]

The College adopted the policy that assistants at surgery should receive an amount equal to 20 percent of the fee paid to the primary surgeon. Implementation of RBRVS resulted in lower fees for surgical services, and this reduced the payments to surgical assistants to 16 percent of the surgeon's payment. Ebert's efforts to maintain the 20 percent were unsuccessful.[24] In 1990, Medicare payments for assistants at surgery were eliminated for procedures that required an assistant less than five percent of the time. The College fought this, and in 1991, 125 procedures were removed from the payment restriction list; in 1993, 700 were removed.[25]

CPT Coding Wars

Because the Medicare fee schedule was based on codes for services in the *Current Procedural Terminology* manual, the timeliness and accuracy of the manual was critical for physicians. Ebert proposed that the College work with groups included in the MVPS for surgical services to develop relative work values for new or revised CPT codes for surgical services. After learning that the AMA/RUC process would not deal with new codes, these were submitted directly to HCFA.[26] As the result of these and other fee schedule refinements and new procedure codes that were added to the fee schedule, HCFA projected that Medicare expenditures for physician services would increase by an additional $450 million. Because the law prohibited such changes to increase or decrease total fee schedule payments by more than $20 million in a single year, HCFA implemented a 2.783 percent across-the-board reduction in all relative values for physician services.[27] Obviously, the surgical community that brought new procedures and technology forward for the benefit of patients was frustrated and angry over this government policy and action.

≈ ✳ ≈

Ebert's Plan Works

In 1993, HCFA announced that based on their performance under MVPS for 1991, procedures performed by surgeons would be subject to a conversion factor of $31.962, whereas the conversion factor for all other physician services will be $31.249. This meant that payment for surgical services in 1993 was about $.71 higher per relative value unit than payment for all other physician services.[27] Clearly, Ebert's and the College's strategy was working. The differentials in conversion factors between surgical services and other physicians' services for subsequent years were as follows:

1993: $31.926 (Surgical); $31.249 (Nonsurgical)
1994: $35.158 (Surgical); $32.905 (Nonsurgical); $33.718 (Primary Care)
1995: $39.447 (Surgical); $34.616 (Nonsurgical); $36.382 (Primary Care)
1996: $40.7986 (Surgical); $34.6296 (Nonsurgical); $35.4173 (Primary Care)
1997: $40.9603 (Surgical); $33.8454 (Nonsurgical); $35.7671 (Primary Care)
1998: $36.6873

Surgeons fared better than other physicians through 1997, when the AMA and the ASIM advocated for a single update for all physicians. Secretary of Health and Human Services (HHS) Louis Sullivan and the PPRC agreed, and Congress established a single conversion factor for all physicians in the Balanced Budget Act of 1997. The single fee schedule conversion factor of $36.69 resulted in a 10.5 percent reduction in Medicare payments for all surgical services beginning on January 1, 1998.[28]

In 1998, Congress replaced the RBRVS with sustainable growth rate (SGR) methodology. The SGR was a budgetary control device. A sustainable growth rate was set by the secretary of HHS, who took into account estimates of the weighted average percentage increase in fees for all physicians services in the fiscal year involved, the percentage change in the number of individuals enrolled in Medicare, the projected percentage growth in real domestic product per capita, and the percentage change in expenditures for all physician services in the coming fiscal year that was expected to result from changes in law or regulations.

If the increase in spending for physician services exceeded the 1.5 percent sustainable growth rate for, say, 1998, the conversion factor established in calendar year 1999 was reduced by the percentage equal to the amount of that excess spending. Conversely, if the spending remained below the 1.5 percent sustainable growth rate, the conversion factor update in 1999 was increased by a corresponding bonus amount. Unlike the Medicare volume performance standards, the sustainable growth rate system was a cumulative one, where the rate of allowable expenditure growth was always calculated back to April 1, 1997. As a result, any excess in actual spending growth would continue to affect how relative performance is measured and is compensated for in the succeeding year by a negative rate of growth.[28]

Under SGR, the conversion factor has declined, and the cumulative effects have led to draconian cuts in physician reimbursement under Medicare. Physician pressure, and the fear that doctors will no longer accept Medicare patients led Congress to pass legislation that suspended the cuts for various periods of time, but repeal of the SGR methodology remained a goal of organized medicine throughout the remainder of the College's first century.

REFERENCES

1. Hanlon, C., *Is there cognition before operation? In The American College of Surgeons. 1970-1986. Directors Memos.* 1986, Chicago: American College of Surgeons.

2. Davis, L., *Fellowship of Surgeons. A History of the American College of Surgeons.* 1960, Chicago: American College of Surgeons.

3. *Minutes of the meeting of the Board of Regents of October 21, 1983.* 1983, Archives of the American College of Surgeons: Chicago.

4. *Minutes of the meeting of the Board of Regents of June 8-10, 1984.* 1984, Archives of the American College of Surgeons: Chicago.

5. Hsiao WC, S., WB, *Toward developing a relative value scale for medical and surgical services.* Health Care Financial Review, 1979(Fall, 1979): p. 23-38.

6. *Minutes of the meeting of the Board of Regents of February 2-4, 1984.* 1984, Archives of the American College of Surgeons: Chicago.

7. *Minutes of the meeting of the Board of Regents of October 19-21, 1984.* 1984, Archives of the American College of Surgeons: Chicago.

8. *Minutes of the meeting of the Board of Regents of June 14, 15, 1985.* 1985, Archives of the American College of Surgeons: Chicago.

9. *Minutes of the meeting of the Board of Regents of February 1-3, 1985.* 1985, Archive of the American College of Surgeons: Chicago.

10. *Minutes of the meeting of the Board of Regents of October 11-13, 1985.* 1985, Archives of the American College of Surgeons: Chicago.

11. *Minutes of the meeting of the Board of Regents of October 18, 1985.* 1985, Archives of the American College of Surgeons: Chicago.

12. *Minutes of the meeting of the Board of Regents of February 7-9, 1986.* 1986, Archives of the American College of Surgeons.: Chicago.

13. *Minutes of the meeting of the Board of Regents of October 17-19, 1986.* 1986, Archives of the American College of Surgeons: Chicago.

14. Sheldon, G., *Interview of Dr. Paul Ebert, May 23, 2008.* 2008, Archives of the American College of Surgeons: Chicago.

15. *Minutes of the meeting of the Board of Regents of February 6-8, 1987.* 1987, Archives of the American College of Surgeons: Chicago.

16. *Minutes of the meeting of the Board of Regents of February 5, 6, 1988.* 1988, Archives of the American College of Surgeons: Chicago.

17. *Minutes of the meeting of the Board of Regents of June 10, 11, 1988.* 1988, Archives of the American College of Surgeons: Chicago.

18. *Minutes of the meeting of the Board of Regents of February 3, 4, 1989.* 1989, Archives of the American College of Surgeons: Chicago.

19. *Minutes of the meeting of the Board of Regents of October 21-23, 1988.* 1988, Archives of the American College of Surgeons: Chicago.

20. *Minutes of the meeting of the Board of Regents of June 9, 10, 1989.* 1989, Archives of the American College of Surgeons: Chicago.

21. *Minutes of the meeting of the Board of Regents of February 2, 3, 1990.* 1990, Archives of the American College of Surgeons: Chicago.

22. *Minutes of the meeting of the Board of Regents of February 2, 1991.* 1991, Archives of the American College of Surgeons: Chicago.

23. *Minutes of the meeting of the Board of Regents of October 18-20, 1991.* 1991, Archives of the American College of Surgeons: Chicago.

24. *Minutes of the meeting of the Board of Regents of October 9-11, 1992.* 1992, Archives of the American College of Surgeons: Chicago.

25. *Minutes of the meeting of the Board of Regents of June 10, 11, 1994.* 1994, Archives of the American College of Surgeons: Chicago.

26. *Minutes of the meeting of the Board of Regents of June 12, 13, 1992.* 1992, Archives of the American College of Surgeons: Chicago.

27. *Minutes of the meeting of the Board of Regents of February 5, 6, 1993.* 1993, Archives of the American College of Surgeons: Chicago.

28. *Minutes of the meeting of the Board of Regents of February 6, 7, 1998.* 1998, Archives of the American College of Surgeons: Chicago.

CHAPTER 19
College Activities Intensify

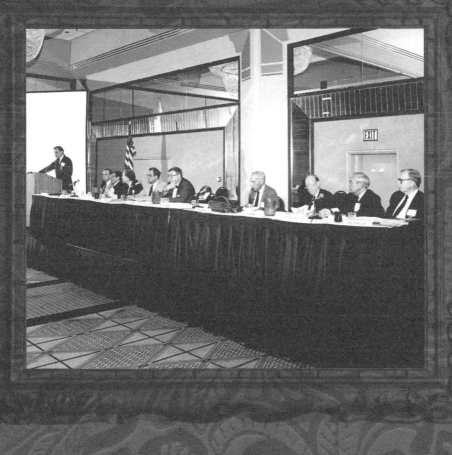

Board of Governors committee chairs giving reports, 1989

When Paul Ebert took over the directorship in 1986, the College was stable and in very good condition. The number of dues paying Fellows in 1990 was 37,374, increasing to 38,819 in 1994. This reflected a gradual upward trend throughout the entire history of the College.[1] The average age of retirement at this time, from the College, was 62.7 years.[2] A survey of College chapters revealed that they were healthy as well. The average chapter membership in 1991 was 596, up from 453 in 1988. The average age of the chapters' elected officers was a surprisingly young 46.2 years, reflecting the influence of young surgeons committees that most chapters had established, following the lead of the College itself.

There had been spectacular growth in the College finances. Total assets grew from $2.3 million in 1942 to $105 million in 1992. More importantly, the endowment fund grew from $932,000 in 1942 to $81 million in 1992. A portion of the interest earned by this fund was used for scholarships and operations, relieving pressure on dues. Nevertheless there was a steady increase in annual dues to $365 in 1990. Mr. Robert G Happ, the controller, retired in 1989 and was replaced by Mr. John Brodson, whose detailed financial reports enabled the Regents to improve their fiduciary oversight.[3]

A development committee was organized in 1988 with Dr. Robert E Hermann, chief of general surgery at the Cleveland Clinic, as chair. They created the Fellows Leadership Society to which donors gained membership if their cumulative contributions were $10,000 or more.[4] Later, the Distinguished Philanthropist Award was established for donors who make exceptional gifts.[3] The first was Dr. Earl H Mayne, who established a trust in 1944 that matured to $1.0 million when it was turned over to the College in 1994. This was the first major gift to the College in its entire history.[5] From 1989 through 1995 the contributions to the College, mostly from Fellows, totaled $9.2 million and averaged $1.3 million annually.[6-8]

The Governors Become a Force

Rollo Hanlon's clarification of the duties of Governors and their subsequent annual reports to the Regents, listing the concerns of the fellowship, developed into an invaluable resource for the College. During Ebert's directorship the main concerns of the Fellows were economic, reflecting the deep involvement of the government in the financing of health care and, more specifically, the reimbursement of physicians for services to Medicare beneficiaries. Private insurers followed the government's lead, especially in the reduction of payments to doctors. Controlling payments to physicians enabled insurers to swell their profits. Given the declining reimbursement per unit of activity, most physicians eliminated waste in their expenses and increased their productivity, seeing more patients in shorter periods of time. The phrase, "working harder and making less," was heard frequently at gatherings of doctors.

Not surprisingly, the main concerns of Fellows, as reported by the Governors during Ebert's tenure, were reimbursement issues, Medicare, professional liability, the impact of alternate delivery systems (managed care, HMOs, PPOs), and payment for assistants at surgery.[9-11] These issues led the Governors' committee on socioeconomic issues to recommend the formation of a College political action committee, but after discussion the Governors rejected it by a two-thirds vote.[12]

The Governors dealt with issues raised by the public. Concern about the HIV/AIDS epidemic led many to demand mandatory testing of health care workers, especially surgeons, who had contact with blood and other body fluids of infected patients. Some surgeons wanted all patients to be tested before operation. The Governors developed a statement on the surgeon and HIV infection that provided background indicating that transmission of HIV between doctor and patient was essentially non-existent and could be completely avoided by the highest standards of infection control. The statement strongly encouraged surgeons to continue to care for HIV-infected patients and to assume the same ethical obligations to them as to other patients.[9] This information, widely circulated, dispelled the fear of surgeons and patients alike, and spurred the use of strict infection control procedures in hospitals throughout the country.

Because transmission of hepatitis from patient to surgeon was also a concern, the Governors prepared a statement on hepatitis that recommended strict infection control procedures throughout health care facilities. The College cosponsored a scientific meeting with the Centers for Disease Control that focused on the evaluation of surgical techniques and devices to minimize the transmission of blood-borne pathogens in the operating room. Later, immunization for hepatitis B became available, and is now required for most health care workers; a vaccine for hepatitis C, however, has not been developed.[13]

Eventually health care facilities were required to meet standards of the Occupational Safety and Health Administration (OSHA) that were designed to protect workers from exposure to viruses causing hepatitis B and AIDS. Standards for gloves and gowns were set forth, masks and eye protectors were required, and sharp, disposable items had to be placed in puncture resistant containers for disposal.[14] These measures greatly reduced the incidence of body fluid contacts and inadvertent needle sticks among health care workers.

A few surgeons were performing procedures in their offices with insufficient personnel and equipment for unexpected complications or emergencies. Concerned about this, the Board of Governors developed a publication called *Guidelines for Optimal Office-Based Surgery*, designed to keep patients safe.

Surgeons and residents were susceptible to the same issues that caused drug and alcohol abuse in the general population. Recognizing this, the Governors produced an educational video dealing with substance abuse by surgeons for distribution to the directors of residency programs in surgery and the surgical specialties, and to the chiefs of surgery at all hospitals.[15]

Through their committees and their deliberations the Governors had become a resource for the College dealing with the wide range of issues that confronted surgeons in daily practice. The dissemination of this information to the entire fellowship had a salutary effect on patient care. The Governors also provided, and continue to provide, information about the real world of surgical practice to the Regents and the College staff, a function of enduring value to the College, and more importantly, to surgical patients.

≈≈✦≈≈

SG&O Becomes *JACS*

Franklin Martin, the founder and owner of the College journal *Surgery, Gynecology, and Obstetrics*, which preceded the formation of the American College of Surgeons (ACS), willed the ownership of the journal to the College. Soon after Martin's death in 1935 the College created the Franklin H Martin Memorial Foundation to own and operate it.

The members of the Foundation were the Regents of the College, and its seven directors were College officials. For several years before 1992 the gross advertising income of the Foundation exceeded the income from subscriptions, creating the concern that the Internal Revenue Service could revoke its not-for-profit tax exemption. Adding the $1.0 million of advertising revenue to the income from operations of the College, however, would not threaten the tax exempt status of the College because the advertising revenue was a very small portion of its total revenue. Accordingly, in 1992 the Regents dissolved the Foundation and moved the operations of the *Journal* into the College.[16]

After Dr. G Thomas Shires, former chair of the Board of Regents and former president of the College, had served 11 years as the editor of *Surgery, Gynecology, and Obstetrics*, Dr. Samuel A Wells, Jr., chair of surgery at Washington University in St. Louis, was appointed editor in January 1994.[5] Simultaneously, the name of the journal was changed to the *Journal of the American College of Surgeons* to more accurately reflect its ownership and its primary audience. In 1998, the management and printing of the *Journal* was contracted to Elsevier, but the College retained ownership and complete editorial control.[17]

❧ ✳ ❧

ACOSOG Is Formed

Near the end of his term Hanlon appointed Dr. David P Winchester, chair of the department of surgery at Evanston Hospital and professor at Northwestern, as part-time medical director of the College cancer department. In 1992, he reported that the Cancer Commission, established in 1922, continued to pursue its goals through the standard-setting and educational activities of its subcommittees, which were approvals and special issues, cancer liaison, education, patient care and research, cancer management course, and the executive committee. As of 1992, there were 91 members of the commission; 62 were College Fellows and 29 were representatives of affiliated professional organizations. The committee on approvals oversaw the survey and approval process for cancer programs. There were 1,245 approved programs and another 1,300 programs working toward achieving approval. Consultants and surveyors completed 431 surveys of cancer programs in 1991. The cancer liaison committee was guiding the activities of more than 2,000 volunteer cancer liaison physicians who provided local leadership.[18]

Winchester moved the statistical support for patient care studies and the collation and analysis of data from the Roswell Park Memorial Institute in Buffalo, New York, to the Community Oncology and Rehabilitation Branch of the National Cancer Institute, under its chief, Dr. Charles R Smart, who was a former director of the College's cancer department. His organization agreed to keypunch and analyze data and assist the patient care and research committee in preparing manuscripts, with College investigators as the primary authors. There was no charge for this service. This was a very satisfactory interim step toward the long-term goal of bringing the entire database and its management in-house.[19]

Winchester engaged the American College of Radiology, the Society of Surgical Oncology (SSO), and the American Cancer Society to develop standards for breast conservation therapy.[9] Later, guidelines for the vexing problem of the diagnosis and management of ductal carcinoma in-situ of the breast were released for clinical use.[20]

Stereotactic breast biopsy had become available and the College was concerned that general surgeons would not be able to perform breast biopsy because the state of the art equipment was located in radiology departments. Through Winchester's work, the College established a joint accreditation program for stereotactic biopsy with the American College of Radiology.[11, 17]

Winchester also reported on the National Cancer Data Base, which was started in 1989 by the Commission on Cancer of the College and the American Cancer Society. The purposes of the database were to assess cancer patient care on a national, regional, state, and local hospital basis and enhance hospital cancer programs throughout the United States. Each contributing hospital would receive a report on patterns of care for their institution. They also would be able compare their tumor-staging practices with other institutions.[9]

In 1988, the Conjoint Council on Surgical Research recommended that the College serve as a coordinating center for clinical trials.[4] Winchester had an outside firm perform a study on surgeons' attitudes about clinical trials. A majority thought that the College should become more involved with clinical trials, and about half the respondents had patients in clinical trials or were participating in clinical trials in one way or another.[3] Winchester explored the possibility of obtaining a planning grant from the National Cancer Institute (NCI) for College-directed clinical trials.[1] Dr. Samuel Broder, Director of the NCI, was ecstatic about this. He noted the paucity of surgical trials and the great need for them. Many surgical procedures for cancer and adjuvant chemotherapy had been selected empirically, and the long term results of different procedures for the same disease had not been compared in a scientific manner. He noted the almost unlimited supply of cancer patients cared for by Fellows of the College.

Subsequently, a group of surgical oncologists, chaired by Dr. Samuel A Wells, chairman of surgery at Washington University in St. Louis, planned for the College involvement in clinical trials. Wells, the immediate past president of the SSO, involved this organization in planning also. Soon thereafter, the College was awarded a $50,000 planning grant by the NCI and the decision was made to organize the American College of Surgeons Oncology Group (ACOSOG).

In 1996, Wells submitted a grant to develop a clinical trials organization, including the infrastructure necessary to conduct trials on a large scale, and to plan clinical trials for breast, colon, and prostate cancers.[12] After a site visit, the grant was funded in 1998, and ACOSOG was established at the College offices in Chicago.[17] This was a singular event in the history of the College, which never before had been directly involved in research. It also would become a challenge for the College's leaders.

⋙ ✳ ⋘

Surgical Research and the Research Committee

In 1985, toward the end of the Hanlon era, Dr. Hiram Polk, the popular chair of surgery at the University of Louisville, proposed that the College, together with the American Surgical Association, the Society of University Surgeons, and the Society of Surgical Chairmen, and later the Association for Academic Surgery, investigate the success and failure of surgeons in obtaining grants from the National Institutes of Health (NIH).[21] Dr. William Longmire was asked to organize and chair a group to work on this, later named the Conjoint Council on Surgical Research. He arranged for the College to maintain the secretariat and proceeded to obtain data from the National Institutes of Health.[22]

The Council gathered extensive data on grants, grant submissions, and success on grants by surgeons. Compared with other fields of medicine, surgery was found wanting. The Council noted that one of the greatest deficiencies in surgery was the lack of adequately trained investigators. Representatives of the Conjoint Council met with the director of the NIH, Dr. James Wynngarden. At his request, the Council developed a model academic surgical research training program, which was submitted to Dr. Wynngarden's office.[23] Subsequently, the NIH used this to develop training grants. The Joint Council encouraged specific surgery departments to apply, and within a year four of five submitted training grant applications were funded.[19]

The Conjoint Council activities were assumed by a new standing committee of the College, the research committee, in 1988.[14] It was staffed by Dr. Olga Jonasson, who initiated the biennial surgical investigators conference, where the intricacies of writing successful grant applications were taught. Later, a clinical trials methods course and an outcomes research course were added. The research committee also sponsored courses and sessions designed to help surgical investigators at the Clinical Congress. Although the number and quality of NIH applications have increased, they have not increased nearly as much as applications from non-surgeons, so the percentage of funded surgical grants has declined relative to other funded grants. Although the percentage of surgical grants funded is about the same as for non-surgical grants, the problem is that not enough surgeons are submitting applications.[24]

The National Trauma Registry Is Founded

The Committee on Trauma proposed the development of a national trauma database and analysis system, later called the National Trauma Registry. This was a computer program into which hospitals would enter data on their trauma patients. The database would be used to determine national trends, and hospitals could compare their work with the work of other hospitals. This project, approved by the Regents, would be a major step for the improvement of the care of trauma patients.[25] The registry was marketed to Level I and II Trauma Centers.[9]

This and other Committee on Trauma projects designed to improve the care of trauma patients were the results of the distinguished trauma surgeons who chaired the committee during the turn of the century, including Drs. Donald Trunkey, Erwin Thal, A Brent Eastman, John Weigelt, David Hoyt, J Wayne Meredith, John Fildes, and Michael Rotondo.

The Plight of General Surgeons

During the 1970s and 1980s general surgeons developed an insidious discontent with their standing in the medical profession and among the public. In the College's early years, almost all operations were performed by general surgeons, those broadly based specialists who could perform most of the existing procedures. There were early exceptions, of course, such as ophthalmology and otolaryngology. Specialization within surgery involved splitting off segments of the original general surgeons' armamentarium, such as orthopaedic, urologic, cardiothoracic, and neurosurgical procedures.

By the second half of the 20th century, general surgeons were left with surgery of the abdomen, the vascular system, the breast, the endocrine glands, pediatric surgery, and trauma surgery. But then, general surgery continued to fragment, with vascular surgery achieving its own training programs and pushing for separate board certification. Colorectal surgeons began to claim better results than general surgeons who performed colon and rectal surgery.

Gastroenterologists were performing procedures through endoscopes that previously required procedures by general surgeons, such as the removal of colon polyps. Transplantation required additional training beyond the general surgery residency. Interventional radiologists, guided by imaging equipment, were able to drain abdominal abscesses using catheters inserted through the skin, eliminating "open" operations. As the scope of their specialty shrank, general surgeons wondered if they were headed for extinction. Would they lose their source of livelihood?

Another vexing problem was the poor reimbursement of general surgeons relative to the other specialties of surgery, the result of a quirk in the development of the Medicare fee schedule, during which HCFA designated inguinal herniorraphy, a relatively simple procedure and one that was valued very low for reimbursement, as the reference procedure for many other general surgery procedures.[18] This established the value of many complex general surgery procedures below the value of relatively simple procedures in the other surgical specialties. The incomes of general surgeons were the lowest of the surgical specialties.

General surgeons, the core of the College, began to be solicited by a new organization, the American Society of General Surgeons (ASGS), for membership.[7] The Society asserted that it was the advocate and voice for all general surgeons. This caused general surgeons to question how aggressive the College had been in speaking and advocating for general surgery, and soon many general surgeons became disenchanted with the College. There was concern that the College was not doing much to improve reimbursement for general surgeons or to prevent the fragmentation of general surgery.

Dr. George E Block, the likeable and straight-talking chief of general surgery at the University of Chicago, was chairman of the advisory council for surgery; he outlined the problems of general surgeons to the Regents in no uncertain terms.[25] Subsequently the Executive Committee recognized and reaffirmed that the College was the main representative of general surgery,[3] but this did little to appease general surgeons.

A meeting of representatives of the American Board of Surgery, the Association of Program Directors in Surgery, the Residency Review Committee for Surgery (RRC-s), and the Surgery Advisory Council was held to discuss methods to identify solutions to strengthen general surgery.[26] The Board of Governors also studied the issue, concluding that poor reimbursement and the turf issues were the major problems.[27]

At the 1990 spring meeting, the General Surgery Advisory Council arranged a program entitled "The role of general surgery within the College and other organizations." Speakers were representatives of the regulatory and certifying bodies and the societies within general surgery. A panel discussion on "Where is general surgery going in the 1990s?" included the image of the general surgeon, physician reimbursement and CPT codes, credentials and franchises in general surgery, and the role of the ACS in relation to general surgery. During the long discussion period many general surgeons took the opportunity to vent their frustrations.[28]

Soon thereafter, having heard enough, the College began to act. The Advisory Council for Surgery was expanded by adding five practicing general surgeons. Fortunately, 91 percent of the general surgery CPT codes for which the College recommended changes and additions were accepted by HCFA.[29] Thereafter the CPT/Relative Value Update Committee (RUC) developed recommendations for relative work values for these new and revised general surgery CPT codes.

The College organized regional workshops throughout the country for general surgeons and their office staffs about the intricacies of coding that improved reimbursement. A coding consultation hotline was established for all surgeons at the College with coding experts available to assist office staff in coding issues, which were often complex and confusing. Previously, many surgeons failed to take advantage of codes simply because the process was difficult and time consuming.[27]

A newsletter in the form of a newspaper for general surgeons was initiated.[5] The College department of communications also produced a brochure entitled, "What does the College do for you?" Although it was sent to all surgeons, it had particular relevance to general surgeons.[18] The College wanted general surgeons to know that it was paying attention to them.

In 1992, the Advisory Council for Surgery, noting that ASGS was active in the AMA, requested that the Regents take action to resume its seat in the AMA House of Delegates.[18] A majority of the Governors also voted in favor of this.[30] The Board of Regents agreed, and appointed Dr. George Block to fill the seat.

These measures improved the contentment of general surgeons with the College, but it was an unforeseen development that gave these specialists new status with the profession and the public. Between 1985 and 1990 surgeons in Europe had been experimenting with the use of rigid scopes, tiny video cameras, and special instruments to remove the gallbladder through a few 1cm incisions in the abdomen. By the early 1990s laparoscopic cholecystectomy was sweeping the United States. General surgeons hustled to get into short courses run by a few surgeons; these cost thousands of dollars. The teachers, most of whom were not faculty from universities, had learned the technique in Europe and worked with instrument manufacturers to expand and improve the armamentarium. Although the availability of instruments and equipment was at a premium, courses were set up at hospitals and medical centers using pigs, and the saying went, "a pig over the weekend and a patient on Monday."

Almost every first laparoscopic cholecystectomy in a community was the subject of a news story, and soon patients were demanding the procedure that almost eliminated hospitalization and pain. Within a decade many standard abdominal procedures were performed laparoscopically. Laparoscopic surgery fellowships began to proliferate for general surgeons who had completed their residencies. General surgeons were lauded by the profession and the public for these truly remarkable achievements, and they no longer believed that general surgery was the forgotten specialty.

Managing the Technology Tsunami

The College staff was besieged with requests from surgeons for courses on laparoscopic techniques, but the College was not equipped to develop hands-on courses using animals in an operating room environment. The best it could do was to provide didactic courses and seminars at the Clinical Congress, which were helpful, but insufficient. Surgeons needed to actually work with the new scopes and instruments, and learn how to use them in the clinical setting. Expecting that the same problem would confront the College by another technologic advance, the staff asked the Regents to create a committee on emerging surgical technology and education (CESTE).[30] CESTE was charged to assess and/or reassess the use of emerging technology with respect to appropriateness, safety, effectiveness, and outcome; to develop methods to enhance and accelerate the acquisition of new surgical skills that did not involve the use of animals; to recommend methods of surgical education and practical training; and to recommend how surgeons who use new technology may be judged. Dr. C James Carrico, chairman of the department of surgery at University of Texas-Southwestern and a future president of the College, was named chairman of the committee.[5] (Figure 19.1)

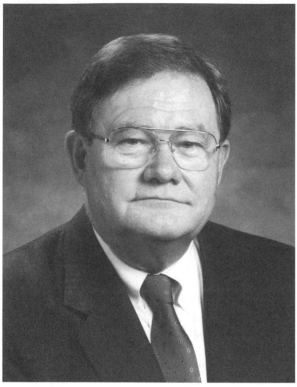

FIGURE 19.1 Dr. C James Carrico, Chairman of CESTE and Chair, Board of Regents, 1999–2000.

The committee developed a statement asserting that the development of a new technology had to be accompanied by scientific assessment of safety, general efficacy, and need. The committee also said that diffusion of technology into clinical practice required appropriate education of surgeons and evaluation of their use of the new technology. Finally, widespread application of new technologies had to be continually assessed and compared with alternate therapies to assure appropriateness and cost effectiveness through outcomes studies.[15]

CESTE wanted the College to work with companies engaged in the development of human computer simulation programs for teaching surgical techniques. The committee also recommended that the College consider establishing a program to educate surgeons in new technology at a fixed learning site or a traveling facility, but this proved too expensive. A hernia trial was to compare trans-abdominal pre-peritoneal repair and laparoscopic extra peritoneal repair with conventional hernia repair. The committee also issued a statement on endovascular procedures in the aorta and major arteries.[31]

Responding to the committee, a hands-on course using work stations with ultrasonographic and stereotactic equipment, live models, and phantom breast moulages were used at the 1992 spring meeting to develop image-guided breast biopsy skills.[12] Later, the committee sponsored an exhibit at the 1997 Clinical Congress that demonstrated computer assisted surgical simulation.[20]

The pervasive influence of the CESTE was exemplified by the program for the 1997 Clinical Congress, which included "The role of the general surgeon in image guided breast biopsy;" "Intraoperative abdominal ultrasound;" "New surgical techniques: what's proven, what's not;" "Endovascular stents: the role of the surgeon;" and "Virtual reality: where do we stand?"[32]

Young Surgeons Become a Force

Begun during Hanlon's directorship, the committee on young surgeons was growing in its activities and influence. Because their representatives attended Regents' meetings, which included lunches and dinners where the participants got to know one another, young surgeons were increasingly appointed to College committees. For example, committee on young surgeons representative Dr. Irving Kron, later to be the chairman of surgery at the University of Virginia, was appointed to the committee on ethics.[7]

In 1993, the committee on young surgeons issued a white paper, recommending appointment of young surgeons to each of the Advisory Councils and many other important committees of the College. They also recommended regional workshops on practice management, a study on why only 32 percent of surgeons achieving American Board of Surgery certification later became Fellows of the College, and several initiatives to further the interest of medical students in surgery.[29] Almost all these recommendations were approved by the Regents and eventually implemented by the College.

The young surgeons' committee met in Washington, DC, in 1994 and visited congressional representatives under the direction of the Washington staff of the ACS.[1] This began their intense, lasting interest in the advocacy efforts of the College, both at the chapter and central College levels.

The technologic marvel called the Internet was receiving attention all over the world and the committee on young surgeons recommended using it to promote the activities of the College and to disseminate information about the College. The Regents created an "informatics" committee, chaired by Dr. David Krusch of the University of Rochester, New York, to examine this possibility.[33] At its recommendation, an internet node was created at the College, electronic mail was begun, and staff was hired to develop an ACS homepage and web-based services.[2]

The attention to young surgeons through the young surgeons' committee was one of the Regents' most consequential decisions during the first century of the College, ranking with the appointment of young Evarts Graham to the Board of Regents and listening to him. Young surgeons, now firmly rooted in the machinery of the College, would strongly influence its decisions, and therefore its future. As the College turns 100, it fully understands that the future belongs to its younger members, and that they must have the opportunity to chart it.

Other Issues

The College had to deal with other issues during Ebert's leadership, including the restriction on work hours for residents proposed by the Accreditation Council for Graduate Medical Education (ACGME). The College objected on the basis that specific hours could not be defined for each surgical specialty and that residents needed to learn continuity of care, which practicing surgeons deliver. Nevertheless, responding to congressional pressure, the ACGME imposed restrictions on duty hours.

Under the leadership of Dr. Paul Nora, director of the professional liability program, a book, *Professional Liability/Risk Management. A Manual for Surgeons*, was mailed to all active U.S. and Canadian Fellows.[9]

When the Agency for Health Care Policy and Research, later the Agency for Research and Quality, issued its first federally sponsored clinical practice guideline in 1992 it was clear that the issue of quality in health care would be thrust on the profession.[18] The Joint Commission emphasized that hospitals should improve organizational performance through continuous monitoring of functions affecting patient outcomes and use these data to improve outcomes.[29]

The Advisory Council chairmen recommended that the College serve as a national repository for outcomes data, and that the College take a leadership role in developing computer programs for outcomes studies.[31] Specific proposals to measure outcomes from committees of the Board of Governors, however, were not approved by the Regents because of liability and cost

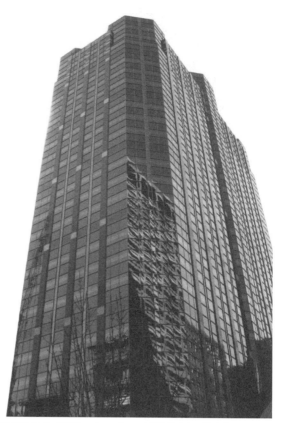

FIGURE 19.2 ACS headquarters at 633 N Saint Clair Street, Chicago.

concerns.[10, 17] The emphasis on quality and outcomes measurement had not yet reached the stage of compelling the College to act, and it put the College and its Fellows behind in this arena.

Managed care organizations had sprung up after the Clinton health care plan failed in Congress, and the College convened two groups of 100 practicing surgeons for advice. The surgeons believed that managed care could serve patients well but feared that the art of medicine was being replaced by the business of medicine. They believed that the most important issues they faced were restrictions on services to patients and loss of autonomy in decision making, which they thought eroded the quality of care. Nevertheless, they displayed a great sense of idealism and a concern for ethics.[2, 34]

Ebert's Legacy

Paul Ebert, working with the controller, Robert Happ, became concerned about the amount of money and effort required to maintain the College's buildings, which spanned the north and south sides of an entire block of Erie Street, two blocks west of the "Magnificent Mile" segment of Michigan Avenue in downtown Chicago. The former house on the Northeast corner of Erie and Rush streets had been rented to the Chez Paul restaurant. The Martin Memorial Building to the west of it housed the journal offices, and the adjacent Murphy Auditorium, in which some offices were located, was not ideal for the daily work of the College. The Nickerson Mansion, to the west of the Murphy, was leased to the RH Love Galleries.[3] This left the administration building at 55 East Erie, on the south side of Erie Street, opposite the other College properties, to house many, but not all, of the College operations, and it had become too small for the growing staff, forcing some operations into nearby rented property. This fragmentation of the staff hindered efficient operations.

When Happ retired and John Brodson was appointed controller, he and Ebert began a two-year search for another building in downtown Chicago. Fortuitously, they found an empty, new, 28-story building at 633 St. Clair, three blocks east of the College properties. Ebert and Brodson, with Regental approval, negotiated the purchase of this attractive, glass enclosed structure,

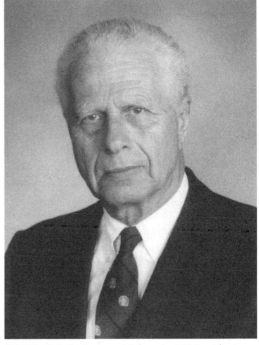

FIGURE 19.3 Dr. Seymour I Schwartz, ACS President 1997–98.

owned by two banks, for the bargain sum of $20.295 million. The College used a bond issue to build out its space on the top seven floors, leased three floors to an advertising firm, and a portion of the ground floor to the Capital Grille, an upscale restaurant. Fortunately, the Wyndham Hotel leased the remaining 16 floors and built it out without financing from the College. The income from the leases to the Wyndham Hotel and the advertising firm initially totaled $5,026,000 annually. The continuing income from the leases has underpinned the financial stability of the College.[35] (Figure 19.2)

Meanwhile, the Chez Paul restaurant building and the Martin Memorial Building were sold for $1.5 million, and the building at 55 East Erie Street was sold for $9.15 million.[12, 17] The College retained the Murphy Auditorium and the Nickerson Mansion.

Paul Ebert retired in 1998. Dr. Seymour Schwartz, Chair of the Board of Regents, chaired the search committee for his successor. (Figure 19.3) The President, Dr. David G Murray, announced the nomination, and the Board of Regents approved the appointment of Dr. Samuel A Wells, Jr as the next Director of the College, effective in June 1998.[36]

Paul Ebert died in 2008 at age 76 in California, where he had retired to be near his family. His legacy in surgery, especially the surgery of infant cardiac anomalies, is extraordinary by any standard. But Ebert's second career, directing the College during its most vulnerable period, when the federal involvement in health care threatened to marginalize all professional organizations, was probably more important. Ebert showed the College and many other organizations how to deal with the federal government. He not only obtained for surgery what rightfully belonged to surgery, but also helped the leaders of Congress, Medicare, and other agencies shape the Medicare system for the benefit of patients. He did so in plainspoken language, without regard for himself, and with simple, clear convictions of what made sense and what did not.

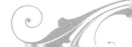

REFERENCES

1. *Minutes of the meeting of the Board of Regents of October 7-9, 1994.* 1994, Archives of the American College of Surgeons: Chicago.
2. *Minutes of the meeting of the Board of Regents of June 9, 10, 1995.* 1995, Archives of the American College of Surgeons: Chicago.
3. *Minutes of the meeting of the Board of Regents of June 9, 10, 1989.* 1989, Archives of the American College of Surgeons: Chicago.
4. *Minutes of the meeting of the Board of Regents of June 10, 11, 1988.* 1988, Archives of the American College of Surgeons: Chicago.
5. *Minutes of the meeting of the Board of Regents of June 11, 12, 1993.* 1993, Archives of the American College of Surgeons: Chicago.
6. *Minutes of the meeting of the Board of Regents of February 2, 3, 1990.* 1990, Archives of the American College of Surgeons: Chicago.
7. *Minutes of the meeting of the Board of Regents of February 7, 8, 1992.* 1992, Archives of the American College of Surgeons: Chicago.
8. Hermann, R., Thompson, JC, *The ACS development program and surgical research and education.* Bulletin of the American Colllege of Surgeons, 1993. **78**: p. 33-48.
9. *Minutes of the meeting of the Board of Regents of October 18-20, 1991.* 1991, Archives of the American College of Surgeons: Chicago.
10. *Minutes of the meeting of the Board of Regents of October 4-6, 1996.* 1996, Archives of the American College of Surgeons: Chicago.
11. *Minutes of the meeting of the Board of Regents of October 9-12, 1997.* 1997, Archives of the American College of Surgeons: Chicago.
12. *Minutes of the meeting of the American College of Surgeons of February 9, 10, 1993.* 1993, Archives of the American College of Surgeons: Chicago.
13. *American College of Surgeons. Statement on the surgeon and hepatitis.* Bulletin of the American College of Surgeons, 2004. **89**: p. 35-39.
14. *Minutes of the meeting of the Board of Regents of October 21-23, 1988.* 1988, Archives of the American College of Surgeons: Chicago.
15. *Minutes of the meeting of the Board of Regents of February 4,5, 1994.* 1994, Archives of the American College of Surgeons: Chicago.
16. *Minutes of the meeting of the Board of Regents of October 16, 1992.* 1992, Archives of the American College Surgeons: Chicago.
17. *Minutes of the meeting of the Board of Regents of February 6, 7, 1998.* 1998, Archives of the American College of Surgeons: Chicago.
18. *Minutes of the meeting of the Board of Regents of June 12, 13, 1992.* 1992, Archives of the American College of Surgeons: Chicago.
19. *Minutes of the meeting of the Board of Regents of February 5, 6, 1988.* 1988, Archives of the American College of Surgeons: Chicago.
20. *Minutes of the meeting of the Board of Regents of June 6, 7, 1997.* 1997, Archives of the American College of Surgeons: Chicago.
21. *Minutes of the meeting of the Board of Regents of February 1-3, 1985.* 1985, Archive of the American College of Surgeons: Chicago.
22. *Minutes of the meeting of the Board of Regents of June 14, 15, 1985.* 1985, Archives of the American College of Surgeons: Chicago.
23. *Minutes of the meeting of the Board of Regents of February 6-8, 1987.* 1987, Archives of the American College of Surgeons: Chicago.
24. Mann M, T.A., Birger N, Howard C, Ratcliffe MB., *National Institutes of Health funding for surgical research.* Annals of Surgery, 2008. **247**: p. 217-221.

25. *Minutes of the meeting of the Board of Regents of February 3, 4, 1989.* 1989, Archives of the American College of Surgeons: Chicago.
26. *Minutes of the meeting of the Board of Regents of October 13-15, 1989.* 1989, Archives of the American College of Surgeons: Chicago.
27. *Minutes of the meeting of the Board of Regents of October 8-10, 1993.* 1993, Archives of the American College of Surgeons: Chicago.
28. *Minutes of the meeting of the Board of Regents of February 2, 1991.* 1991, Archives of the American College of Surgeons: Chicago.
29. *Minutes of the meeting of the Board of Regents of February 5, 6, 1993.* 1993, Archives of the American College of Surgeons: Chicago.
30. *Minutes of the meeting of the Board of Regents of October 9-11, 1992.* 1992, Archives of the American College of Surgeons: Chicago.
31. *Minutes of the meeting of the Board of Regents of February 2,3, 1990.* 1990, Archives of the American College of Surgeons: Chicago.
32. *Minutes of the meeting of the Board of Regents of October 17, 1997.* 1997, Archives of the American College of Surgeons: Chicago.
33. *Minutes of the meeting of the Board of Regents of June 10, 11, 1994.* 1994, Archives of the American College of Surgeons: Chicago.
34. *Minutes of the meeting of the Board of Regents of June 7, 8, 1996.* 1996, Archives of the American College of Surgeons: Chicago.
35. *Minutes of the meeting of the Board of Regents of October 27, 1995.* 1995, Archives of the AMerican College of Surgeons: Chicago.
36. *Minutes of the meeting of the Board of Regents of October 11, 1996.* 1996, Archives of the American College of Surgeons.: Chicago.

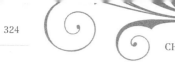

CHAPTER 20
A Difficult Time

Board of Regents October 9, 1999, San Francisco

Dr. Samuel A Wells, Jr, the new Director, was one of the most respected and admired leaders in American surgery. He was a product of Dr. David Sabiston's research-based, grueling residency program at Duke that produced many surgical leaders. Wells stayed on at Duke as a faculty member and made advances in the field of endocrine surgery. He was best known for his brilliant idea to implant a sliver of parathyroid gland tissue into the muscle of the forearm when all four glands were removed from the neck because they produced too much of the parathyroid hormone, parathormone. The implanted tissue was just enough to keep patients from suffering the ravages of hypoparathyroidism because they lacked parathormone. Wells' elegant solution left other researchers wondering why they had not thought of this simple procedure that was a lifesaver for parathyroid

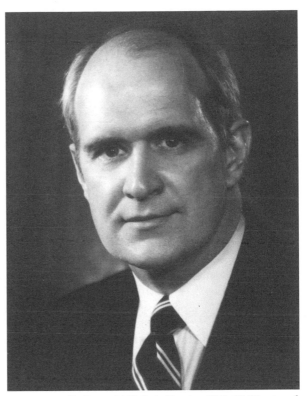

FIGURE 20.1 Dr. Samuel A Wells Jr, Director, 1998–99; Director of ACOSOG.

surgery patients. Wells went on to take the chairmanship once held by the great College leader, Dr. Evarts Graham, at Washington University in St. Louis. (Figure 20.1)

In 1996, at the request of the Regents, Wells had applied for a grant to create the infrastructure for the American College of Surgeons Oncology Group (ACOSOG). The grant was funded in 1998, so as he was beginning his new job as Director of the College he also was very busy with the recruitment of statisticians, grant managers, nurse coordinators, and a host of others necessary to initiate clinical trials, an activity entirely new to the staff of the College.

Having essentially taken on two jobs, he decided to make major changes in the management team at the College. Mr. James Haug, the director of socioeconomic affairs, had retired with Dr. Ebert, and Wells replaced him with Dr. Henry R Desmarais, a principal with Health Policy Alternatives, the Washington consulting group retained by the College.[1] Dr. Frank Padberg, the long-time director of the fellowship department and the graduate education programs, retired and was replaced by Dr. Karen Guice, a surgeon with a master's degree in public health policy who had worked on the staff of the Senate Committee on Labor. Dr. David Winchester, the part time director of the cancer department, was replaced by Dr. Monica Morrow, an equally well-respected surgical oncologist. Ms. Rosemary Clive, who managed the cancer department for many years, took early retirement.

Early in 1999, Wells created the positions of chief operating officer and chief general counsel. The creation of these positions, the arrival of new executives, and the growing number of new appointees in the ACOSOG unit were upsetting to the College staff, who had worked within a different management model.

The Work Continues

Despite the changes that concerned the College staff, they persevered. Their work and that of College committees went on. Outsourcing publication of the *Journal of the American College of Surgeons* to Elsevier turned significant losses into significant profits.[2] The finance committee brought more order to the budget process by establishing a spending rate of five percent on all operating, endowment, and certain restricted fund balances, beginning in 1999. Increasing numbers of Fellows were retiring in their mid-sixties, so the Regents lowered the limit for dues exemption from 70 to 65 years of age.[3]

Most importantly, the finance committee decided to seek the advice of individuals experienced in management of investment portfolios in large institutions to advise the committee and the Board of Regents on strategies for managing College investment portfolios.[2, 3] They engaged Cambridge Associates as investment consultants,[3] a move that brought the College into the multifaceted, sophisticated world of institutional investing, and resulted in large returns on College funds.

The graduate education committee was concerned that medical schools were not properly preparing students for training in surgery. Accordingly, they prepared and the College published and distributed 15,000 copies of *Prerequisites for Graduate Surgical Education: A Guide for Medical Students and PGY-1 Surgical Residents*.[1, 3]

A major effort to engage residents and young surgeons who had not yet applied for College fellowship was undertaken by Dr. Olga Jonasson, whose ideas resulted in several programs that engaged young surgeons. With help from the Committee on Young Surgeons, she formed the Resident and Candidate Society, later called the Resident and Associate Society. Its members had access to College activities and programs, and met during the Clinical Congress. An educational session at the Clinical Congress was devoted to their interests and needs.[2-4] This organization has been instrumental in encouraging and assisting residents during training, and in developing future leaders of the College.

The Internet-based directory of Fellows and associate Fellows was launched in January 1999. Surgeons were beginning to use computers for some business functions, and applications were becoming available to assist surgeons in their practices, such as formularies and drug interaction information. Basic and advanced courses in informatics, given at the Clinical Congress, were extremely popular.[2]

The Committee on Emerging Surgical Technology and Education (CESTE) also staffed by Dr. Jonasson, continued to bridge the education gap for surgeons trained before certain new technologies were available. For example, the committee offered a course in sentinel node biopsy, a new procedure to determine the extent of breast cancer, using telemedicine techniques. Eight developers of surgical simulation technology were available for consultation during the Clinical Congress. The breast biopsy and ultrasound courses continued to be very popular.[5]

The rapidly changing health care environment continued to create difficulties for practicing surgeons. The Clinton health plan, which had featured managed care competition, failed in Congress, but insurance companies and entrepreneurs created managed care organizations that created problems for patients and doctors alike. Managed care emerged as the primary concern of Fellows in the 1999 Governor's report.[2] Limitations placed on length of stay in the hospital and the requirement to perform many procedures in less expensive outpatient facilities led to headlines such as "Drive-through Mastectomies." Physicians were penalized for keeping patients in the hospital longer than the managed care stipulations, and a "take it or leave it" attitude prevailed in contract negotiations with doctors. The College advocated for legislation that eventually obviated some of these abuses.[5]

Responding to the Fellows who complained that the College was not working hard enough for them in the socioeconomic arena, the College organized practice management workshops throughout the country. Twenty-five workshops were presented in 1999, a huge undertaking.[6]

Dr. Wells and Dr. Desmarais held quarterly meetings with the surgical specialty societies. The discussions were almost exclusively socioeconomic, centering on Medicare reimbursement. But proposals that would increase reimbursement for one specialty often affected another specialty adversely, so it was difficult to obtain consensus around socioeconomic issues.[6]

In October 1998, Dr. Wells reported that the ACOSOG would soon begin three clinical trials. In addition, protocols for 24 trials that spanned the entire field of surgery and its specialties were in various stages of development, a remarkable achievement in just a few months.[3]

Trouble Brewing

By early 1999, the staff was greatly disturbed by the changes in management of the College. The anxiety created by change was compounded by rumors about a list of individuals who would be fired. Staff was grousing, and most senior staff believed they were unappreciated. Many talked about leaving. Most of them had worked closely with one or more Regents or officers while staffing College committees. They used these relationships to vent their frustrations to Regents at their meetings, or even by telephone. News of the unrest and the problems of employees were passed on to Board Chairman Harvey Bender and President George Sheldon. Bender and Sheldon had extensive interactions with College staff over many years, and recognized that the unrest was uncharacteristic.[7]

For the first time in the College's history, Bender convened a meeting of the College's Presidents' Advisory Committee, created in the 1930s in case the advice of wise elders was needed. Collectively, the past presidents were regarded as the wisest and most respected College resource. The issues were presented to them, and Dr. Wells was invited to speak as well. After discussion, the consensus of the President's Advisory Committee and the Executive Committee was that the College should make a change.[8]

The Regents Act

At a meeting of the Board of Regents on June 5, 1999 the Executive Committee asked for an affirmative vote to eliminate Dr. Wells' position as Director and to appoint him as Director, Center for Clinical Trials and Evidence-Based Medicine. A majority of the Regents voted in the affirmative.[7]

Subsequently, in the absence of a Director, the Executive Committee met by conference call or in person on six occasions to deal with College administrative and transitional matters. At a three-day "workshop" in late July they decided to change the title of the Director to Executive Director and to more clearly delineate his or her duties. They also agreed that the comptroller, who according to the bylaws reported exclusively to the Regents, should report to both the Regents and the Executive Director. Department heads, who would be called directors, should be hired or fired by the Executive Director with the advice and consent of the Board of Regents, whereas the comptroller should be hired or fired by the Board of Regents with the advice and consent of the Executive Director. They organized a search committee for the new Executive Director and agreed to hire an interim Director.[2] A few days later Wells agreed to assume the position of director of the Center for Clinical Trials and Evidence-based Medicine.

≈✳≈

The College Moves On

Bender then asked Dr. David L Nahrwold, the recently retired chair of surgery at Northwestern University, and a Regent, to serve as interim Director.

Nahrwold had frequent group and individual meetings with the department heads to assist and supervise them. He also met with all College employees in small groups, where they expressed their frustrations and concerns about the College. These ventings and Nahrwold's reassurances that the College leadership was committed to their well-being helped to restore morale and obviated an exodus of employees.

With the consent of the Executive Committee he hired Ms. Gay Vincent as comptroller, to replace Mr. John Brodson, whose contract had expired, and he also hired Mr. Frederick Holtzrichter as director of the development office. Nahrwold's meetings with employees convinced him that the College needed a comprehensive strategic plan. He developed a plan to carry this out, but the Executive Committee decided to delay it.

≈✳≈

A Perspective

Wells had tried to establish a different management model within the College. He could not attend to all the details of developing a multimillion dollar clinical trials operation and simultaneously manage all aspects of the College operations. He believed a chief operating officer was needed to manage the day-to-day activities of more than 200 employees, who staffed dozens of committees and had to be responsive to the needs of more than 50,000 Fellows. He hired legal counsel to provide legal advice for the clinical trials operation and other business of the College and to obviate outsourcing every legal question.

Wells' hiring of a chief operating officer and general legal counsel was appropriate, but his strategy diverged from the fairly consistent pattern of management established after the death of Franklin Martin in 1935. The Regents at that time had decided not to replace Martin; instead, they made almost all operational and strategic decisions, and the Chairman of the Board of Regents, George Crile, communicated these decisions to the senior staff. The Regents actually managed the College. Remnants of that basic model have persisted throughout the remaining history of the College. After 15 years without a Director, General Paul Hawley was hired to implement the will of the Regents. Whenever he stepped beyond that role, he was reminded of his subservience to them.

Subsequently, John Paul North, Rollo Hanlon, and Paul Ebert understood that the Regents made decisions and the Director implemented them. Because Board Chairmen rotated every one or two years, there were modest variations in this pattern that depended on the degree of involvement of the Board Chair. Most Chairs worked in partnership with the Director, but occasionally the Chair delved more deeply into managing, leading to disagreements and friction between the Board Chair and the Director, and even some members of the Board of Regents. Wells' management of the College fell outside the traditional pattern in place since 1935. The question of whether or not the College could (or should) adapt to another model of Board and management relationships remains unanswered.

⌦✳⌫

ACOSOG Survives and Flourishes

Wells' expertise and brilliance in developing ACOSOG were obvious to the leadership. They liked his idea of engaging Fellows in clinical trials, an important activity to advance the science and practice of surgery. For this reason they wanted to keep him on as the Director of the Center for Clinical Trials and Evidence-Based Medicine. Eventually, Wells became convinced that the College did not have the in-house academic and infrastructure support necessary for a large clinical trials operation, and the Regents realized that the College could not afford the necessary expenditures and space. After exploring several options, Wells elected, with the Regents' concurrence, to move himself and the ACOSOG operations to Duke University.

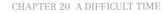

New Leadership

Dr. Bender, chair of the search committee for a new Executive Director, reported to the Regents in October 1999. The committee had interviewed almost a dozen well-qualified candidates, all of whom had spectacular credentials. The room fell silent when he announced the selection: Dr. Thomas R Russell, a colorectal surgeon in private practice who also served as chief of surgery at California Pacific Medical Center in San Francisco. Russell was completing his second term as a Regent. The Regents expected an extroverted, high-profile academic. What they got was exactly what they needed: a kind, outgoing man who listened to the fellowship and returned the College to its basic mission of fostering the ethical and competent practice of surgery for the benefit of the public. (Figure 20.2)

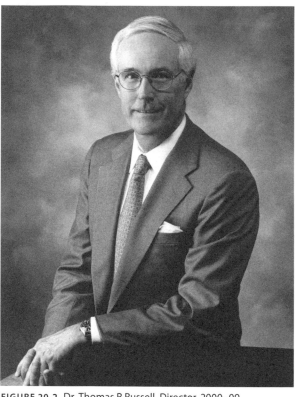

FIGURE 20.2 Dr. Thomas R Russell, Director, 2000–09.

REFERENCES

1. *Minutes of the meeting of the Board of Regents of June 5, 6, 1998.* 1998, Archives of the American College of Surgeons: Chicago.
2. *Minutes of the meeting of the Board of Regents of October 8-10, 1999.* 1999, Archives of the American College of Surgeons: Chicago.
3. *Minutes of the meeting of the Board of Regents of October 25, 1998.* 1998, Archives of the American College of Surgeons: Chicago.
4. *Minutes of the meeting of the Board of Regents of June 4, 5, 1999.* 1999, Archives of the American College of Surgeons: Chicago.
5. *Minutes of the meeting of the Board of Regents of October 23-25, 1998.* 1998, Archives of the American College of Surgeons: Chicago.
6. *Minutes of the meeting of the Board of Regents of February 5, 6, 1999.* 1999, Archives of the American College of Surgeons: Chicago.
7. *Dr. David Nahrwold personal recollection of June 5, 1999.* 1999.
8. Sheldon, G., *Historical recollections of the American College of Surgeons.*, Archives of the American College of Surgeons: Chicago.

CHAPTER 21
Emphasis on
the Fellowship

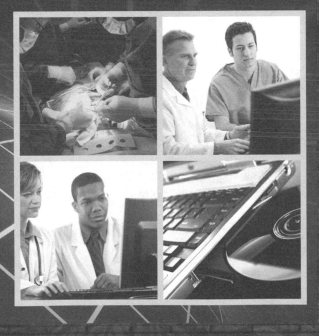

D
r. Russell found that years of program expansion and new activities without changes in organizational structure had created a difficult management problem. Thirteen directors of various departments and programs reported directly to him, leaving little time for anything else.[1] The overall direction of the American College of Surgeons (ACS) was unclear to many employees, and this was reflected in their work. Many policies needed review because they were outdated. Russell and the Regents concurred that a major strategic planning process was necessary.[2]

Russell proposed to reorganize the College into four divisions: education; research and optimal patient care; advocacy and health policy; and member services.[3] A fifth function, administrative services, supported the entire enterprise. He appointed a task force of Regents, officers, and staff for each of the four divisions, and charged them with creating a strategic plan for their respective divisions. The task forces, led by a Regent or pair of Regents, produced a vision statement, mission statement, and goals and objectives for each division. Russell's brilliant strategy ensured that the Regents, officers, and staff, would support the plans they had created; in fact, they were eager to monitor them and see progress.[4] Eventually, committees of the College were aligned with the appropriate divisions. The process also led to a new overall mission statement for the College: "The American College of Surgeons is dedicated to improving the care of the surgical patient and to safeguarding standards of care in an optimal and ethical practice environment."[4]

Within a year Russell recruited leaders for the new divisions. Dr. Paul E Collicott, a Regent who had been in private practice and was a founder of the Advanced Trauma Life Support (ATLS®) Course, replaced Dr. Karen Guice as director of the division of member services.[5] Regent Alden Harken was appointed director of the division of research and optimal patient care on a part-time basis until the position was filled permanently by Dr. R Scott Jones after he completed his term as president of the College in 2002. Dr. Olga Jonasson left the College, and Dr. Ajit Sachdeva was recruited to head the newly created division of education. Ms. Cynthia Brown, who had been a member of the Washington, DC office staff, was appointed director of the division of advocacy and health policy.[6]

This team managed the daily activities of the College, enabling Russell to travel extensively, especially to chapter meetings. Unlike the custom of some College representatives in the past, Russell participated in entire chapter meetings, listening to the Fellows, making friends, identifying leaders, and formulating his plans to support the Fellows through College programs. He continued this outreach to the chapters, the most efficient way to interact with Fellows, throughout his tenure. In 2006, Russell or other officers of the College attended 43 chapter meetings.[7] No other director, save the founder Franklin Martin, had reached out to the fellowship as extensively and so truly knew about their daily work, their aspirations, and their problems.

Russell believed the College should not only embrace surgeons, but also those who supported them in their work. He engaged anesthesiologists, nurses, and operating-room technicians, offering their organizations affiliate membership in the College and making them welcome at the Clinical Congress.

Russell also met with the leadership of the American Society of General Surgeons (ASGS), the organization that had created a vexing situation for the College by seemingly advocating for general surgery more strongly than the College. Previous Directors had regarded the Society as anti-College, but Russell engineered its acceptance by the Board of Governors as an organization entitled to a Governor. This effectively neutralized the Society as a competing organization and brought it under the umbrella of the College, which embraced its goals of advocacy for general surgeons.[1]

The Governors Promote Volunteerism

The goal of support for volunteerism was a product of the strategic planning process in 2000. Russell recognized that Fellows of the College routinely provided uncompensated care worth millions of dollars, but they received no recognition from the College. Under the leadership of Drs. Andrew Warshaw and Robert Stephens, the Governor's committee on socioeconomic issues surveyed the fellowship and found that an astonishing 80 percent of Fellows had volunteered their services in settings that ranged from hospital emergency rooms filled with uninsured and underinsured patients through organized, not-for-profit volunteer missions in poor Third World countries. They spent an average of four weeks annually in volunteer activities. One-half of the respondents had volunteered internationally. When asked why they volunteered, a majority said it was "the right thing to do" or "it is part of what it means to be a physician."[5]

The committee on socioeconomic issues recommended that the College develop a clearinghouse of information about volunteer opportunities and organizations. The program was dubbed Operation Giving Back, and Dr. Kathleen M Casey was appointed its director. More than 1,000 surgeons quickly enrolled in the database of volunteers. Today, a wide range of volunteer resources, including more than a hundred partnering organizations, is provided on an ACS Operation Giving Back website (*http://www.operationgivingback.facs.org*).[8, 9] By 2011, approximately 1,750 surgeons had provided profiles for the database and 2,300 indicated they wanted to receive alerts and newsletters. After the disastrous earthquake in Haiti in early 2010, almost 1,000 surgeons and supporting personnel indicated their willingness to volunteer.[10] From 2004 on, volunteers in several categories have received the American College of Surgeons/Pfizer Surgical Volunteerism and Humanitarian Awards, generously funded by Pfizer.[11]

After the terrorist attacks on September 11, 2001, the blood-borne infection and environmental risk committee of the Board of Governors sponsored a general session on unconventional acts of civilian terrorism and developed a slide set and text available on the College's website to inform Fellows about this subject and to enable them to teach their communities about responses to terrorism with agents of mass destruction.[12]

Dr. J Patrick O'Leary, Chairman of the Board of Governors in 2001 and 2002, radically changed the process used for the annual Governors' reports, replacing them with an

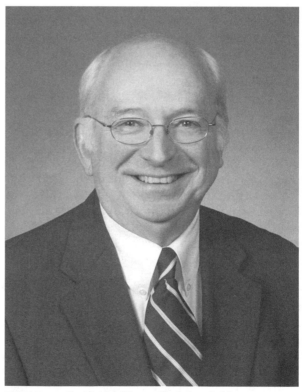

FIGURE 21.1 Dr. J Patrick O'Leary, Chair, Board of Governors, 2001–03; First Vice President, 2005–06.

electronic survey that allowed for statistical analysis. For example, a typical Governors' report might state that 92 percent of the Governors ranked the importance of tort reform at six or above, resulting in an overall average ranking of 8.9. The overall ranking was then used to rank the issues of tort reform, Medicare reimbursement, and health care reform, among others.

O'Leary also changed the structure of the Governors' committees, aligning them with the College's activities. The number of committees was reduced from eight to six; mission statements, goals, and objectives were created for the committees. These were major improvements that increased the value of the input from the Board of Governors and its committees to the College. A Governors' handbook was developed to extend their knowledge about the College and its operations.[12] A performance checklist was developed that helped chapters improve and expand their activities.[13] Dr. O'Leary's leadership improved the activities of the Governors and their committees. (Figure 21.1)

To deal with professional liability, the number one issue in the annual Governors' survey of Fellows in 2004 because of rising premiums, the College joined and eventually chaired the Health Coalition on Liability and Access, a consortium of 75 organizations supporting federal medical liability reform. The Coalition used public relations activities to highlight the importance of reform. Coalition dues, which funded these activities, were paid by the American College of Surgeons Professional Association (ACSPA), the College's 501 (c) 6 entity created when its political action committee (PAC) was formed.[14]

Association Management

Among his efforts to make the resources of the College more widely available to the surgery community was Russell's offer to house the offices of surgical organizations and to provide society and association management services. These services also included joint investment and Continuing Medical Education (CME) programs, travel services, and meeting and exhibit management. Among the 17 organizations that contracted for one or more of these services were the American Board of Surgery (ABS), the Southeastern and Southwestern Surgical Congresses, the Pacific Coast Surgical Association, and the Society for Vascular Surgery.[8, 11, 15]

The expanded medical education requirements of the Accreditation Council for Continuing Medical Education (ACCME) frustrated medical organizations that wanted to provide official credit to their members for attendance at their scientific and educational meetings. After receiving complaints from governors who represented surgical societies that the new requirements were onerous, the College introduced a joint sponsorship program in 2001 that reduced the burden for the societies. The College, as the ACCME-accredited sponsor, assigned credit hours for the educational activities of surgery organizations and allowed them to use the College logo to promote their meetings. Ironically, the inaugural joint sponsorship program was with the ASGS for their annual meeting. Joint sponsorship proved to be a very popular program, because it made it easy for surgery organizations not ACCME accredited to offer approved continuing medical education credits.[5]

The Foundation and Scholarships

The College created the American College of Surgeons Foundation in 2005 to support its charitable and educational work. The Foundation assumed the activities of the development office and the committee on development.[16] This move, and the addition of several development officers, resulted in a dramatic increase in fundraising, from approximately $1.2 million in 1999[2] to almost $2.1 million in 2009.[17] The leadership hoped to increase giving to help fund the constant growth in College programs.

A significant portion of donated funds was for scholarships. For example, Joan L and Dr. Julius H Jacobson II announced an endowment fund of $500,000 to support an award to recognize outstanding surgeons engaged in research advocating the art and science of surgery who had shown through their research early promise of significant contribution to the practice of surgery and the safety of surgical patients. This became known as the promising investigator award.[18] A new traveler exchange program with the German Society of Surgery was established at a cost of $18,000 for three years.[12]

Although the number varies, the scholarships committee has offered approximately 10 faculty research fellowships at $40,000 per year for each of two years. On an annual basis the total budget has been $800,000. Resident research scholarships have also been awarded. For 2007–2009, six were approved at $30,000 for each of two years.[7, 9] Eight specialty organizations and the College cosponsor health policy scholarships for the health care policy program offered at Brandeis University.[19] The Nizar N Oweida MD, FACS scholarship supports attendance at the Clinical Congress by a Fellow or associate Fellow under the age of 45 who is serving a rural U.S. community with a population of approximately 15,000 or less.[7]

The College Deals with its Archives and its Properties

A working group on archives and properties recommended moving the many records, portraits and artifacts stored in the Nickerson Mansion and the Murphy Auditorium to the better environment and security of the 633 St. Clair building. In 2000, the College hired an experienced archivist, Ms. Susan Rishworth, to establish and administer an archives and records program.[1, 2] Renovated space was made available on the 27th floor and a program of oral histories was initiated.[20] By 2008, various digital collections of the Archives were available on the College website[11] and efforts were being made to digitize the memoirs of Franklin Martin and the invaluable notebooks of Martin's assistant, Ms. Eleanor Grimm.

The Nickerson Mansion, in need of repair, and the deteriorating Murphy Auditorium, neither of which was used regularly, were a financial drain on the College. Dr. C Rollins Hanlon, Executive Consultant since retiring as Director, worked with Dr. Russell to sell the Nickerson Mansion to Hanlon's friend, Mr. Richard Driehaus. A philanthropist and collector interested in neoclassical architecture and objects, Mr. Driehaus was the founder and chairman of Driehaus Capital Management. He purchased the Nickerson from the College in 2004 and renovated it to the Richard H Driehaus Museum of the Decorative Arts as a fine example of neoclassical architecture and to house a portion of his collection. The financial arrangements also enabled his experts to restore the Murphy Auditorium to its original splendor, allowing the auditorium to remain the property of the College. The Murphy is rented by the College as an increasingly popular venue for weddings, receptions, and other events. The sale of the Nickerson ended the College's ownership on one of Chicago's most valuable and interesting properties, but it preserved and extended its role in Chicago's rich architectural history.

≈ ✳ ≈

The National Surgical Quality Improvement Program (NSQIP®)

The strategic plan was shaped in part to deal with compelling external pressures the College could not ignore. The Institute of Medicine report, *To Err is Human: Building a Safer Health System,* released in 2000,[21] showed that hospitals were dangerous places, where patients acquired infections, developed complications, and died due to error much more frequently than the medical profession and the public had realized. A large proportion of deaths was related to surgical procedures and their complications. It was clear that the College needed to respond to these issues. One such program was immediately available. Under the leadership of surgeon Dr. Shukri Khuri, the Veterans Administration (VA) had developed the National Surgical Quality Improvement Program (NSQIP), and had shown that collecting, analyzing, and feeding back risk-adjusted data on surgical patients led to improved patient outcomes.

After its introduction at 128 VA medical centers in 1991, there was a 27 percent decrease in the 30-day postoperative mortality rate and a 45 percent decrease in lengths of stay related to a decline in morbidities. A 1999 pilot study at three medical centers outside the VA system substantiated the risk-adjustment and predictive outcome models of the VA NSQIP, as well as its positive impact on the quality of surgical care.

Doctors Thomas Russell and R Scott Jones and others recognized the potential of this program to improve the safety of surgical patients and to respond to public criticism of the profession after *To Err is Human* was published. They and Dr. Khuri convinced the VA to allow the College to introduce NSQIP into non-VA hospitals. The Agency for Healthcare Research and Quality (AHRQ) gave the College's division of research and optimal patient care a $5.25 million grant to do this, and the College's finance committee allocated an additional $250,000.[13] By 2011, approximately 400 hospitals were enrolled in the program and evidence continued to mount that the program effectively reduced the mortality and morbidity of surgical procedures.[22, 23] NSQIP has significantly improved care of the surgical patient in the United States and has become one of the College's most important programs in its efforts to improve the quality of surgical care.

ACS NSQIP became a centerpiece of the division of research and optimal patient care, which was led by Dr. Jones until 2007, when he retired and Dr. Clifford Ko was appointed director. This division also provided oversight for ACOSOG, which under Dr. Wells' leadership was moved to Duke University to take advantage of Duke's extensive research infrastructure. ACOSOG's funding by the National Cancer Institute (NCI) continued, with intermittent supplementation by the College. Drs. David Ota and Heidi

Nelson, at Duke University and the Mayo Clinic, respectively, were appointed co-chairs of the group in 2005.[16]

Another program developed under the Division of Research and Optimal Patient Care was the ACS bariatric surgery center network accreditation program,[11] undertaken to provide peer evaluation of bariatric surgery facilities against rigorous, nationally recognized standards. Documentation of outcomes and continuous quality improvement are required. More than 100 programs were fully accredited by 2010.[17]

The Cancer Program

Dr. Monica Morrow, professor of surgery and director of the breast center at Northwestern University, was the part-time director of the Commission on Cancer when Dr. Russell was appointed Executive Director. She led a redesign of the national cancer data base and the approvals program to incorporate evidence-based measures for an ongoing assessment of quality cancer care, information that was then fed back to the approved hospitals.[1] The Joint Commission approved the cancer program of a hospital if the program was approved by the Commission on Cancer of the College, lending prestige and value to the Commission on Cancer and promoting its growth. In 2000, 1,638 hospital registries reported 872,722 cases to the College's national cancer database, and data was available on 1,014,364 breast cancers.[3]

Dr. Morrow, who had replaced Dr. David Winchester during the Wells era, left the College in 2001, and Dr. Winchester returned to direct the program. He modernized the programs through web-based technology and developed the College's national accreditation program for breast centers. Its purpose has been to improve the quality of care and measure outcomes for patients with diseases of the breast.[5]

The Trauma Program

Russell appointed a work group for strategic planning in trauma. Communication between the Committee on Trauma and the College leadership had been less than optimal. This was solved by the appointment of a director for the trauma department, Dr. David Hoyt, who reported directly to the executive director.[24] Under Hoyt's direction the trauma registry and the national trauma databank were converted to web-based programs, which greatly expanded the trauma program. Between 2001 and 2006, the number of patient records in the databank grew from 180,000 to 1,500,000, and during the same period the number of participating trauma centers increased from 67 to 564. All 50 states were represented.[19]

Dr. Hoyt stepped down as chair of the Trauma Committee in 2006 and was replaced by Dr. J Wayne Meredith, who introduced the trauma quality improvement program, designed to provide risk-adjusted benchmarking of participating trauma centers to track outcomes and improve patient care, using the infrastructure of the national trauma data bank.[25]

The ATLS course has been given to an estimated 25,000 to 30,000 individuals annually all over the world.[19] The lifesaving impact of this course was one of the College's greatest achievements during its first 100 years. Courses in trauma evaluation and management, advanced trauma operative management, and optimal trauma center organization and management are also provided by the trauma department.[26]

The Board of Governors expressed concern that hospitals were having difficulty staffing emergency departments with surgical specialists, especially at night and on weekends. The risk of malpractice suits from trauma victims, inadequate reimbursement, insufficient trauma experience of some specialists, and other factors contributed to this problem. Although some hospitals sufficiently compensated on-call surgeons, others did not, and the care of trauma patients in small hospitals and rural areas continues to be vexing issues for the College's trauma department.[27]

Education

The College had never had a leader of its education programs who had formal training in education and whose career was in education until Dr. Ajit Sachdeva took over the Division of Education in 2001. (Figure 21.2) The results were spectacular. Sachdeva discerned that external forces were influencing the educational paradigm, and he implemented programs that enabled the fellowship to meet the new requirements. The American Board of Medical Specialties, the umbrella organization of the certifying boards, implemented a maintenance of certification (MOC) program that required diplomates of the boards to demonstrate competencies expected of the contemporary physician beyond the medical knowledge and patient care measured though the examination processes of the certifying boards.

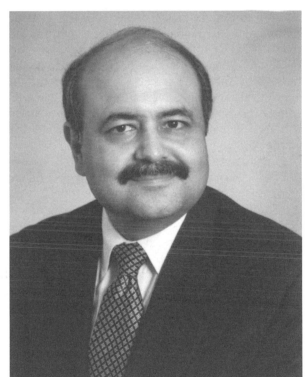

FIGURE 21.2 Dr. Ajit K Sachdeva, Director, Division of Education.

The competencies added were interpersonal and communication skills, professionalism, systems-based practice, and practice-based learning and assessment. The MOC programs of each board were designed to include evaluation of diplomates for lifelong learning and self-assessment, cognitive expertise, and assessment of practice performance. The Council of Medical Specialty Societies (CMSS), of which the College was a prominent member, provided expertise and endorsed the maintenance

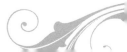

of certification model, and its constituent organizations revamped their educational offerings to help their members meet the new requirements.

These requirements, which continue to affect almost all Fellows of the College, introduced the need for new programs and curricula. For example, courses on professionalism and how surgeons should function in the multiple systems entailed in the care of a patient were not offered by organizations that provided continuing education. Sachdeva appointed a task force for each of the six general competencies. The task forces generated ideas and programs to educate the Fellows in the competencies. The centerpiece of the College's education activities, the annual Clinical Congress, was filled with offerings on professionalism, methods of practice assessment, and interpersonal skills information that Fellows welcomed and used in their practices.[26]

Sachdeva and the talented education experts he hired modernized and extended many existing College activities. For example, electronic submission of Surgical Forum abstracts was introduced, the lengths of didactic courses and general sessions were reduced to make them more focused, the resident ethics curriculum was revised and manuals were prepared for instructors and residents.[6]

Bariatric surgery was becoming increasingly popular, but bariatric surgeons tended to determine their own indications for the operations they performed, giving rise to the need for evidence-based standards. The division of education, working with the American Society for Bariatric Surgery (ASBS) and the Society of American Gastrointestinal Endoscopic Surgeons, developed education courses on bariatric surgery presented at the Clinical Congress, and an electronic primer on a CD-ROM.[26]

The College's focus on bariatric surgery led to the development of the American College of Surgeons bariatric surgery center network.[25] In 2005, the center network accreditation program was initiated.[19] The validity of the standards for accreditation was reinforced shortly thereafter, when Medicare announced that it would pay for bariatric procedures only if they were performed in a facility accredited by the College or the ASBS.

Surgeons were brought into the relatively new field of palliative care when a surgical palliative care task force, supported by the Robert Wood Johnson Foundation, developed priorities and projects, beginning with a workshop on the subject.[26]

During its first ten years, the division of education introduced webcasts of College educational offerings, a series of practice management courses, a code of professional conduct for surgeons, a popular course on surgeons as leaders, and a series of teleconferences on implementation of the confidentiality requirements of the Health Insurance Portability and Accountability Act (HIPAA).[20]

Because of the increasing emphasis on practice outcomes, the College developed an Internet and personal digital assistant program that enabled surgeons to keep and monitor a database of patients and their outcomes and to compare them with benchmarks.

The division of education also produced skills-oriented postgraduate courses such as the bedside procedures workshop, health care leadership, and laparoscopic and hand-assisted laparoscopic colon resection. Also, review courses in urology, pediatric surgery, and cardiac and thoracic surgery were provided. Dozens of internet-based education programs from previous Clinical Congresses were made available.[16] A major initiative in 2006 was the development of a College web portal, which gave Fellows access to specialty, subspecialty, and subject communities for postings and discussions.[25]

The *Journal of the American College of Surgeons* instituted an Internet-based CME program, allowing Fellows to obtain Category I credit for studying selected articles and completing tests.

The 2007 meeting in Las Vegas was the last of the spring meetings. Its demise was related to increasing expenses and decreasing attendance. Fellows were increasingly reluctant to be absent from their practices and travel long distances for continuing education.[7] In an attempt to alleviate these problems and make quality continuing education more accessible to Fellows, the College developed a program to accredit regional educational institutes sponsored by hospitals and other organizations that met the program's standards. Instruction in new skills and procedures and support of surgeons for MOC were provided. By 2009, 47 education institutes were accredited.[17]

≈ ✻ ≈

Graduate Medical Education

In 2003, the American Surgical Association (ASA) created a blue ribbon committee to address residency education in general surgery in partnership with the College and the ABS. The committee reported its concern about a possible shortage of surgeons and about the number of women in surgery. Women comprised fewer than 30 percent of the total number of students entering surgical residencies even though they were 50 percent of all graduating medical students. The committee recommended more faculty involvement in medical student education in surgery, a standardized, national curriculum for surgical education and training, and a fundamental curriculum for all residents before entering respective surgical specialties. They also advocated support for education through faculty development at the departmental level, more mentoring in resident training and surgical research, and introducing residents to continuous professional development. The committee was supportive of the ACGME-proposed 80-hour work week for residents because it would encourage elimination of non-educational work and promote efficiencies in education.[13, 20, 28]

The ABS, with the support of the College, the ASA, and other organizations involved in surgical education, collectively called the surgical council on resident education (SCORE) took the lead in creating a uniform, structured curriculum for residents. The Board hired Dr. Richard Bell, chair of surgery at Northwestern, as assistant executive director to develop the program.[16] The curriculum, still very much in use, is accompanied by modules on medical knowledge, patient care, and systems based practice; textbook content; narrated operative videos; a radiologic image library; and multiple choice questions. In 2011, the number of residents and residency programs enrolled were 8,960 and 263 respectively.

Under the direction of Dr. Lewis Flint, the College supported education of residents and its Fellows by acquiring *Selected Readings in General Surgery,* a topic-specific collection of reprints and summaries of articles, published eight times each year. Recognized by the ABS to fulfill MOC requirements, the program includes posttests in the format used in board examinations. The first issue of *Selected Readings* from the College was mailed in February 2008. An electronic version is also available.[11]

In 2000, the Candidate and Associate Society of the American College of Surgeons (CAS–ACS) developed its council of representatives and formed committees, including education, career opportunity and communications issues, and membership. The Society had 6,258 members.[1] The purpose of CAS was to support residents and recent residency graduates and to engage them in College activities, bringing them into fellowship seamlessly. Some of their activities included creating a job bank for surgeons completing their residencies, taking positions on resident work hours, and developing educational activities such as Surgical Jeopardy and spectacular case presentations.[11,24] The name of the Society was changed to the Resident and Associate Society (RAS) of the ACS in 2004 to more accurately reflect its membership.[14]

The success of engaging residents in College activities led the College to renew its emphasis on engaging young surgeons, an effort in the 1960s that led to the development of many College leaders. In 2009, the Young Fellows Association was formed. Its goals were to promote the needs of young physicians within the College's legislative agenda, to increase the awareness and involvement of young Fellows in the College, and to promote programs and initiatives that serve the needs of young Fellows.[17]

The College was growing. A total of 1,285 domestic and international candidates applied for fellowship in 2009, of which 170 were international. There were 3,245 associate Fellows, 8,550 resident members, 1,448 medical student members, and 347 affiliate members, for a total membership of 74,342.[11, 17]

Patient Safety and Quality of Care

The publication of *To Err is Human* led to many efforts to improve patient safety and the quality of care. Eliminating wrong-site surgery and surgical complications such as infection and venous thromboembolism became the goals of many organizations.

Continuing media reports of surgery performed on the wrong patient and the wrong site, plus an increasing number of such instances reported to the Joint Commission, stimulated the College, the Joint Commission, the American Academy of Orthopaedic Surgeons (AAOS), and the AMA to convene a large number of organizations at a conference to address this problem.[6] The Joint Commission used the results to develop standards requiring preoperative marking of the surgical site, enhanced patient identification procedures, and a "time out" before beginning an operation to ensure that the correct operation was about to be performed on the correct patient.[26]

The AMA physician consortium for performance improvement appointed a work group chaired by Dr. R Scott Jones, representing the College, and a representative from the American Society of Anesthesiologists. The group developed a set of six physician performance measures in the areas of antibiotic and venous thromboembolism prophylaxis. They were submitted to the National Quality Forum for further refinement and approval, and were later made part of Medicare's Pay for Performance program.

The Surgical Quality Alliance, a coalition of 20 surgical specialty societies and anesthesiology, was organized by the College to respond to the call for patient safety and improved quality. The Alliance developed a set of performance measures for use by various subspecialties, which were submitted to Medicare for inclusion in its physician voluntary reporting program. The Alliance has collaborated on many projects and commented on quality and safety issues to Medicare, the National Quality Forum, and the Ambulatory Quality Alliance.[9] The Ambulatory Quality Alliance approved the perioperative care measures set developed in the Surgical Quality Alliance. It consisted of six measures in the areas of prophylactic antibiotic timing, selection, and discontinuation, and venous thromboembolism prophylaxis. These were sent to the National Quality Forum for review and endorsement.[7] Eventually, a version of the measures developed by these organizations was used by Medicare for pay-for-reporting and pay-for-performance programs.[9]

Recognizing that the safety and quality of modern surgery requires a high performing team from various educational backgrounds and disciplines, Russell formed a Council on Surgical and Perioperative Safety (CSPS) that began meeting informally in 2004 and since 2007 has been an independent, incorporated, organization with an executive director. The Council consists of the American Association of Nurse Anesthetists, the American Association of Surgical Physician Assistants, the ACS, the Association of periOperative Registered Nurses, the American Society of Anesthesiologists, the Society of PeriAnesthesia Nurses, and the Association of Surgical Technologists. They developed vision and mission statements and goals and objectives. The CSPS continues to be dedicated to promoting safety and excellent care by an integrated team in the surgical and perioperative environment.[11]

The Revitalized College

Russell's directorship was focused on the Fellows, individually and collectively. In his practice he had experienced the need for evidence-based information in dealing with patient problems. He too needed to learn how to use technology that did not exist during his training. He understood that the College could provide help to the Fellows in the daily conduct of their practices. His reorganization of the College and recruitment of effective leaders allowed them to innovate, and to develop new ideas and new programs that would serve the fellowship and help them improve the care of their patients. The number of new programs and activities introduced during the decade of Russell's tenure exceeded those introduced in any other decade of the College's history. More importantly, true to the mission of the College, they enabled the members to improve the care of the surgical patient within an optimal and ethical practice environment.

REFERENCES

1. *Minutes of the meeting of the Board of Regents of June 9, 10, 2000.* 2000, Archives of the American College of Surgeons: Chicago.

2. *Minutes of the meeting of the Board of Regents of February 11, 12, 2000.* 2000, Archives of the American College of Surgeons: Chicago.

3. *Minutes of the meeting of the Board of Regents of February 9, 10, 2001.* 2001, Archives of the American College of Surgeons: Chicago.

4. *Minutes of the meeting of the Board of Regents of June 8-10, 2001.* 2001, Archives of the American College of Surgeons: Chicago.

5. *Minutes of the meeting of the Board of Regents of October 5-7, 2001.* 2001, Archives of the American College of Surgeons: Chicago.

6. *Minutes of the meeting of the Board of Regents of February 8, 9, 2002.* 2002, Archives of the American College of Surgeons: Chicago.

7. *Minutes of the meeting of the Board of Regents of February 9, 19, 2007.* 2007, Archives of the American College of Surgeons: Chicago.

8. *Minutes of the meeting of the Board of Regents of October 15, 16, 2005.* 2005, Archives of the American College of Surgeons: Chicago.

9. *Minutes of the meeting of the Board of Regents of October 7, 8, 2006.* 2006, Archives of the American College of Surgeons: Chicago.

10. *Personal communication from Dr. Kathleen Casey to Dr. David Nahrwold, July 7, 2011.* 2011.

11. *Minutes of the meeting of the Board of Regents of June 4-6, 2009.* 2009, Archives of the American College of Surgeons: Chicago.

12. *Minutes of the meeting of the Board of Regents of February 6, 7, 2004.* 2004, Archives of the American College of Surgeons: Chicago.

13. *Minutes of the meeting of the Board of Regents of October 18, 19, 2003.* 2003, Archives of the American College of Surgeons.: Chicago.

14. *Minutes of the meeting of the Board of Regents of October 9, 10, 2004.* 2004, Archives of the American College of Surgeons.: Chicago.

15. *Minutes of the meeting of the Board of Regents of February 7, 8, 2003.* 2003, Archives of the American College of Surgeons.: Chicago.

16. *Minutes of the meeting of the Board of Regents of February 11, 12, 2005.* 2005, Archives of the American College of Surgeons: Chicago.

17. *Minutes of the meeting of the Board of Regents of October 9, 10, 2009.* 2009, Archives of the American College of Surgeons: Chicago.

18. *Minutes of the meeting of the Board of Regents of June 10-12, 2004.* 2004, Archives of the American College of Surgeons: Chicago.

19. *Minutes of the meeting of the Board of Regents of June 9, 10, 2006.* 2006, Archives of the American College of Surgeons: Chicago.

20. *Minutes of the meeting of the Board of Regents of June 5-7, 2003.* 2003, Archives of the American College of Surgeons: Chicago.

21. Kohn LT, C.J., Donaldson MS. Institute of Medicine Committee on Quality of Health Care in America, *To Err is Human. Building a Safer Health System.* 2000, Washington: National Academies Press.

22. Hall BL, H.B., Richards K, Bilimoria KY, Cohen ME, Ko CY., *Does surgical quality improve in the American College of Surgeons Quality Improvement Program? An evaluation of all participating hospitals.* Annals of Surgery, 2009. **250**: p. 363-376.

23. Hollenbeck CS, Boltz MM, Wang L, Shubart J, Ortenzi G, Zhu J, Dillon PW, *Cost-effectiveness of the National Surgical Quality Improvement Program (NSQIP)*. Annals of Surgery, 2011. 254: p. 619-624.

24. *Minutes of the meeting of the Board of Regents of October 20-22, 2000*. 2000, Archives of the American College of Surgeons: Chicago.

25. *Minutes of the meeting of the Board of Regents of February 10, 11, 2006*. 2006, Archives of the American College of Surgeons: Chicago.

26. *Minutes of the meeting of the Board of Regents of June 7,8, 2002*. 2002, Archives of the American College of Surgeons: Chicago.

27. *Minutes of the meeting of the Board of Regents of June 13, 14, 2008*. 2008, Archives of the American College of Surgeons: Chicago.

28. Debas HT, B.B., Brennan MF, et al., *American Surgical Association Blue Ribbon Committee report on surgical education*. Annals of Surgery, 2005. **241**: p. 1-8.

CHAPTER 22
Women Impact Surgery and the College

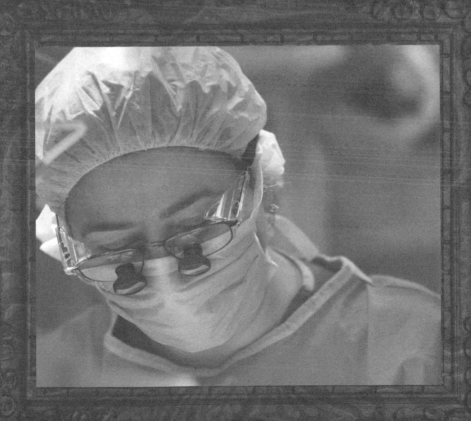

Surgeon at work

Women and Medical School

Elizabeth Blackwell was the first woman to graduate from a formal U.S. medical school. She received her degree in 1849 from Geneva Medical College in upstate New York, which later became Upstate Medical University. Hoping to become a surgeon, she went to Paris to study surgery, but was denied access to hospitals there because of her gender. Instead, she enrolled at La Maternité, a highly regarded midwifery school. Unfortunately, an ophthalmic infection left her blind in one eye, dashing her hopes of becoming a surgeon. Later, she helped establish the New York Sanitary Commission, the New York Hospital for Women and Children, and a medical school for women in New York.[1]

Women were a small minority of medical students until approximately 1970. For example, only four women were among the 131 students who graduated in 1960 from the Indiana University School of Medicine, then one of the largest in the country. After the publication of Betty Freidan's *The Feminine Mystique* in 1963,[2] which signaled the beginning of the contemporary women's movement, many young women sought careers in business and the professions that were traditionally male-dominated. The number of female medical school applicants began to rise in the late 1960s, but the acceptance rate remained small, even after the Association of American Medical Colleges (AAMC) recommended that schools accept women who had credentials comparable to those of men. Title IX of the Education Amendments of 1972 stipulated that "no person shall, on the basis of sex, be excluded from participation in, be denied the benefits of, or be subjected to discrimination under any education program or activity receiving Federal financial assistance...", which included universities and their medical schools. Subsequently, the acceptance rate for women increased until approximately 1990, when parity with men was reached. Since then, approximately half of medical school applicants and matriculants have been women.[3]

Women and Surgical Residencies

The increase in the proportion of women in medical schools was not accompanied by an increase in the proportion of women in surgical residencies until recently. Clearly, women have concern about childbearing and childrearing, but the reasons they have tended to avoid surgical careers, and therefore surgical residencies, are complex. A major problem is an insufficient number of women surgeons on medical school faculties who can mentor, advise, and serve as role models for female medical students.[5] A concerted effort by the College, surgery specialty societies, certifying boards, program directors, and surgical leaders to encourage women to pursue surgical careers has been successful. The requirement of an 80-hour work week for residents was also helpful. In general surgery, recent data show that when international medical graduates (IMG) are excluded, the entering residency class in 2000 was 32 percent female, increasing progressively to 40 percent by 2005. IMGs accounted for 11 to 18 percent of entering residents during this period, but few IMGs are female, so women comprised only 33 percent of all applicants to general surgery programs in 2005.[4] However, by 2011, 42 percent of general surgery residents were women.

Women and the College

At least five women were listed in the membership directory in 1914, a year after the College was founded. Thereafter, a woman was occasionally admitted to fellowship, but there were few women in medicine and hardly any in surgery before 1970. Most women admitted to the College were obstetricians-gynecologists, because of the predilection of women medical school graduates for this specialty and pediatrics. It was not until 1950 that Helen Octavia Dickens, director of the Mercy Douglass Hospital's department of obstetrics and gynecology in Philadelphia, became the first African American woman admitted to fellowship.

Women who were Fellows of the College did not feel that they were truly a part of the fellowship. Women surgeons were often asked if they were nurses or wives of surgeons as they toured the exhibition area at the Clinical Congress, and sometimes no one sat next to them during lectures or other sessions. They felt isolated in a College that described its members as a fellowship. In 1981, Dr. Patricia Numann, a young surgeon at SUNY Upstate Medical University in Syracuse, put up a sign inviting women surgeons and residents to an informal breakfast at the Clinical Congress in San Francisco. She recalls that approximately 18 attended, and that they shared common experiences of feeling isolated, without mentors, and were all very happy to meet other women in surgery. The breakfasts continued and the group grew, leading to its incorporation as the Association of Women Surgeons (AWS) in 1986.[6] By 1988 there were almost 1,000 members and a formal meeting program was established. (Figure 22.1)

In 1995, the College recognized the AWS as an organization entitled to be represented by a Governor. In addition to a mentoring program and other activities to support women surgeons, the AWS and its members advocate for women as members of surgical organizations, the American Board of Surgery (ABS), and committees of the College. The goals of the organization are to advance the highest standards of competence and ethical behavior, to foster an environment supportive of personal values and individual diversity, to enhance and facilitate interaction

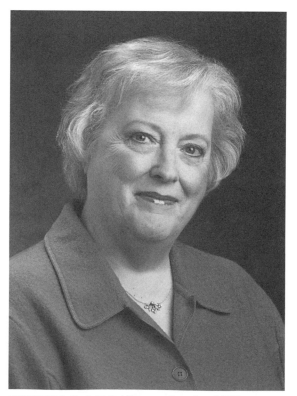

FIGURE 22.1 Dr. Patricia J Numann, founder of AWS; ACS President, 2011–12.

among women surgeons throughout the world, and to promote professional growth and development.[6] This organization and its members have stimulated, and sometimes goaded, the College into integrating women into its activities and its leadership.

Because residency training is required for full fellowship in the College, the pool of potential female initiates is the number of women completing surgical residencies, now the main rate-limiting step for the number of women in the College. In 2011, only 11 percent of dues-paying Fellows of the College were women. Although there is no documentation of bias against admitting women currently, it undoubtedly existed in the past. Many women surgeons who have completed training are extremely busy with starting their practices, having children and caring for them, and managing households. They simply do not have much time left to devote to organizations, the value of which may not be obvious. Furthermore, many have no mentors to encourage them to join or help them in the process.

The College Hires a Woman Executive and Creates a Committee on Women's Issues

No female surgeon had held an executive position with the College until Director Paul Ebert hired Dr. Olga Jonasson, who had been the chairman of the department of surgery at Ohio State University and the first woman to chair a surgery department, as director of research and education in 1993. Dr. Jonasson, a celebrated transplant surgeon, was the first female member of the American Surgical Association (ASA) and the Society of University Surgeons (SUS), and the first female director of the ABS. She was admired by the small, but growing number of women in surgery, and her appointment and advocacy for women helped to advance the cause for women and open other leadership positions in the College for them. (Figure 22.2)

One of Jonasson's responsibilities was oversight of the longitudinal study of surgical residents, a system of tracking surgical residents to document future surgical manpower. Fortuitously, this gave her access to data on residents by gender, which she used effectively in advocacy for women. In 1998, noting that women accounted for 42 percent of medical students, but that only five percent of women entered a surgical residency other than obstetrics and gynecology, Johansson proposed that the Board of Regents create a standing committee on women's issues. She informed the Regents that women did not have effective mentoring, did not possess adequate negotiating skills, and tended to assume nurturing roles in institutions, such as participation in committees that demanded time and effort with little reward.

For example, she said, women are often clerkship directors and assistant program directors. The Regents had a lengthy debate over whether or not to form a standing committee on women's issues. Eventually, they agreed to form an ad hoc committee on women's issues. As usual, there was concern that every "minority group" would want their own Regental standing committee.[7]

A year later, Dr. Johansson reported to the Regents that appointments to the committee on women's issues had been made. They were all members of the Board of Governors and the advisory councils. Nine were women and two were men. None of the Regents noticed then or later that she had removed the "*ad hoc*" from the "committee on women's issues," and if anyone had, he or she was unwilling to challenge the formidable Dr. Jonasson.[8]

A major problem for advocates of women was that the College database did not include the gender of the Fellows. Dr. Amilu Rothhammer, the first female Chair of the Board of Governors, reported to the Regents in 1998 that the Governors requested the College to explore means of collecting gender and ethnic data on its Fellows, believing that the success or failure of diversity programs depended on the analysis of data. She was joined in this request by the Secretary, Dr. Kathryn Anderson, but the Regents took no action.[7] A year later the Regents authorized Dr. Karen Guice, director of the fellowship department, to obtain gender and ethnicity data on the fellowship after the Board of Governors developed a survey tool for this purpose.[9]

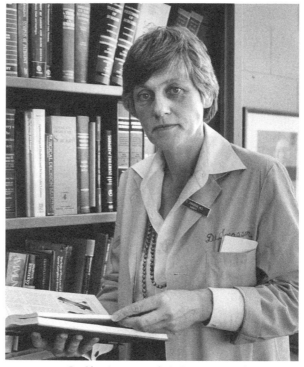

FIGURE 22.2   Dr. Olga Jonasson, chair, Department of Surgery, The Ohio State University; Director, Education and Surgical Services, ACS, 1993–2004.

The committee on women's issues held its first meeting in October 2000. Four areas of focus were identified. They were College membership recruitment and retention, professional development, society membership, and leadership roles.[10] The committee decided to gather data on women in surgery, to include medical school recruitment, graduate medical education, working environment, and issues associated with work hours, academic careers, surgical practice, and career guidance.[11]

The committee has implemented policies and programs that meet the needs of women surgeons and advance their cause. For example, the committee contributed to College statements on diversity and the code of conduct included in the College's statement on principles.[12] Partnering with the AWS, the committee created an ongoing mentoring program for women faculty in surgery, launched in 2004.[13, 14]

Other College committees also have advanced the cause of women surgeons. The Commission on Cancer program committee openly sought diversity of ethnicity, gender, and age in the presenters of its programs. The chapter activities committee of the Board of Governors, chaired by the noted surgical oncologist Dr. Margaret Kemeny, successfully prodded the College program committee to increase the number of presenters from underrepresented groups.[15]

In 2007, the name of the committee on women's issues was changed to the women in surgery committee, with the goals of promoting the recruitment and retention of women in the surgical specialties, and aiding the development and enhancement of leadership roles for women in the College and other surgical and medical organizations.

There has been a definite awareness of the need for women on College committees, where much of the basic work of the College originates. In 2011, eight of the 29 committees of the College were chaired by women, as were two of the six committees of the Board of Governors.

Women in College Leadership Positions

Although slow progress has been made through the College committee structure, the opportunities for women to work in major College leadership positions were sparse until very recently. It was not until 1993 that the first woman to hold office in the College, Dr. Kathryn Anderson, was elected Secretary, a position she held for eight years. In 2001, she became First Vice President, and in 2005 she was the first woman elected President of the College. (Figure 22.3) Dr. Margaret Longo became the first female Regent in 1993. The second was Dr. Mary McGrath, a distinguished plastic surgeon, who was elected Vice Chairman of the Board of Regents in 2006. Since 2001, at least three women have been members of the Board of Regents simultaneously, increasing to five in 2010-2011. The committee on young surgeons, spawned during Dr. Hanlon's tenure as Director, was the first committee to operate outside the "old boy" network of the College. Dr. Martha McDaniel, a vascular surgeon who became the first chairman of a department (anatomy) at Dartmouth Medical School in 2001, was appointed chair of this committee in 1994.[16]

A major problem has been the lack of a majority of women on committees that nominate Regents and College officers. For example, until 1995 no woman had served on the nominating committee of the Board of Regents, which nominates the Board's officers. Between 1998 and 2003, inclusive, only three women were members of the nominating committee of the Board of Regents. During the same period of time, 75 men served on the nominating committee.[17]

Several women were elected First or Second Vice President of the College after Dr. Patricia Numann was the first female Second Vice President in 1999. Dr. Numann was also the first woman to receive the College's Distinguished Service Award. In 2010, she was the First Vice President, and was elected President of the College in 2011 after Dr. Lazar Greenfield resigned as President Elect.

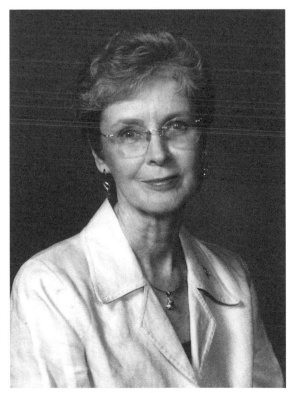

FIGURE 22.3 Dr. Kathryn D Anderson, ACS Secretary, 1993-2001; ACS President, 2005–06.

A Portent of the Future Relationship between Women and the College

Dr. Greenfield, the retired chairman of surgery at the University of Michigan, was editor in chief of *Surgery News*, a monthly publication of the College. He wrote a Valentine's Day editorial for the February 2010 issue that offended many surgeons, especially women. Their reaction spread through the Internet and social media and was reported by the *New York Times*.[18] Dr. Greenfield, long a supporter of women in surgery, publicly apologized and resigned as editor in chief. Subsequently, he resigned as president elect, denying himself one of the highest honors in American surgery.

The incident released latent sentiments among many women surgeons that they had not achieved equality and were still not valued as Fellows of the College. In their opinions, the discrimination they experienced in medical school, residency programs, and the workplace continued. These reactions transcended the editorial itself, and exposed the leadership of the College to the serious gender issues still extant for the profession of surgery and the College.

REFERENCES

1. Totenberg, N., *Olga M. Jonasson Lecture: Women in the professions.* Bulletin of the American College of Surgeons, 2011. **96**: p. 12-23.

2. Friedan, B., *The Feminine Mystique.* 1963, New York: William Norton and Co.

3. Cooper RA., *Medical schools and their applicants: An analysis.* Health Affairs, 2003. **221**: p. 71-84.

4. Davis EC, R.D., Blair PG, Sachdeva AK., *Women in surgery residency programs: Evolving trends from a national perspective.* Journal of the American College of Surgeons, 2011. **212**: p. 320-326.

5. Neumayer LA, C.A., Melby BS, Foy HM, Wallack MK., *The state of gereral surgery residency in the United States. Program director perspectives.* Archives of Surgery, 2002. **137**: p. 1262-1265.

6. *Association of Women Surgeons website.* September 10, 2011]; Available from: www.womensurgeons.org.

7. *Minutes of the meeting of the Board of Regents of October 25, 1998.* 1998, Archives of the American College of Surgeons: Chicago.

8. *Minutes of the meeting of the Board of Regents of October 15, 1999.* 1999, Archives of the American College of Surgeons: Chicago.

9. *Minutes of the meeting of the Board of Regents of October 8-10, 1999.* 1999, Archives of the American College of Surgeons: Chicago.

10. *Minutes of the meeting of the Board of Regents of June 8-10, 2001.* 2001, Archives of the American College of Surgeons: Chicago.

11. *Minutes of the meeting of the Board of Regents of October 5-7, 2001.* 2001, Archives of the American College of Surgeons: Chicago.

12. *Minutes of the meeting of the Board of Regents of February 8, 9, 2002.* 2002, Archives of the American College of Surgeons: Chicago.

13. Butcher L., *Mentorship program designed to advance women in academic surgery.* Bulletin of the American College of Surgeons, 2009. **94**: p. 6-10.

14. *Minutes of the meeting of the Board of Regents of October 18, 19, 2003.* 2003, Archives of the American College of Surgeons.: Chicago.

15. *Minutes of the meeting of the Board of Regents of February 6, 7, 2004.* 2004, Archives of the American College of Surgeons: Chicago.

16. *Minutes of the meeting of the Board of Regents of October 14, 1994.* 1944, Archives of the American College of Surgeons: Chicago.

17. *Minutes of the meeting of the Board of Regents of February 7, 8, 2003.* 2003, Archives of the American College of Surgeons.: Chicago.

18. Chen PW., *Sexism charges divide surgeons' group.*, in *New York Times.* 2011: New York.

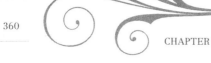

CHAPTER 23
Health Policy,
A New Building,
and a New Director

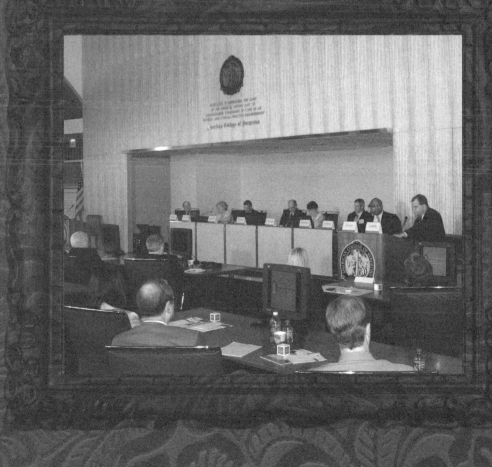

After Dr. Paul Ebert and Mr. James Haug, the director of socioeconomic affairs, retired, Dr. Wells appointed Dr. Henry R Desmarais to succeed Haug. Desmarais had been a principal with Health Policy Alternatives, the Washington, DC, consulting and lobbying firm used by the College for many years. The Regents were not well-versed in how Washington worked, and did not give him specific directions about which issues he should address with Congress and regulators, nor did they indicate what the positions of the College might be. Finally, Desmarais requested that the College form a Regental committee on public policy and government affairs that would provide him and the Washington office with direction. The Executive Committee, reluctant to take public positions on legislative issues and mindful that the Board of Governors voted against developing a political action committee (PAC) in 1988, did not approve his proposal.[1] Instead, Dr. James Carrico, Chair of the Board of Regents, appointed a committee to determine whether or not a health policy committee was needed.[2]

The Regents Act

In 2001, acting on the strong recommendation of this committee, the Regents established a health policy steering committee to identify and prioritize public policy issues affecting surgeons and their patients, and select those on which the College should focus. The committee was to recommend positions and initiatives, develop action plans to address the issues, and expand and monitor mechanisms by which the College makes surgeons, patients, and the public aware of the College's health policies and agendas.[3, 4] This formidable undertaking was led by the committee's chair, Dr. Josef Fischer, an outspoken, hands-on Regent who was chair of surgery at Harvard's Beth Israel New England Deaconess Medical Center. The Vice Chairman was Dr. LaMar McGinnis, an Emory University surgical oncologist who had been president of the American Cancer Society and would later be a President of the College. Both were well-versed in government's activities in health care.

Access to federal legislators was increasingly difficult without making campaign contributions. To facilitate access the health policy steering committee quickly recommended that the Regents form a 501(c)(6) organization for the purpose of establishing a PAC,[5] which could make contributions to political campaigns. The Board of Governors concurred. The College itself was barred from political activity because of its status as a 501(c)(3) tax-exempt organization, so the Regents established the ACSPA as a 501(c)(6) organization, permitted to operate a PAC and to offer a broader range of activities to benefit surgeons and their patients than is the College. The PAC raised and appropriated $2.6 million to political candidates of both parties and legislative initiatives from 2003 through 2008.[6]

Henry Desmarais resigned as director of socioeconomic affairs in 2001, and Dr. Russell appointed Ms. Cynthia Brown as director of the newly named department of health policy and advocacy.[5] Many organizations were developing measures of quality and systems to report quality because they believed that physicians needed financial incentives to improve health care quality. Eventually, it was hoped, they would be used in the pay for performance schemes of payers, including Medicare. The health policy steering committee developed a proposed set of principles to guide surgeons and surgical organizations in this process. The principles addressed issues such as an environment for safety, confidentiality, legality, risk adjustment, and collaboration. Surgeons were asked to encourage their hospitals and other facilities to track and use risk-adjusted outcomes to continuously improve the quality of care.[7]

The issue of tort reform was a high priority of the fellowship because of the high cost of medical liability insurance and the increasing frequency of lawsuits, many of which were frivolous. But Congress had no enthusiasm for enacting nationwide tort reform. More successful were efforts of state medical societies and state specialty societies to support caps on liability payments.

The testimony of College leaders before Congress and federal agencies on issues such as chronic wound care and silicone gel-filled breast prostheses was very successful, but their fervent requests for major reforms in the payment system were ignored. Instead, Congress enacted temporary annual "fixes" to obviate the draconian cuts in reimbursement required by the sustainable growth rate (SGR) methodology.[8]

By 2004, the SGR methodology for Medicare reimbursement was progressively decreasing the incomes of physicians and surgeons; private insurers were following suit. The National Health Care Act, which called for a single payer, was introduced in Congress in 2004, and although it did not pass, its introduction was frightening to physicians. Single payer health care schemes were introduced into the legislatures of 18 states. Physicians were called on by legislators, bureaucrats, health policy experts, and the public to practice evidence-based medicine, create patient safety procedures, and eliminate expensive complications, especially infections.

During his travels to chapter meetings, the Fellows, fearing "socialized medicine," pleaded with Dr. Russell to "do something." The Regents and staff held another strategic planning exercise in June 2004, and identified advocacy and health policy as their highest priority.[9] The need for legislative action by the College had never been greater. The College needed a plan of action.

Dr. Josef Fischer, chair of the health policy steering committee, believed the Washington office needed to be strengthened. On his strong recommendation, the College contracted with the Duberstein Group of Washington, DC, which he believed had the reputation of opening doors to key people in Washington and could help secure the College at a place at the table to influence the debate over health care public policy. The Group was to complement the activities of the College's Washington office on important issues.[10,11] Unfortunately, this led to questions of authority and responsibility in the Washington office and the office of the Executive Director. The Duberstein Group's contract was not renewed. Ms. Brown accepted the prestigious position of vice president of government affairs

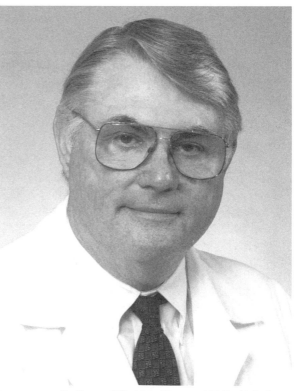

FIGURE 23.1 Dr. George F Sheldon, Director, ACS Health Policy Research Institute; ACS President, 1998–99.

at the AMA in April 2008 and was replaced by Mr. Christian Shalgian, a long-time member of the Washington staff.[12]

Although the College did not find it difficult or inappropriate to take positions on socioeconomic issues such as Medicare reimbursement, its altruistic leaders felt the need to identify issues related to the well-being of the patients that surgeons serve. They believed the College would be true to its mission by advocating for patients, and would be seen by its constituencies as an altruistic organization interested in something more than the financial remuneration of its members. Research was necessary, however, to identify emerging problems and to generate solutions. Scholarly, well thought-out policies would be based on the best evidence that could be generated, facilitating constructive participation in health care reform. The health policy steering committee recommended establishment of a health policy research institute to carry out this research.[8]

The Health Policy Research Institute was eventually launched in early 2008, an election year that featured debate over public health policy. Dr. George Sheldon, a past President of the College and distinguished professor of surgery at the University of North Carolina, was named director of the Institute, and Thomas J Ricketts, PhD, deputy director of the University of North Carolina Shep's Center for Health Policy Research, was named administrative director. (Figure 23.1) The Shep's Center served as the Institute's headquarters. The Institute immediately began to study surgery workforce projections, tracking surgical sub-specialization, trends in utilization of surgical services in North Carolina and the United States, and the surgical workforce in rural areas.[12, 13]

⋙✻⋘

The Affordable Care Act

President Barack Obama took office in January 2009 and soon made health care reform his legislative priority. The College issued a general statement about the impending legislation, advocating for measures that would improve the quality and safety of care, improve the public's access to health care, correct physician workforce imbalances, and reduce health care costs.[14] During the debate the College and a large coalition of physician organizations called for repeal of the SGR methodology and replacement by a system that would set a new baseline for reimbursement and use multiple conversion factors based on the category of service.

The College and its coalition members were opposed to funding increased primary care reimbursement by reducing payments made to surgeons.[13] In various congressional hearings and roundtable discussions the College presented data showing a shortage of general surgeons, advocated for trauma and emergency medical systems support and financing, and opposed the creation of an independent Medicare advisory commission with unprecedented authority to regulate Medicare payment policy. In general, the College avoided strong statements on proposals to regulate insurance company activities and make medical care more accessible to the uninsured or underinsured, both of which were prominent features of the proposed legislation.[6, 14, 15]

The final product, signed into law in March 2010, would be phased in over four years and contained hundreds of requirements and changes in health care financing and in delivery systems. The more important provisions were that the uninsured population would be markedly reduced, insurance companies would be unable to deny insurance, and Medicaid would cover more individuals. Doctors would be incented to form "accountable care organizations" (ACOs) to better coordinate care and receive bundled payments for services rather than payments to individual providers. In 2015, Medicare will be required to create a physician payment program based on quality of care rather than volume.

The act specifies that general surgeons practicing in "health professional shortage areas" would receive a 10 percent bonus from Medicare, and more federally funded resident positions would be allocated to general surgery. Funding for trauma centers and emergency medical care was also included. But the College leadership and the fellowship were disappointed that there was no provision for repeal of the SGR methodology or federal tort reform. These continue to be high priorities for the legislative agendas of the College and other surgery organizations.

The College Moves to F Street

The Washington office, opened in 1979, had been housed in a small building in Georgetown that was adequate for the early, low-key advocacy efforts of the College. But by the turn of the century the necessary staff could not be hired because of insufficient space. Capitol Hill was an hour away, virtually precluding visits from legislators and their staffs and making it difficult and inefficient for College staff to attend meetings there. As the frequency and importance of health care legislation increased, Ms. Cynthia Brown, then director of the division of advocacy and health policy, recommended that the College seek other space.[16]

Comptroller Ms. Gay Vincent, with help from the real estate firm Jones Lang LaSalle, analyzed available properties and recommended purchase of a building site at 20 F Street, NW, in Washington, for construction of an office building. The site was ideally located, within a short walk to the U.S. Capitol and Union Station. A hotel was next door. In 2006, the Regents approved purchase of the site and construction of a 10 story building for approximately $114 million.[17-19] The building, which has ample space for

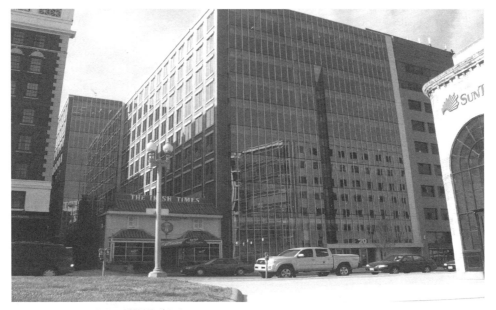

FIGURE 23.2 20 F Street NW, Washington, DC.

meetings, receptions, and entertaining, opened in 2010, as the Affordable Care Act was being debated. The College occupies the top floor and the other floors are leased, providing an income stream for amortizing debt. (Figure 23.2)

≈✦≈

Preparing for the Second Century

One of the factors in the decision to build the impressive F Street building was the desire by College leadership to enhance the visibility of the College to the fellowship and its stakeholders. Some of the surgical specialties, especially orthopaedics, neurosurgery, and ophthalmology, had grown and established their own advocacy programs, sometimes believing that the College did not represent them adequately or was too focused on general surgery. Paradoxically, general surgeons were restive, believing that the College needed to do more for them. Leaders worried that the College was losing its clout and identity.

At the recommendation of a newly established public profile and communications steering committee chaired by Regent Jack McAninch, the College hired the public relations firm Weber Shandwick to help the College expand and enhance its visibility.[17-20] A fifth division of the College, the division of integrated communications, under Ms. Linn Meyer, was created to help implement the plan to raise the College's profile.

With Weber Shandwick's help, the steering committee developed a plan that focused on reaching health care policy leaders, the broader medical community, and the surgical community. The plan revolved around three goals. The first was to build the public profile of the College and its leadership based on quality, measurement, and patient safety, targeting health care influencers, top-tier news media, leading health care patient advocacy organizations, and consumers. The second was to increase College credibility by targeting health plans and hospitals, with a marketing plan to drive the visibility of ACS NSQIP, the committee on cancer, ATLS, trauma verification, and the National Trauma Database. The third goal was to reconnect with Fellows and drive the growth of new members.[21]

≈✦≈

Russell Retires from the College

Dr. Russell retired as Executive Director on December 31, 2009. In addition to his extraordinary efforts to connect with the fellowship, his reorganization of the College into four, later five, divisions modernized and streamlined its operations. He improved the morale of the 243 College employees and reduced employee turnover rate from 27 to about 5 percent. Through Chief Financial Officer Gay Vincent and the wise counsel of Treasurer Dr. John Cameron, he improved control over the budget and established business policies that had been lacking. The investment balance grew from $201 million in 2000 to $294 million after the recession, with a high point of $387 million before the recession.

The underused Nickerson Mansion was in effect exchanged for a total renovation of the Murphy Memorial, now a venue for Chicago events and College activities.[6] The ACS PAC raised and appropriated $2.6 million to political candidates and initiatives from 2003 through 2008. But Russell's most striking accomplishment was the massive expansion of the College education program.[6] Numerous courses, seminars, lectures and other educational activities were added and made available in a wide array of electronic media. Surgeons could keep current on the latest scientific, clinical, and business advances through the College. Everything they needed to maintain their board certification was provided. The College could not have been more productive during Russell's ten years of leadership.

A New Executive Director

A broadly based search committee selected Dr. David B Hoyt to succeed Russell. A 1976 medical school graduate of Case Western Reserve University, Hoyt was trained in surgery at the University of California, San Diego, where he remained as a member of the faculty until 2006, when he was appointed chair of surgery and the John E Connolly Professor of Surgery at the University of California, Irvine. A trauma surgeon, he had chaired the Committee on Trauma, and was an active leader in many College activities. (Figure 23.3)

Hoyt immediately began to implement the recommendations of the public profile and communications steering committee and the plan developed by Weber Shandwick. Cast as the "Inspiring Quality Initiative," the College made a national effort to encourage collaboration among health care leaders and to urge them to share best practices on quality programs proved to improve outcomes and add value to our health care system. The initiative was kicked off at a health care forum in Chicago in July 2011.

Another important element of the plan was for surgeons to explain through videos what inspired them to elevate their standards and strive for better outcomes. A video for hospitals and other delivery organizations explained that ACS NSQIP, the cancer and trauma programs, and the College's accreditation programs have improved care and produced better outcomes at reduced cost.

Ms. Linn Meyer, who had developed effective means through which the College communicated with its Fellows and stakeholders, retired in 2011 and was succeeded by Ms. Lynn Kahn, who had more than 25 years of experience as a communications professional. Dr. Paul "Skip" Collicott, generally regarded as the father of the Advanced Trauma Life Support

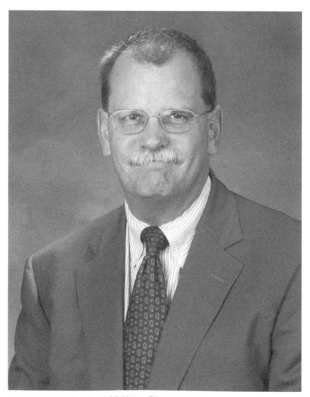

FIGURE 23.3 Dr. David B Hoyt, Director, 2010–.

(ATLS) Course, retired after ten years as director of the division of member services. Dr. Patricia Turner was appointed to succeed him.

Through his extensive experience with the trauma programs Hoyt captured the elements of programs necessary to improve care and has promulgated them in meetings with other organizations and in testimony before congressional committees. They include setting standards, building the right infrastructure to support the program, using the right data, and verifying that the program is functioning as intended and is improving the quality of care. This innovative approach undoubtedly will help the College develop new programs that actually improve the quality and value of health care.

REFERENCES

1. *Minutes of the meeting of the Board of Regents of February 11, 12, 2000.* 2000, Archives of the American College of Surgeons: Chicago.
2. *Minutes of the meeting of the Board of Regents of June 9, 10, 2000.* 2000, Archives of the American College of Surgeons: Chicago.
3. *Minutes of the meeting of the Board of Regents of October 20-22, 2000.* 2000, Archives of the American College of Surgeons: Chicago.
4. *Minutes of the meeting of the Board of Regents of February 9, 10, 2001.* 2001, Archives of the American College of Surgeons: Chicago.
5. *Minutes of the meeting of the Board of Regents of June 8-10, 2001.* 2001, Archives of the American College of Surgeons: Chicago.
6. *Minutes of the meeting of the Board of Regents of October 9, 10, 2009.* 2009, Archives of the American College of Surgeons: Chicago.
7. *Minutes of the meeting of the Board of Regents of June 5-7, 2003.* 2003, Archives of the American College of Surgeons: Chicago.
8. *Minutes of the meeting of the Board of Regents of June 10, 11, 2005.* 2005, Archives of the American College of Surgeons: Chicago.
9. *Minutes of the meeting of the Board of Regents of October 9, 10, 2004.* 2004, Archives of the American College of Surgeons.: Chicago.
10. *Minutes of the meeting of the Board of Regents of February 11, 12, 2005.* 2005, Archives of the American College of Surgeons: Chicago.
11. *Personal communication from Dr. Josef Fischer to Dr. David Nahrwold of March 1, 2010.* 2010: Chicago.
12. *Minutes of the meeting of the Board of Regents of June 13, 14, 2008.* 2008, Archives of the American College of Surgeons: Chicago.
13. *Minutes of the meeting of the Board of Regents of June 4-6, 2009.* 2009, Archives of the American College of Surgeons: Chicago.
14. *American College of Surgeons statement of healthcare reform.* 2009, American College of Surgeons: Chicago.
15. *Workforce issues in health care reform: Assessing the present and preparing for the future. Statement of the American College of Surgeons to the Committee on Finance, United States Senate.* March 12, 2009, Archives of the American College of Surgeons: Chicago.
16. *Minutes of the meeting of the Board of Regents of February 6, 7, 2004.* 2004, Archives of the American College of Surgeons: Chicago.
17. *Minutes of the meeting of the Board of Regents of June 9, 10, 2006.* 2006, Archives of the American College of Surgeons: Chicago.
18. *Minutes of the meeting of the Board of Regents of October 7, 8, 2006.* 2006, Archives of the American College of Surgeons: Chicago.
19. *Minutes of the meeting of the Board of Regents of October 12, 2006.* 2006, Archives of the American College of Surgeons: Chicago.
20. *Minutes of the meeting of the Board of Regents of February 10, 11, 2006.* 2006, Archives of the American College of Surgeons: Chicago.
21. *Minutes of the meeting of the Board of Regents of February 9, 19, 2007.* 2007, Archives of the American College of Surgeons: Chicago.

APPENDIX

Presidents of the American College of Surgeons

1913–1916	John MT Finney, Baltimore		1968–1969	Preston A Wade, Concord
1916–1917	George Crile, Cleveland		1969–1970	Joel W Baker, Seattle
1917–1920	William J Mayo, Rochester		1970–1971	Howard Mahorner, New Orleans
1920–1921	George E Armstrong, Montreal		1971–1972	Jonathan E Rhoads, Philadelphia
1921–1922	John B Deaver, Philadelphia		1972–1973	William P Longmire, Jr, Los Angeles
1922–1923	Harvey Cushing, Boston		1973–1974	Claude E Welch, Boston
1923–1924	Albert J Ochsner, Chicago		1974–1975	Charles W McLaughlin, Jr, Omaha
1924–1925	Charles H Mayo, Rochester		1975–1976	H William Scott, Jr, Nashville
1925–1926	Rudolph Matas, New Orleans		1976–1977	George R Dunlop, Worcester
1926–1927	WW Chipman, Montreal		1977–1978	Frank E Stinchfield, New York
1927–1928	George David Stewart, New York		1978–1979	William A Altemeier, Cincinnati
1928–1929	Franklin H Martin, Chicago		1979–1980	William H Muller, Jr, Charlottesville
1929–1930	Merritte W Ireland, Washington		1980–1981	James D Hardy, Madison
1930–1931	C Jeff Miller, New Orleans		1981–1982	G Thomas Shires, Las Vegas
1931–1932	Allen B Kanavel, Chicago		1982–1983	John M Beal, Valdosta
1932–1933	J Bentley Squier, New York		1983–1984	Henry T Bahnson, Pittsburgh
1933–1934	William D Haggard, Nashville		1984–1985	Charles G Drake, London
1934–1935	Robert B Greenough, Boston		1985–1986	David C Sabiston, Jr, Durham
1935–1936	Donald C Balfour, Rochester		1986–1987	W Dean Warren, Atlanta
1936–1937	Eugene II Pool, New York		1987–1988	C Rollins Hanlon, Chicago
1937–1938	Frederic A Besley, Waukegan		1988–1989	Oliver H Beahrs, Rochester
1938–1939	Howard D Naffziger, San Francisco		1989–1990	MJ Jurkiewicz, Atlanta
1939–1940	George P Mullor, Philadelphia		1990–1991	Frank C Spencer, New York
1940–1941	Evarts A Graham, St Louis		1991–1992	Ralph A Straffon, Cleveland
1941–1946	W Edward Gallie, Toronto		1992–1993	W Gerald Austen, Boston
1946–1947	Irvin Abell, Louisville		1993–1994	Lloyd D MacLean, Montreal
1947–1948	Arthur W Allen, Boston		1994–1995	Alexander J Walt, Detroit
1948–1949	Dallas B Phemister, Chicago		1995–1996	LaSalle D Leffall, Jr, Washington, DC
1949–1950	Frederick A Coller, Ann Arbor		1996–1997	David G Murray, Syracuse
1950–1951	Henry W Cave, New York		1997–1998	Seymour I Schwartz, Rochester
1951–1952	Alton Ochsner, New Orleans		1998–1999	George F Sheldon, Chapel Hill
1952–1953	Harold L Foss, Danville		1999–2000	James C Thompson, Galveston
1953–1954	Fred W Rankin, Lexington		2000–2001	Harvey W Bender, Jr, Nashville
1954–	Frank Glenn, New York*		2001–2002	R Scott Jones, Charlottesville
1954–1955	Alfred Blalock, Baltimore		2002–2003	Richard R Sabo, Bozeman
1955–1956	Warren H Cole, Asheville		2003–2004	Claude H Organ, Jr, Oakland
1956–1957	Daniel C Elkin, Lancaster		2004–2005	Edward R Laws, Charlottesville
1957–1958	William L Estes, Jr, Bethlehem		2005–2006	Kathryn D Anderson, San Gabriel
1958–1959	Newell W Philpott, Westmount		2006–2007	Edward M Copeland III, Gainesville
1959–1960	Owen H Wangensteen, Minneapolis		2007–2008	Gerald B Healy, Boston
1960–1961	IS Ravdin, Philadelphia		2008–2009	John L Cameron, Baltimore
1961–1962	Robert M Zollinger, Columbus		2009–2010	LaMar S McGinnis, Jr, Atlanta
1962–1963	Loyal Davis, Chicago		2010–2011	LD Britt, Norfolk
1963–1964	J Englebert Dunphy, San Francisco		2011–2012	Patricia J Numann, Syracuse
1964–1965	James T Priestley, Rochester		2012–2013	A Brent Eastman, San Diego
1965–1966	Howard A Patterson, New York			
1966–1967	Walter C MacKenzie, Edmonton			
1967–1968	Reed M Nesbit, El Macero			

*Succeeded to Presidency on death of Dr. Rankin, May 22, 1954

Chairs of the Board of Regents

1913–1939	George Crile, Cleveland
1939–1949	Irvin Abell, Louisville
1949–1951	Arthur W Allen, Boston
1951–1954	Evarts A Graham, St Louis
1954–1960	IS Ravdin, Philadelphia
1960–1962	Loyal Davis, Chicago
1962–1964	James T Priestley, Rochester
1964–1967	Preston A Wade, New York
1967–1969	Jonathan E Rhoads, Philadelphia
1969–1971	William P Longmire, Jr, Los Angeles
1971–1973	J Englebert Dunphy, San Francisco
1973–1976	Frank E Stinchfield, New York
1976–1978	William H Muller, Jr, Charlottesville
1978–1980	G Thomas Shires, New York
1980–1982	John M Beal, Chicago
1982–1984	David C Sabiston, Jr, Durham
1984–1987	Oliver H Beahrs, Rochester
1987–1989	Frank C Spencer, New York
1989–1991	W Gerald Austen, Boston
1991–1993	Alexander J Walt, Detroit
1993–1994	David G Murray, Syracuse
1994–1997	Seymour I Schwartz, Rochester
1997–1999	Harvey W Bender, Jr, Nashville
1999–2001	C James Carrico, Dallas
2001–2003	Edward R Laws, Jr, Charlottesville
2003–2005	Edward M Copeland III, Gainesville
2005–2006	Gerald B Healy, Boston
2006–2008	Josef E Fischer, Boston
2008–2009	LD Britt, Norfolk
2009–2010	A Brent Eastman, San Diego
2010–2011	Carlos A Pellegrini, Seattle
2011–2012	J David Richardson, Louisville

INDEX

C

F

G

M

S

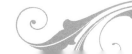

T

U

V

W

◦—✳—◦

Y

◦—✳—◦

Z